CONTENTS

INTRODUCTION

THIS book has been written in order to explain to the student nurse the anatomical and pathological abnormalities of infancy and childhood in so far as their surgical correction is concerned. Before you can apply your nursing care and technique in the best interests of your patient it is essential that you have a clear idea of these matters: that is to say what is wrong, why it is wrong and how it may be put right. In addition to this basic knowledge we shall also consider the observations that you yourself will be required to make, for whereas the surgeon in charge is able to visit his patient for the most part only on certain set occasions, you the nurse are the permanent companion and mentor to the child and it is upon your observations that he will depend in order to assess the state and progress of his case; just as it is upon your care that he will rely in order to ensure the success of his skill. Never forget this. If at times you feel that your full worth and necessity is not acknowledged, remember that you are just as essential as any other member of the surgical team and although the limelight may not always be yours, it is upon you that the success of all the definitive surgical manoeuvres will ultimately depend.

Before we embark upon this study, however, let us first consider a few remarks about the people to whom your work and interest are subscribed—the child and the parents.

Children show a considerable variation in the way that they accommodate themselves to hospital life. Whereas some proclaim their immediate displeasure in a loud voice others merely take a reluctant but consuming interest in all that goes on around them. The majority, however, settle down very rapidly but it is essential that as far as possible they be allowed to do so in their own time. Never overwhelm a newly admitted child with a theatrical show of affection, yet never ignore them completely; the correct approach lies somewhere between these two extremes and is one which you will only come to learn by continual experience. In many ways children are like all other young animals—once they are ready to make friends they will come to you for that friendship but first they

1

must be confident that their trust is well placed. For this reason never delude a child. If some minor procedure such as a venepuncture is about to be performed, tell the child what to expect ; never say that it won't hurt when you know full well that it will; similarly never say that an uncomfortable dressing is nearly over when it has only just begun. If you do these things the child will have the best grounds in the world for distrusting everything else you ever say. Providing you are scrupulously honest in your dealings with a child you will be rewarded by a natural affection and fortitude that would be otherwise unobtainable, for honesty is an infectious quality. Always remember that in their assessment of people, children are often more penetrating and profound judges than mature adults, and while you are wondering what sort of problem they are likely to become don't forget that they are regarding *you* with the same quiet consideration.

Children suffering from acute pyogenic infections are often notoriously difficult to manage. Never fail to appreciate that their recalcitrant behaviour is due to the associated toxaemia (see Chapter I) and not to an ' hysterical ' predisposition, for there is no such thing as hysteria in a young child. Once the infection has been overcome or almost immediately following the evacuation of pus, you will be astounded at the sudden change in the child's demeanour, for whereas they were previously fractious and unreasonable the passing of the toxaemia allows them to return to their normal placid and friendly disposition.

Sometimes you will no doubt be perplexed by the vagaries of behaviour of parents but always remember that they, like their children, are at first liable to feel out of place in a hospital ward, and at times it may be difficult for you to understand their feelings towards the nurse who has temporarily supplanted them in the care of their own children. Therefore be prepared to treat the natural anxieties of parents with sympathy and solicitude rather than with distant interest and cold efficiency. Occasionally you will be required to nurse an infant who to you may appear to be hideously deformed. Whatever your own feelings, never forget that the majority of the parents of such children have become accustomed to the appearance of the child to whom they still bear a considerable degree of affection and for whose comfort and safety they are still deeply concerned.

SURGICAL TERMS

When a child is returned to the ward from the operating theatre the student nurse is not infrequently perplexed by the length of the word that has been used to describe the operation. With the exception of proper names (such as Rammstedt's operation and Elmslie's operation) these terms are composite in nature and consist firstly of the name of the organ that has been attacked and secondly the procedure that has been carried out, and it is this latter half of the word that is usually the most difficult to understand. Although many of the terms have been in use for a long while and have, with the years become more loose in their application, they none the less offer a fair description of the procedure that has been carried out.

(i) -otomy: This merely means a temporary opening; for instance, the time-honoured word for an abdominal exploration is laparotomy which merely means a temporary opening (-otomy) of the lapar (the belly). Similarly tracheotomy is an operation designed to procure a temporary opening between the trachea and the exterior.

(ii) -ostomy: This term refers to a permanent opening which has been fashioned either between a hollow organ and the exterior (such as gastrostomy) or between two hollow organs such as gastro-jejunostomy (i.e. a permanent communication between the stomach and the jejunum), this latter term sometimes being substituted by gastro-enterostomy, the fraction entero- coming from the word entera meaning intestines. Similarly the operation designed to overcome a congenital blockage of the bile duct (see Chapter VIII) is known as choledochoduodenostomy. Formidable as this term may at first appear, it is quite simply broken down into its component parts and means a permanent opening (-ostomy) established between the bile (chole-) duct (-docho-) and the duodenum.

(iii) -ectomy: This simply means 'removal of'; for instance, lobectomy (the removal of a lobe of the lung) and tonsillectomy (the removal of a tonsil).

(iv) -orrhaphy: This ending refers to an operation in which *repair* is a predominant feature. For instance the operation of herniorrhaphy is one in which, once the hernial sac itself has been removed, surgical repair is then performed about the hernial orifice in an attempt to prevent the recurrence of the hernia.

PRE-OPERATIVE AND POST-OPERATIVE MEDICATION

PRE-OPERATIVE MEDICATION

The administration of a general anaesthetic in a child is accompanied by two principal effects. Firstly, there is a natural disinclination on the part of the child to breathe into a rubber mask, and secondly the inhalation of anaesthetic gases causes an increase in the secretion of saliva in the mouth and of mucus in the bronchi, and it is in order to allay the former and inhibit the latter that pre-operative medication is employed.

Sedation

In infants and very young children pre-operative sedation is seldom employed, as a rapid induction of anaesthetic can be obtained by only a few breaths of Ethyl Chloride, a gas which is practically harmless at this age, but which may be accompanied by serious complications in older children. In children between two and eight years of age pre-operative sedation is most commonly carried out by the use of the barbiturate group of drugs. The dose, time and mode of administration depend to a large extent upon the particular preferences of the individual anaesthetist and you must always make sure that you are carrying out his detailed instructions when giving the sedative drug that he has ordered. Some authorities prefer Pentobarbitone or Seconal given by mouth in doses of 0·6 grams per stone body-weight given about two hours before the operation, whereas others prefer the administration of Pentothal via the rectal route; Pentothal powder in doses of 0·1 grams per 5 lb. of body-weight up to a maximum dose of $1\frac{1}{2}$ grams is dissolved in 10 to 20 cubic centimetres of warm tap water and run into the rectum through a small rubber catheter about half to three-quarters of an hour before operation. Occasionally you will come across anaesthetists who prefer paraldehyde given by the same route (60 minims per stone of body-weight made up in five to ten times its volume of normal saline). All these methods are designed to send the child to sleep before reaching the operating theatre so that no apprehension or mental distress is occasioned and so that anaesthesia may be induced smoothly

and easily. Eminently satisfactory as these methods may be for the immediate problem of an anaesthetic, you will sometimes find that children who have been sedated in this fashion may suffer from 'insomnia' for the next few months and frequently awake at night screaming with fear. If you try to explain this fact from the child's point of view you will appreciate that on the day of operation he went comfortably to sleep only to wake with the pain and discomfort of an operation wound. It does not seem surprising, therefore, that a number of children are thereafter both suspicious and afraid of the sleep that they had previously trusted to ' knit-up the ravelled sleeve of care '. Children from eight to ten years of age and upwards are most satisfactorily sedated by the intramuscular injection of Omnopon (1/30 grain per stone body-weight) three-quarters of an hour before operation. Although this drug does not cause the child to go to sleep it is sufficient to allay apprehension and it is usually followed by an intravenous injection of Pentothal immediately prior to the administration of the inhalation anaesthetic.

Inhibition of Secretions

Unless the secretions of saliva and bronchial mucus are inhibited they are liable to be aspirated into the lungs with subsequent blockage of one or more bronchi. Anaesthetics of very short duration employing non-irritant gases such as Nitrous Oxide do not cause increased secretions and in such instances pre-operative medication is not usually employed. On all other occasions, however, an intramuscular injection of Atropine (1/200 grain for small infants, 1/150 grain for children from six to eighteen months and 1/100 grain for all other age groups) should be given three-quarters of an hour before operation. In very apprehensive children who are likely to be unduly distressed by an injection some authorities give twice this dose by mouth about an hour before the operation. In much older children Scopolamine (Hyoscine hydrobromide), which is a drug very similar in its action to Atropine, may be given in its place in doses of 1/150 grain per stone body-weight and it is frequently made up in the same solution as Omnopon so that only one injection is necessary for the administration of both drugs.

Post-operative Medication

Children vary enormously in their sensitivity and tolerance to pain but, even so, the majority need some form of post-operative sedation. The drugs most commonly employed in the immediate post-operative period are Papaveretum (minims 1 plus minims 1 for each year of life) or Nepenthe (minims 1 per year of life) both of which are administered by intramuscular injection. Neither drug should be given more frequently than at four hourly intervals, but it is unusual for more than two or three doses to be required. Minor discomfort, especially at night time, may be relieved by Codeine (1 to 3 grains by mouth) or Aspirin or Dispirin (1 to 5 grains by mouth), in order to help to get the child to sleep.

Children, particularly those who had an elevated temperature at the time of the operation, are liable to perspire freely during the course of an operation. If severe, this fluid loss should be replaced by the rectal administration of warm tap water. This should be run slowly into the rectum through a small rubber catheter, the water reservoir never being held more than one foot above the level of the child, and the sooner that this is done after the operation the better, for once the child begins to regain consciousness the water is liable to be returned.

DEHYDRATION

The term dehydration is used to describe a clinical condition in which the loss of water from the body exceeds both in rate and amount the volume of the intake (a negative water balance). It is potentially a most dangerous condition and one which requires early recognition and prompt and effective treatment. This is particularly so in infancy due to the fact that the infant's normal fluid loss (via the lungs, skin and urine) is proportionally much greater than in older children and thus an additional loss of fluid due to disease is liable to effect a much more rapid depletion of the body fluid.

The state of dehydration may accompany a wide variety of conditions but from the surgical point of view it most commonly occurs in association with three principle types of disorder:

(1) Obstructive conditions of the alimentary tract, in which there is excessive fluid loss due to profuse and protracted vomiting.

(2) Extensive burns and scalds, in which there is excessive fluid loss through the burned area of skin.

(3) Rapid haemorrhage in which there is an excessive loss of the fluid fraction of the blood. In this condition, however, the signs of dehydration are largely over-shadowed by the picture of exsanguination.

As the body fluid contains a varying number of dissolved salts (the electrolytes) it follows that the conditions we have mentioned will of necessity be accompanied by an inevitable *electrolyte loss*. This latter aspect of dehydration is of particular importance especially with sodium chloride, the excessive loss of which, by reducing the volume of the circulating plasma results in the rapid onset of shock and collapse. This in turn reduces the blood flow to the kidneys with the result that there will be a fall in the urinary output (oliguria) and an accumulation of the waste products of metabolism in the blood. In such an eventuality there will be a marked increase in the value of the blood urea and unless the condition is rectified by the speedy restoration of the volume and the electrolyte content of the blood, a rapid decline and death will be the inevitable outcome.

Clinical Features

In the early stages of the condition the infant appears noticeably more restless and fretful than usual, the feeds are taken with enthusiasm and avidity due to the marked degree of thirst, the face is flushed and the lips appear unusually red. A rapid loss of weight is always present and although this may be difficult to estimate in infants when seen for the first time, the daily weight charts of hospital in-patients may furnish valuable information in this respect. It is most important to stress that, slight though these early signs may be, the nurse should train herself to recognize them accurately and immediately and to regard them as potentially dangerous omens, for there is no telling in a given case how rapidly the condition is likely to progress.

As the degree of dehydration increases the infant becomes

progressively restless, the expression has an apathetic or anxious look about it and a thin, high pitched wail replaces the usual lusty cry. The lips are cracked, pale and faintly cyanosed, and the eyes and the fontanelle become increasingly sunken. The skin invariably loses its normal degree of elasticity but you must remember that this may be less obvious in a well nourished child with an abundance of sub-cutaneous fat than it is in a thin child. Oliguria is always present and although thirst may be extreme it may in certain instances be absent altogether.

In the final stages, the baby rapidly becomes desperately ill. The fontanelle and the eyes are deeply sunken, the corneae being faintly dulled due to the absence of tears, and whereas the skin of the face and trunk is deathly pale the lips and extremities are deeply cyanosed. The infant shortly becomes moribund and lies limp and silent in the cot.

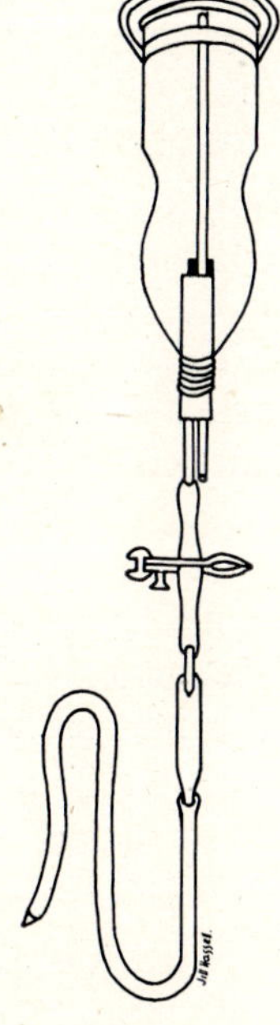

FIG. 1

The standard drip apparatus.

Treatment

The whole aim of treatment is firstly to restore and thereafter to maintain the volume and composition of the body fluid, and for this reason all cases of suspected dehydration should at once be placed upon an intake and output chart. In the early stages of the condition when the degree of dehydration is slight, and providing vomiting is absent, correction may be obtained by the oral administration of fluid. Milk, either half or full strength, is without doubt the best fluid for replacement as it contains both electrolytes and calories, but if it is not tolerated then water, glucose or specially prepared electrolyte solutions are quite suitable. In infancy the amount given at each feed should be calculated on the basis of $2\frac{1}{2}$ ounces per pound of body-weight to which, for the first twenty-four hours of treatment, should be added an additional volume calculated as $2\frac{1}{2}$ ounces per pound of between 5 and 10 per cent of the body-weight, in order to make up the fluid loss already incurred. If this amount is not well tolerated some authorities prefer to

plement the intake by the administration of water or saline by the rectal route, given either by continuous infusion or by the injection of 1 to 2 ounces at six-hourly intervals.

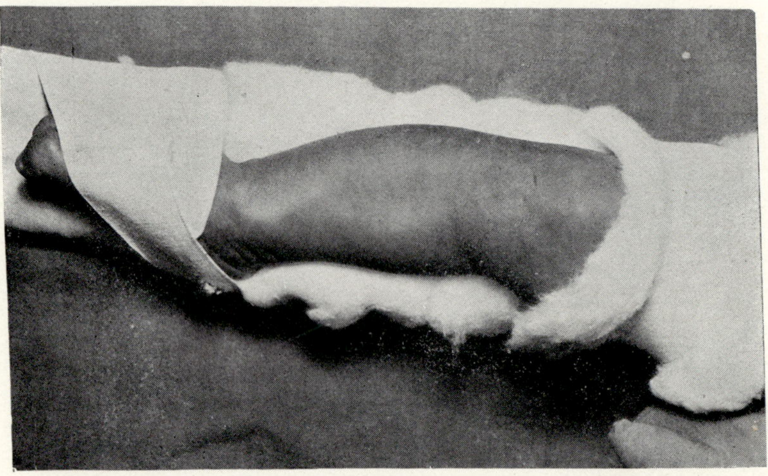

FIG. 2

To demonstrate a satisfactory method of immobilizing the leg.

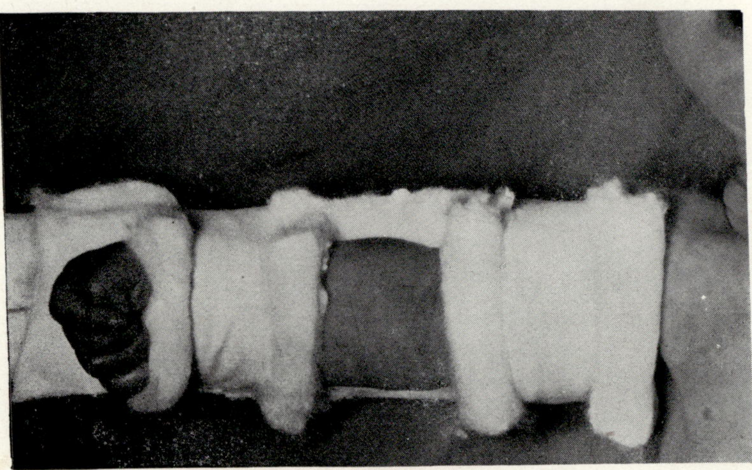

FIG. 3

Immobilization of the arm.

If the degree of dehydration is more severe, then the urgency of the situation demands that fluid be replaced via the intravenous route. Owing to the small size of the superficial veins

in children it is usually impossible to introduce a needle directly
into them through the skin, and for this reason it is necessary
to expose a vein under local anaesthetic.   You will come across
a wide variety of cannulae and special needles which are used

WESTMINSTER CHILDREN'S HOSPITAL   INTRAVENOUS FLUID CHART

Name _______________________________   Birth Weight ___________   Present Weight ___________
Date _______________________________

TIME	PULSE	AMOUNT IN HOUR	RATE OF DRIP	READING ON SCALE	REMARKS	FEEDS BY MOUTH	VOMITS	STOOLS	URINE	
a.m. 1										
2										
3										
4										
5										
6										
7										
8										
9										
10										
11										
12										
p.m. 1										
2										
3										
4										
5										
6										
7										
8										
9										
10										
11										
12										
TOTALS										

TOTAL INTAKE FOR 24 HOURS

Fig. 4

The intravenous fluid administration chart.

for intravenous infusions but quite the most satisfactory expedient is a short length of polythene tubing which after being
connected to a standard drip apparatus (Fig. 1) may be introduced an inch or so into the vein and secured to the limb with
adhesive strapping.   In infants and very young children the

arm or leg should be immobilized as shown in Figs. 2 and 3, but it is important that the proximal restraining band should not be too tight, otherwise compression of the superficial veins will prevent the flow of the infused fluid. In older children, restraint of the limb by a splint is not usually necessary, for the polythene and a few inches of the delivery tube may quite simply be coiled up and secured to the skin with strapping, thus allowing the child additional movement and less discomfort.

The type of fluid used for the infusion is dictated by a variety of considerations which are not our present concern, but it is the nurse's responsibility to see that the flow proceeds regularly and at the rate prescribed. The number of drips per minute together with the reading of the scale on the side of the bottle should be carefully checked at hourly intervals and entered on the intravenous fluid administration chart (Fig. 4), and in addition a quick glance should be given in between, as the fluid rate is liable to speed up from time to time. This is of particular importance in infants, when the sudden rush of fluid may well be too much of a strain on the heart. A careful watch should be maintained on the skin incision for the presence of infection and the urine output should be estimated as accurately as possible in infants and measured directly in older children.

THE THEORY OF BLOOD TRANSFUSION

The grouping of human blood is dependent upon two main facts:

(1) The *red blood corpuscles* of human blood may contain a substance known as an *agglutinogen*.

(2) Human *serum* may contain an anti-substance to the agglutinogen which is known as an *agglutinin*.

Now there are two types of agglutinogen known as A and B and their respective agglutinins in the serum are called *a* and *b*. If red blood corpuscles containing the agglutinogen A are mixed with serum containing its agglutinin *a*, then clumping or *agglutination* of the corpuscles occurs (Fig. 5). On the other hand, if corpuscles containing agglutinogen A are mixed with serum containing agglutinin *b* no agglutination occurs (Fig. 6). It goes without saying, therefore, that the blood of any one individual cannot contain both the agglutinogen A in

the corpuscles and the agglutinin *a* in the serum, nor can it contain B and *b*. It is upon this basis that the blood of all human beings has been grouped according to the agglutinogen or combination of agglutinogens that are present in the corpuscles, and it follows that in each group the corresponding

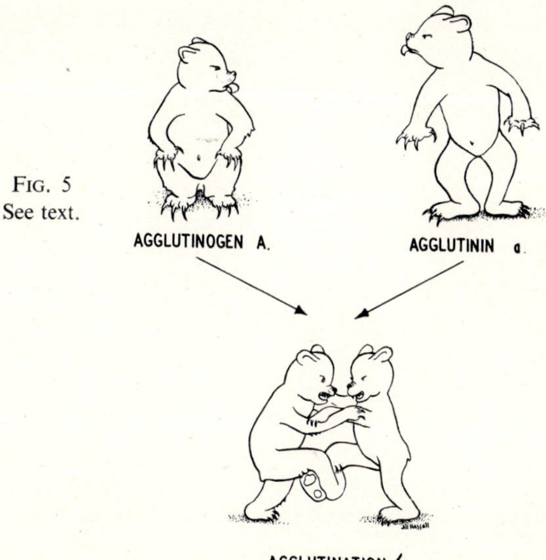

Fig. 5
See text.

agglutinins will be absent from the serum. Thus the four groups that are possible are:

Group Name		Agglutinogens (*in the corpuscles*)	Agglutinins (*in the serum*)
A	containing	A	*b*
B	containing	B	*a*
AB	containing	A and B	neither *a* nor *b*
O	containing	neither A nor B	*a* and *b*

The particular blood group to which any one individual belongs is determined by mixing a sample of the individual's corpuscles with two samples of specially prepared serum, one containing agglutinin *a* and one containing agglutinin *b*. After twenty minutes the mixtures are inspected and if agglutination is present in both samples then the blood group of the individual must be AB; if neither sample is agglutinated then the blood must be group O (i.e. that group which contains no agglutino-

gens); if agglutination is present in the sample containing *a* the blood must be group A and similarly if the sample containing *b* shows agglutination then the group must be B. In so far as blood transfusion is concerned the blood of individuals of *different* groups are referred to as being *incompatible*, whereas

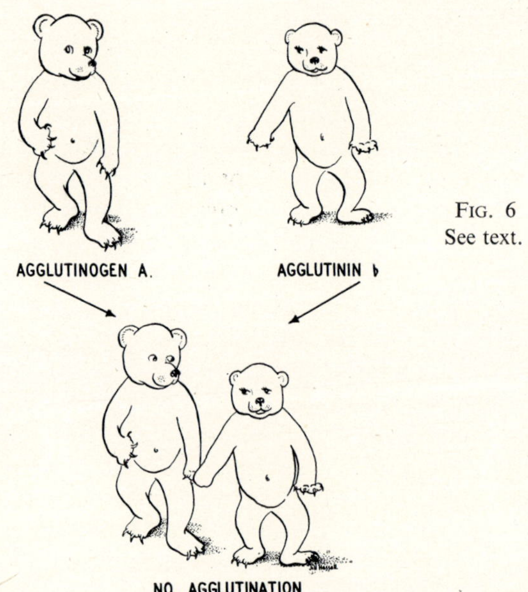

FIG. 6
See text.

those belonging to the *same* group are called *compatible*. The method of blood grouping that we have described is not infallible however, and as an extra safeguard against incompatible transfusion a further test known as a *direct compatibility test* or *cross-matching* is always performed. A few drops of the blood of the donor is mixed with the serum of the patient and if no agglutination occurs the blood of the donor and that of the patient are pronounced *directly compatible*.

The Effects of Incompatible Blood Transfusion

If blood belonging to a person of one group is administered by transfusion to a child of a different group then agglutination of the red blood corpuscles will inevitably ensue. Should this catastrophe occur the child within a few minutes of the commencement of the transfusion experiences acute pain either

beneath the sternum or in the loin. The agglutinated red blood corpuscles disintegrate and the haemoglobin that is consequently liberated is partly excreted in the urine and partly converted into *bilirubin,* causing an intense degree of jaundice. The output of urine is greatly decreased, the blood urea concentration increases and unless the secretion of urine is reestablished the child will die of uraemia within the course of a week or ten days.

Incompatible blood transfusion is fortunately rare but when it does occur it is invariably due to a mistake in the labelling of the bottle of blood, and its effects must impress upon you the necessity of eliminating all possible chances of error so that the correct bottle of blood is *always* administered to the child for whom it was intended. When blood is withdrawn from your patient for the purpose of determining the blood group it should be placed in a specimen bottle and as soon as this has been done you must see that it is *clearly labelled* with the child's name and age and also the name of the ward. Before putting the bottle down make sure that the appropriate form is *fully completed* and that it agrees with the information you have written on the label. Once this has been done the bottle and the label must *not* part company and should be dispatched at once to the pathological laboratory. When the labelled bottle of blood for transfusion is sent back to the ward it is the responsibility of the nurse to make sure that the details on the label agree with those of her patient. This information must then be checked either by the staff nurse or the ward sister and *on no account* may the label be removed from the bottle until the transfusion has been administered. Incompatible blood transfusion is a potentially fatal happening and in guarding against it in the extra precautions that we have mentioned, the nurse as well as the doctor also carries a high degree of responsibility.

The Rhesus Factor

Some years ago it was discovered that human red cells may contain an agglutinogen the incidence of which is independent of the classification we have considered. This agglutinogen is known as the Rhesus factor (Rh) and is estimated to be present in 85 per cent of individuals (Rh +) and absent in the remaining 15 per cent (Rh −). It is of the greatest importance in the following circumstances:

(1) If a Rh — mother conceives a Rh + foetus then the Rh agglutinogen passes through the placenta from the foetal to the maternal circulation where *anti-substances* are made against it. These anti-substances in their turn enter the foetal circulation where they cause agglutination and disintegration of the red blood corpuscles of the foetus. The pronounced degree of anaemia which follows may be sufficient either to kill the foetus or cause it to be born with severe anaemia and jaundice (erythroblastosis foetalis).

(2) As we have just seen the Rh — mother of a Rh + child will produce an anti-substance to the Rh factor. If at any subsequent time she should receive a blood transfusion of Rh + blood her Rh anti-substances will agglutinate the cells she has received with the same grave consequences that we have mentioned when dealing with incompatible transfusions.

It is for these reasons that in addition to determining the A, B, AB, or O groups that we have already described, Rh grouping is nowadays always performed as well.

HAEMANGIOMATA

A haemangioma consists of a mass of intertwining blood-vessels which takes no active part in the general circulation and which is supplied with blood by numerous small branches from the neighbouring normal vessels. Such a malformation occurs more commonly in girls than in boys and although it is usually present at birth there may be a delay of several months before the condition becomes apparent. In the majority of instances it is situated in the skin but more rarely it may occur in deeper tissues such as the meninges, the brain and the vertebrae, and in these latter situations attention is not usually drawn to the presence of the malformation until such time as it begins to cause pressure effects on the surrounding tissues.

For the purposes of description the haemangiomata are usually divided into the following three varieties:

(1) The Port-wine Stain

This type of haemangioma is always present at birth and appears as a diffuse, mottled, red and purple discoloration of the skin. It most commonly occurs in the skin of the face, the

neck or the upper arms, and remains constant in size throughout life.

(2) The Capillary Haemangioma

A capillary haemangioma as its name implies is composed of a mass of small or capillary blood-vessels. It appears either as a patchy, diffuse, pink discoloration of the skin (a ' strawberry mark ', Figs. 7 and 8) or as a localized swelling, in which

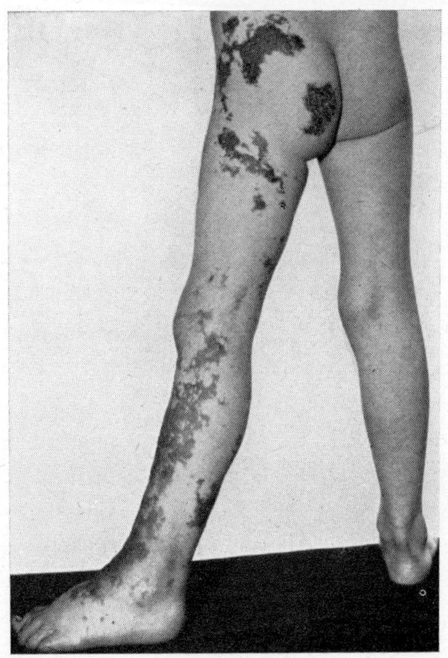

FIG. 7
Multiple haemangiomata of the leg.

instance it is often intermixed with a collection of fatty tissue (a naevo-lipoma).

(3) The Cavernous Haemangioma

A cavernous haemangioma consists of a mass of large, thin walled blood vessels which, if not present at birth appears shortly afterwards as a well localized, deep red swelling projecting above the surface of the surrounding skin (Fig. 8). As a rule it exhibits a rapid increase in size during the first year of life but thereafter it shows a gradual tendency to regress. Unlike the other types of haemangioma that we have mentioned it is particularly prone to injury and consequent haemorrhage

due to the ease with which its vessels may be ruptured, and it is for this reason that treatment for a cavernous haemangioma is more imperative than it is for the other forms.

Treatment

In the case of the port-wine stain, treatment is directed primarily to improvement of the cosmetic appearance. If the

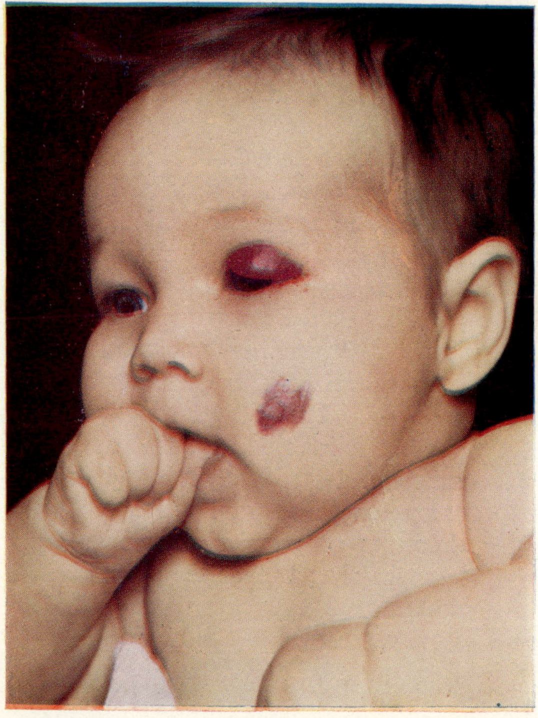

FIG. 8

A cavernous haemangioma of the eyelid suitable for diathermy coagulation, and a capillary haemangioma of the cheek.

lesion is very small then excision with primary suture of the wound may sometimes be carried out. More often than not, however, the size of the lesion precludes this form of treatment and resort to excision and skin grafting will have to be made, but it is important for you to realize that from the cosmetic point of view, the grafted area may appear just as conspicuous as the original disfigurement, especially when the face is involved.

2

In the case of capillary and cavernous haemangiomata, total excision of the malformation may be carried out whenever and wherever it is practicable. This procedure is, however, only seldom possible and for the most part treatment is directed to inducing thrombosis (clotting of the blood) within the abnormal vessels and the vessels of supply. This may be carried out in a variety of ways but all the methods employed depend for their success upon the production of an aseptic inflammatory process within the malformation. This in turn causes thrombosis which in the course of time is replaced by fibrous tissue which subsequently effects obliteration and shrinkage of the haemangioma.

CARBON DIOXIDE 'SNOW'.—This method is particularly applicable to the cavernous variety of haemangioma and depends for its success upon the production of a thermal burn around the circumference of the malformation. A thin pencil of solid carbon dioxide (which has a temperature of $-70°$ C.) is applied to the edges of the haemangioma for about twenty seconds. As soon as the pencil is removed the site of application appears dead white in colour but after an hour or so a blister begins to form. This blister usually subsides in the course of a week but it is important that during this time it should be adequately protected by a dressing in order to prevent the access of secondary infection. After a few weeks the haemangioma becomes progressively more pale and steadily begins to decrease in size; but as the process of thrombosis and fibrous replacement that has been initiated is liable to continue for some while, a period of from three to six months should be allowed to elapse before considering a second application.

DIATHERMY COAGULATION.—Diathermy coagulation is an equally effective method of inducing thrombosis within the abnormal vessels. In the capillary variety, under a general anaesthetic the overlying skin is touched in a number of places with a diathermy electrode, each application being for one second or less. In the cavernous type the electrode should be thrust deeply into its substance and a coagulating current passed for between two and three seconds. As in the case of carbon dioxide snow, this method merely initiates the process of thrombosis which should then be allowed to proceed for a number of months before a second application is considered.

SALINE INJECTIONS.—This method is particularly applicable to cavernous haemangiomata. A few minims of 30 per cent saline solution are injected into the *deepest* part of the malformation and in a large number of cases a satisfactory and progressive thrombosis is obtained. The only disadvantage to the method is that should the injection not be sufficiently deep, then breakdown of the overlying skin with subsequent secondary infection and profuse haemorrhage is liable to occur.

IMPLANTATION OF RADON SEEDS.—A radon seed is a small metal container about 3/16 inch long and 1/8 inch wide which is filled with a gaseous emanation of radium known as Radon, and one or more of them may be introduced into the substance of a cavernous haemangioma in order to initiate the process of thrombosis. The precise length of time that they should be allowed to remain in the haemangioma is calculated beforehand and when this time (usually about thirty-six hours) has expired the seeds should be withdrawn by gently pulling on the thread which is attached to each of them. Once removed the seeds should be counted and checked in the presence of a trained nurse and then placed in a lead container that will be supplied to you and promptly returned to the radiotherapy department. This method has, like the injection of 30 per cent saline solution, the disadvantage that breakdown of the overlying skin is occasionally liable to occur.

HIGH VOLTAGE X-IRRADIATION.—This method of treatment is reserved for those cases in which the haemangioma is deeply situated and where surface applications are consequently impossible. Its use is reserved almost exclusively for haemangiomata of bone.

LYMPHANGIOMATA

Lymphangiomata are very much less common than haemangiomata and although occasionally obvious at birth the majority do not become apparent until the child is a few months old. They are usually classified into those which consist of a multitude of capillary lymphatic vessels (which are invariably *diffuse* in extent) and those which are made up of large lymphatic cysts (which present as a localized swelling).

The Diffuse or Capillary Lymphangioma

This type may occur in a variety of situations. It may cause a diffuse, incompressible, firm swelling in a limb or more rarely it may infiltrate the lip (macrochelia) or tongue (macroglossia) causing gross swelling and disfigurement. As the lymphangiomata are notorious for their resistance to surface

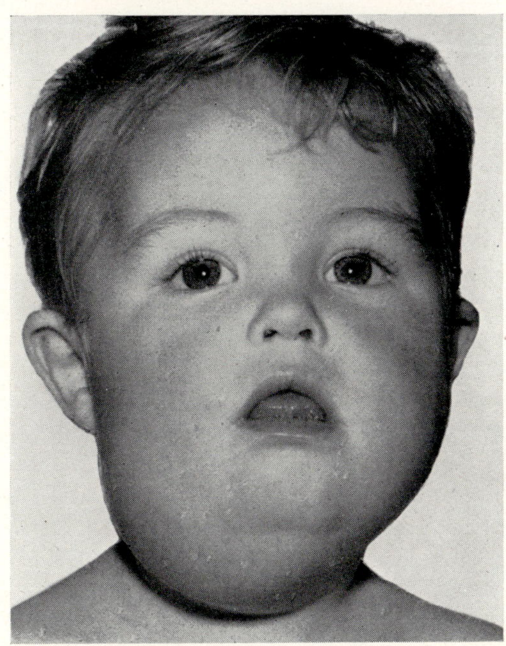

Fig. 9

A cystic hygroma. Note the associated capillary lymphangioma of the anterior two-thirds of the tongue. (See Chapter iv.)

applications or to radiotherapy the only treatment available is surgical excision, and in the case of macrochelia and macroglossia this invariably has to be followed by plastic repair.

The Localized or Cavernous Lymphangioma (Cystic Hygroma)

A cystic hygroma is seldom present at birth but usually becomes apparent within the first year of life though its appearance may more rarely be delayed until later childhood or adolescence. It consists of a localized collection of thick-walled lymphatic cysts and may be situated either in the upper cervical

region of the neck (Fig. 9), the supra-clavicular region or less commonly in the apex of the axilla. As the cysts themselves are firmly embedded in the surrounding tissues, surgical removal is a long and tedious procedure and it is for this reason that instead of surgical excision, treatment is most commonly directed to the production of an aseptic inflammation within the cysts so that the subsequent fibrous contraction will effect obliteration of the cysts and a reduction in the size of the swelling. A wide variety of irritant fluids, such as a weak solution of iodine or sodium morrhuate are sometimes injected into cystic hygromas in order to produce this effect, but the chief drawback to their use is the fact that once an irritant fluid has been introduced into the cysts there is no way of retrieving it. Barbaric as it may sound the injection of boiling water into the cysts is one of the safest and most satisfactory methods available. Under a general anaesthetic the skin of the neck is thickly spread with sterile vaseline as a precaution against scalding should the syringe leak, and then a few cubic centimetres of boiling water, taken straight from the sterilizer, are injected directly into the cysts comprising the hygroma. Postoperatively there is often a mild reactionary swelling but this causes the child little or no discomfort and usually disappears in the course of a day or so. In order to produce the maximum amount of shrinkage this procedure often has to be repeated a number of times at three or six monthly intervals.

CYSTS

Cystic swellings are not common findings in childhood and are invariably due to the persistence of some embryological structure.

Dermoid Cysts

With the exception of the external angular dermoid (see Chapter IV), dermoid cysts always occur in the mid-line of the body, the commonest situations being the sub-mental region and immediately above the upper end of the sternum. The cyst is usually first noticed as a painless swelling which gradually increases in size and, in view of this progressive enlargement and the fact that secondary infection is a frequent complication, surgical excision of the swelling is always advisable.

2*

THYROGLOSSAL CYSTS

ANATOMY.—The tongue is originally formed from two principal components, one of which forms the anterior two-thirds and the other the posterior third. Before they unite to form the tongue, however, they are separated by a lump of tissue which is destined to become the thyroid gland (Fig. 10 A).

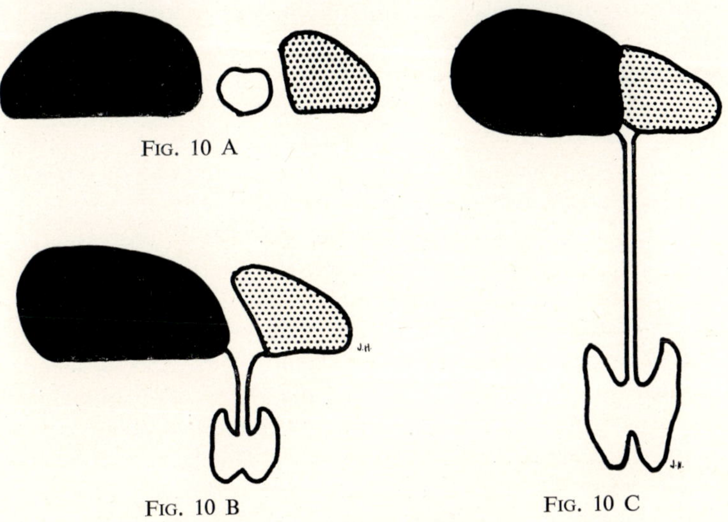

FIG. 10 A

FIG. 10 B   FIG. 10 C

The development of the thyroid gland. The anterior two-thirds of the tongue are coloured black and the posterior third is stippled.

As the two components of the tongue come together so the thyroid tissue leaves its original position and descends to a lower position in the neck (Fig. 10 B). Normally this primitive association between the thyroid gland and the tongue disappears but occasionally it remains in the form of a narrow channel connecting the thyroid gland with the junction of the posterior third and the anterior two-thirds of the tongue (see Fig. 10 C), and a cystic dilatation occurring in this tract is known as a thyroglossal cyst.

Thyroglossal cysts may occur in either boys or girls and they present as a swelling in the mid-line of the neck usually just above the thyroid cartilage. Apart from their unsightliness, the chief complication associated with them is that they may rupture through the skin and leave behind a small hole which persistently discharges a glairy fluid (a thyroglossal

fistula). Treatment of the cyst consists of surgical excision and as the thyroglossal track is always in intimate connection with the mid portion of the hyoid bone this piece of bone should also be removed in the course of the operation. Providing the whole track is excised in this manner the swelling does not recur.

A thyroglossal fistula is a more difficult condition to treat as its lower reaches are chronically infected and adherent to the surrounding tissues, and this renders dissection of the track a more difficult proposition. For this reason a dye, such as methylene blue, is usually injected up the fistula so that during the course of the operation, if the track is cut across, it will be revealed by a discharge of blue dye into the wound. Under a general anaesthetic administered from an endotracheal tube, an elliptical incision is made round the opening of the fistula and after the track has been dissected upwards to the root of the tongue, it is removed together with the mid portion of the hyoid bone.

Branchial Cysts

Branchial cysts are most uncommon in childhood and occur more frequently in adolescents and young adults. They are believed to originate from remnants of one of the primitive gill clefts that are present in early embryological existence and they present as a smooth, cystic swelling which protrudes from beneath the anterior border of the upper third of the sternomastoid muscle. As they invariably continue to increase in size, surgical excision of the swelling is always indicated.

TUMOURS

Tumours are uncommon conditions in infancy and childhood, but none the less it is important for you to know the basic facts about them and the course they are liable to pursue. In the following paragraphs we shall consider the classification of tumours together with the characteristics of one or two individual types, the remainder being described in the relevant chapters dealing with the various systems in which they are prone to occur.

For our present purposes a tumour is best defined as an abnormal mass of tissue, the growth of which exceeds and is

unrelated to that of the normal tissues. It exists at the expense of the body as a whole yet provides no useful contribution in return, and although the word tumour is often applied to any swelling, irrespective of its nature, it is best to reserve its use in order to confirm with the above definition. For the most part tumours may be broadly classified into those that are *benign* and those that are *malignant*, though very rarely there are examples in which it is difficult to obtain such a satisfactory or clear-cut distinction.

BENIGN TUMOURS

Benign tumours are so called because they always remain localized to the situation in which they have arisen and, apart from local pressure effects that they may exert on the neighbouring tissue, they do not threaten the health or integrity of the body as a whole. The individual benign tumours that you should know about are considered in the relevant chapters but the following are those which may occur in almost any situation or system.

Lipoma

A lipoma is an abnormal collection of fatty tissue which, although it may occur in any tissue of the body (except the brain) is most commonly encountered in the region of the back and the shoulders. Lipomata may be large or small and in certain instances may contain varying amounts of fibrous or haemangiomatous tissue. Although they seldom become painful, or tender or in any way a liability to the individual, most parents are anxious that they should be removed and surgical excision may easily be carried out.

Fibroma

A fibroma is an abnormal collection of fibrous tissue which arises for no apparent cause and without a previous episode of acute inflammation. It presents as a firm swelling just beneath the skin and is not infrequently rather tender. It may quite easily be removed by surgical excision.

Neurofibroma

A neurofibroma is a tumour of the peripheral nerves and is composed of an intimate admixture of both fibrous and

nervous tissue. In the generalized condition of neurofibromatosis (Von Recklinghausen's Disease) large numbers of neurofibromata are present on the cutaneous nerves and appear as multiple small, firm swellings beneath the skin. In addition, the skin itself shows irregular patches of fawn discoloration (café au lait spots), and occasionally polydactyly (more than five digits on the hands or feet) may be an associated finding. Treatment for the general condition is of no avail and surgical intervention is confined to the removal of such individual swellings that may become unduly painful.

Malignant Tumours

Malignant tumours differ from the benign variety in that they fail to remain localized to the site of origin. Instead they spread into the surrounding structures, and in addition, malignant cells become disseminated by the lymphatic system or the blood-stream (or both) into more remote tissues and organs. Such secondary deposits of the original tumour (metastases) continue to grow in whatever tissue they may have lodged until finally, after progressive wasting, death is the inevitable outcome.

Principles of Treatment

There are two principle methods available in the treatment of malignant tumours, both of which are frequently used in conjunction with each other. Providing there is no evidence that dissemination has taken place then wide surgical excision of the primary tumour may be carried out in the hope of eradicating the disease. In a good many cases, however, this is impracticable and resort must therefore be made to High Voltage X-irradiation. This form of treatment is based upon the fact that malignant cells are far more susceptible to the lethal effect of high voltage X-rays than are normal cells and it is therefore employed either as a preliminary to surgery in order to effect shrinkage of a large growth and thus make surgical excision possible; or it may be used as a secondary adjuvant to surgery in order to destroy any malignant cells that may have been unavoidably left behind in the tissues following removal; or it may be used as the only therapeutic measure available in certain situations where the local conditions preclude any form

of surgical intervention. High voltage X-irradiation is unfortunately accompanied by various side effects, the most important of which is a pronounced depressant action on the bone marrow which may cause severe degrees of anaemia and leucopenia (a diminution of the number of circulating white blood corpuscles); and it is for this reason that during a course of treatment, regular examinations of the blood should be carried out at weekly intervals.

Hodgkin's Disease (Lymphadenoma)

Hodgkin's disease is one of those conditions which is difficult to fit into the strict classification of benign or malignant tumours. It is best regarded as being somewhere between the two and also as a disease of the whole of the lymphatic system rather than a single tumour. It occurs in late childhood, adolescence and early adult life and irrespective of the course it may run, is invariably fatal in its outcome. It is twice as common in males as it is in females and is characterized by a progressive painless enlargement of the lymph glands of the body. The disease is frequently first revealed in the cervical lymph glands where it may remain localized for many months, but involvement of other groups of lymph glands throughout the body inevitably follows. Short periods of fever sustained from fifteen to twenty-five days may occur (the Pel-Ebstein fever) and in about a third of the cases there is enlargement of the liver and the spleen. As the disease progresses, severe anaemia and an increasing debility of the child make themselves apparent and there is also an increased susceptibility to secondary infections, particularly pulmonary tuberculosis. Surgery is restricted to removal of one of the glands in order to confirm the diagnosis (a biopsy). High voltage X-ray therapy is of value in reducing the size of the glands but its benefit is only temporary and after a short while the glands once again begin to increase in size. Death usually occurs within five years after the appearance of the first swelling.

CHAPTER I

INFLAMMATION

INFLAMMATION is the term used to describe the changes which occur in the tissues of the body as a result of injury or infection. As injuries and infections are the commonest conditions you will be called upon to deal with, it is essential that you should have a clear impression both of the changes that occur and of the effects that they produce. Inflammatory changes are produced by physical, chemical, radio-active and bacterial agents and although the type of inflammation caused by each of these may vary, the fundamental tissue changes are invariably the same. The whole purpose of these inflammatory changes, or the *inflammatory reaction* as it is called, is firstly to localize the causative agent, secondly to overcome it and thirdly to repair the damage that has been incurred in the process. It is thus most easily thought of as a defence system which is automatically brought into play in response to any physical, chemical or bacteriological threat.

Inflammation caused by physical and chemical agents will be considered in the chapters dealing with injuries and burns, so for the present we will consider the inflammatory reaction induced by bacteria.

Bacterial inflammation may be:

(1) acute, or   (2) chronic.

ACUTE INFLAMMATION

The cardinal signs of acute inflammation were first described nearly 2,000 years ago and have been enumerated in the same order ever since. They are:

(1) Heat.   (2) Redness.

(3) Swelling.   (4) Pain, and

(5) Loss of Function.

Now let us see how these signs are produced. The first reaction on the part of the tissues is initiated by the secretions

of the bacteria themselves (*toxins*) and it consists of an increase in the diameter of the capillary vessels in the neighbourhood of the infection. Soon, both the arterioles and venules which supply and drain the area join in this dilatation and the resulting increase in the blood flow through the area involved accounts for the signs of local *heat* and *redness*.

After a short while the walls of these blood-vessels undergo a most important change. Normally the walls of the capillary vessels allow a certain amount of the plasma constituent of the blood to pass through them. In acute inflammation this permeability is greatly increased with the result that large quantities of plasma pass through the capillary walls and enter the tissue spaces. At the same time the white blood corpuscles (*leucocytes*) in the capillaries begin to stick to the lining of the vessel. They then squeeze themselves through the vessel wall and, having done so, enter the tissue spaces and proceed in the direction of the infecting organisms. This collection of plasma and leucocytes is called the *inflammatory exudate*, and by distending the tissue spaces and stretching the nerve endings in them it causes *swelling* and *pain*.

You will remember that the leucocytes of the blood are of three main varieties:

> (1) Polymorphonuclear leucocytes
>   (granulocytes: phagocytes).
> (2) Lymphocytes.
> (3) Monocytes.

In acute inflammation it is the polymorphonuclear leucocytes that are of primary importance. Some confusion always surrounds the various terms that are applied to them. *Granulocyte* merely means that the substance of the cell is granular in appearance under the microscope; *phagocyte* is the term used to describe their capacity for eating bacteria and *polymorphonuclear* refers to the varying number of lobes that the nucleus of these cells may possess. As far as we are concerned these three terms refer to one and the same cell.

The importance of the inflammatory exudate is as follows:
(1) The bacterial toxins are diluted by the plasma and are also exposed to the antibodies which the plasma contains.
(2) The polymorphonuclear leucocytes
　　(*a*) engulf the bacteria (the process of phagocytosis), and
　　(*b*) secrete anti-bacterial enzymes.

Loss of function depends largely on the site of the inflammation.   For example a boil in the middle of the back does not interfere with movement in any way, but a boil on the eyelid makes it almost impossible to open the eye due to the intense pain and swelling that it causes.

Apart from these local changes there is a constitutional reaction as well.   Some of the bacterial toxins are absorbed into the general circulation, causing a mild *toxaemia* (toxins in the blood).   The degree of this toxaemia depends upon the success with which the inflammatory reaction is dealing with the infection, and also upon the type and the virulence of the bacteria.   A mild toxaemia causes an elevation in the temperature and a raised pulse rate together with the subjective symptoms of feeling generally off-colour, loss of appetite (*anorexia*), and sometimes headache.   In infants and very young children the elevation of the temperature may appear to be out of all proportion to the severity of the infection, and in infants especially, toxaemia may be accompanied by protracted vomiting.   Vomiting in such an instance is referred to as *symptomatic* vomiting which denotes that it is an associated happening and not of primary significance.   Provided the toxaemia is not overwhelming it has two important effects:

(1) it stimulates the body to produce an antibody against the circulating bacterial toxin, and

(2) it stimulates the bone marrow to increase the production of *polymorphonuclear* leucocytes (see Fig. 11).

The response of the bone marrow is called the *leucocyte response* and in conditions of acute inflammation the circulating blood may show an increased number of leucocytes reaching as high as 20-40,000/c.mm. of blood (normal 6-8,000/c.mm.) of which the majority (90-95 per cent) are polymorphonuclear cells.   This *white blood cell count* as it is called may be of diagnostic value in the early stages of infected internal organs where only the pain of inflammation is apparent and the heat, redness and swelling are concealed.

These then are the resources, both local and general, that the body can mobilize in its defence.   The fate of the inflamed area depends largely on the ability of the inflammatory reaction to overcome the infection.   If the bacteria are rapidly overwhelmed then the inflammation subsides without incident.   If the virulence of the organism is sufficiently intense, the body

may be unable to localize the bacteria and a *spreading infection* will ensue. On the other hand, there may be a more or less equal balance between the bacteria and the inflammatory reaction and a *localized infection* will result. In this event large numbers of leucocytes and bacteria are destroyed by each other in the course of the contest, and, in addition, local tissue cells

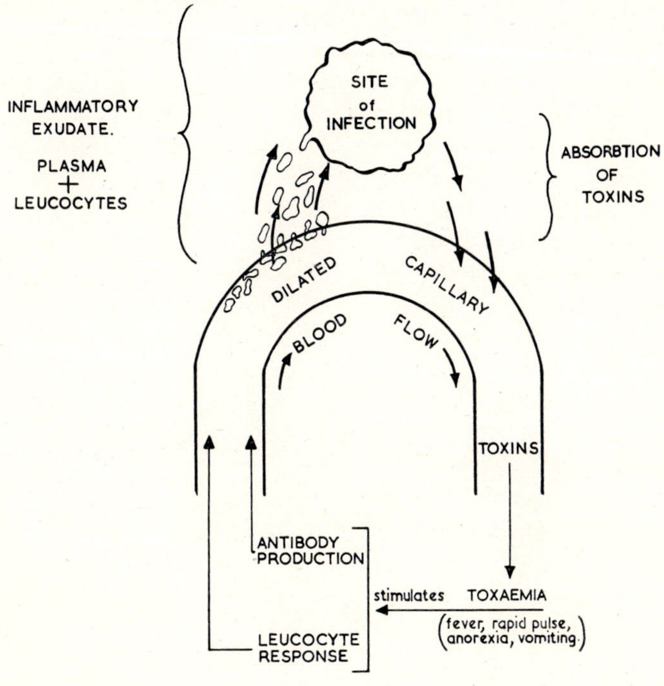

Fig. 11

To illustrate the origin and the effects of toxaemia.

themselves will be destroyed by the toxins of the bacteria. As a result of this, the inflamed area will now consist of a local collection of:

(1) Live and dead bacteria;   (2) live and dead leucocytes;

(3) liquefied dead tissue cells;   (4) plasma;

and this is what is called *pus*. Thus you will see that the production of pus (*suppuration*) is an indication that localization has begun to take place.

The General Treatment of Acute Inflammation

The methods of treating individual cases of acute inflammation will of course be conditioned both by the nature of the infecting organism and the site of the infection, but in general we may say that treatment is directed towards *assisting the inflammatory reaction.* For this reason *heat* in the form of hot poultices and fomentations when applied to the inflamed area will dilate additional numbers of local blood vessels and thus open up further ' routes of supply ' for the defences of the body. The assistance rendered by these measures therefore has the effect of speeding up the inflammatory reaction. In cases of deep-seated inflammation such as in the abdomen and pelvis, short-wave diathermy, which has the property of producing heat at varying distances *beneath* the skin's surface, may be used to promote an increased blood supply to an inflamed organ. Similarly the systemic use of antibiotics such as penicillin, streptomycin and chloromycetin will support and assist the inflammatory reaction by virtue of their lethal (*bacteriocidal*) effect on the bacteria. The sulphonamide group of drugs and also the latest and most powerful antibiotic aureomycin, exert their effect principally by preventing the bacteria from multiplying (a *bacteriostatic* action) and so make the work of the leucocytes easier and more effective.

The pain of acute inflammation is treated most effectively by:

(1) Rest.   (2) Pain relieving drugs (*analgesics*).

(1) **Rest.**—Rest is the oldest and most satisfactory method of treating pain. It allows the inflammatory responses to proceed undisturbed and unhindered by movement. In extensive infections with marked constitutional disturbances complete rest in bed is the first essential in treatment. In local affections such as infection of the pulp of a finger-tip, rest of the affected hand and arm in a sling will afford increased relief from the intense throbbing pain which characterizes this condition.

(2) **Analgesics.**—The only point of treating the pain of an acute inflammation by drugs is to relieve the patient of unnecessary discomfort, especially if it is interfering with sleep. It is most important, however, for you to realize that pain is

also an index of the severity of the local condition. Thus an increase in the degree of pain may indicate an increase in the severity of the condition, and if your patient has been drugged beyond his sensibility to pain, this most valuable sign of increasing danger may pass unnoticed. One of the most satisfactory analgesics for children is small repeated doses of aspirin (2-5 grains every four hours). As well as its pain relieving properties aspirin has an additional beneficial effect in that it causes increased sweating and thus may assist in lowering the child's temperature. More powerful analgesic drugs such as pethidine and the derivatives of morphia are very seldom indicated in acute inflammatory conditions.

The general aspects of treatment in acute inflammation may be summarized as:

 (1) Rest—general or local.
 (2) Local applications of heat.
 (3) Antibiotic drugs.
 (4) Analgesic drugs when required.

CHRONIC INFLAMMATION

Chronic inflammation may best be defined as a state of inflammation in which the acute signs are not in evidence. It is a less dramatic process altogether than acute inflammation and may occur either as a sequel to it, or as the result of an infection by an organism which characteristically does not cause an acute stage (e.g. the organism of tuberculosis).

Whereas the microscopic appearances of acute inflammation are principally the exudate of plasma and the presence of polymorphonuclear leucocytes, in chronic inflammation there is little or no inflammatory exudate and the predominant white blood cells are *lymphocytes*. These lymphocytes accumulate in large numbers and form a defensive zone around the focus of infection. In this zone may also be seen large scavenging cells called *macrophages*, whose main concern is the removal of the dead and dying tissue in the area. This zone of lymphocytes and macrophages merges into a second zone composed of *fibrous tissue cells*. The fibrous tissue formed by these cells acts firstly as a barrier around the focus, and secondly as a means of replacing the damaged tissues by a scar.

Thus we see that *tissue destruction*, which is a rapid and predominant feature in acute inflammation is very much less in evidence in chronic inflammation and is largely overshadowed by the coincident process of *repair* that is proceeding around it.

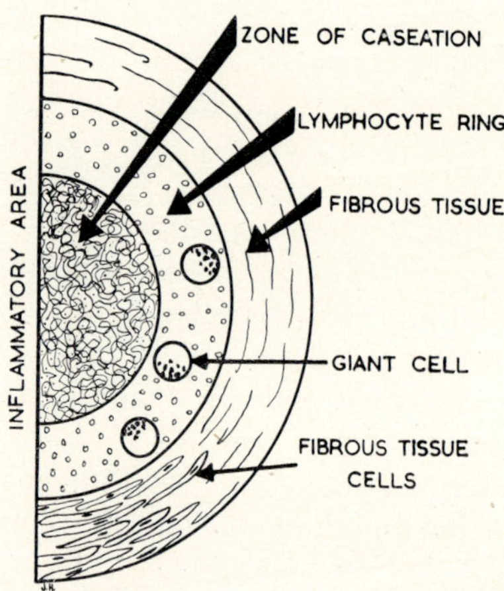

Fig. 12

A diagrammatic illustration of a tubercle.

TUBERCULOUS INFLAMMATION

This is a specific form of chronic inflammation caused by the *tubercle bacillus*.   The reaction of the tissues to the presence of the tubercle bacillus, although basically similar to the one we have just described, is characterized particularly by the presence of *giant cells*.   These are very large, irregularly shaped cells, which contain numerous nuclei (unlike other cells which normally have only one) and they are usually situated on the inner margin of the zone of lymphocytes.

The toxins of the tubercle bacillus in addition to initiating the production of this particular type of tissue reaction also have the effect of causing the obliteration of the adjacent capillaries.   The result of this is that the centre of the focus, being deprived of its blood supply, breaks down into a putty-like substance which, because of its remarkable similarity to cheese is known as *caseous material*.   The disease process that we have described now consists of:

3

    (1) a caseous centre;

    (2) lymphocytes and giant cells;

    (3) fibrous tissue (see Fig. 12).

This focus is known as a *tubercle* and its fate, like all inflammatory conditions, depends upon the virulence of the organism and the success of the defences of the body against it. If the disease fails to progress, the fibrous tissue surrounding the tubercle will finally obliterate it leaving only a dense scar. Subsequently these scars frequently become calcified and as such become visible in X-ray photographs. If, on the other hand, the disease progresses, the caseous material will gradually increase in amount and slowly encroach upon the surrounding tissues, so that if unchecked the whole organ involved (such as a lymph gland or kidney) will eventually be converted into a single caseous mass.

Finally let us summarize the chief differences between the various forms of inflammation that we have mentioned:

TABLE I

	ACUTE	CHRONIC	TUBERCULOUS
Vascularity (heat and redness)	Greatly increased	Very little	None
Inflammatory exudate	Profuse	Minimal	None
Cellular reaction	Polymorphonuclear leucocytes	Lymphocytes Fibrous tissue cells	Lymphocytes Giant cells Fibrous tissue cells
Tenderness of the lesion	Usually intense	Little or none	None
Constitutional disturbances	Fever. Pain. Raised pulse rate. Anorexia. Vomiting (especially in infants)	Little or none	None unless an extensive or rapidly advancing lesion

CHAPTER II

SURGICAL INFECTIONS

As we saw in the previous chapter inflammatory reactions induced by bacteria may be predominantly:

    (1) acute or chronic;

    (2) suppurative or non-suppurative;

    (3) spreading or localized.

By applying these terms to the various conditions we are now about to consider, each infection can be clearly and concisely defined.

A BOIL (furuncle)

A boil is an *acute, localized, suppurative* infection of a hair follicle or sebaceous gland, and is caused either by the staphylococcus albus or aureus. The skin over a boil becomes reddened, hot and acutely tender. After an interval of a few days the boil bursts through the skin with a discharge of thick yellow pus. This discharge continues for a few days after which healing is uneventful. The degree of pain associated with a boil may vary according to the situation of the infection and depends largely on the ability of the local tissues to stretch. For instance, in the external auditory meatus where the skin is firmly attached to the underlying cartilage, there is little or no room for expansion. Thus the greatly increased tension caused by a boil in this situation will produce such an intense degree of pain that incision before the boil is 'ripe' may be necessary in order to relieve it. In other situations surgical incision is seldom called for and treatment is confined to local applications of heat and rest of the affected area. Unless severe constitutional disturbances are present, antibiotics are not advisable as they do not assist early rupture of the lesion. In fact they may do the very opposite. They may so assist the inflammatory reaction (which has already succeeded in localizing the infection)

that a chronic inflammatory state around a collection of semi-sterile pus may ensue.

CARBUNCLE

A carbuncle is an *acute, suppurative, poorly localized, and gangrenous* infection of the subcutaneous tissues and is caused by the staphylococcus aureus. The skin over a carbuncle becomes hot and brawny and is punctuated with several small holes through which the pus from the subcutaneous tissues discharges on to the surface. After a few days the covering skin becomes gangrenous and soon separates from the deeper tissues leaving behind a crater which discharges thick yellow pus and lumps of dead subcutaneous tissue (*sloughs*).

The presence of diabetes should always be excluded by testing the urine for sugar (see p. 184).

Although an uncommon condition in childhood a carbuncle can be none the less a dangerous one. Its chief danger lies in the fact that the walls of the small veins in the subcutaneous tissues may become invaded by the infection. This leads to clotting of the blood on the inside of the vein wall (*thrombosis*). These clots, having become infected themselves, may then become detached from the vein wall and be conducted by the flow of blood into the general circulation. This is of particular significance in the face where the facial veins communicate with a large venous sinus at the base of the brain (the cavernous sinus). Should an infected clot from a carbuncle of the face find its way to the cavernous sinus it will there cause a septic thrombosis of this structure : the result is always fatal.

Treatment of a carbuncle consists of the administration of large doses of penicillin and complete bed rest for the patient. The carbuncle itself should be covered only with a light dressing in order to absorb the pus but apart from this it should not be disturbed in any way in view of the danger of disseminating septic clots. If the skin loss is extensive skin, grafting to the raw area may eventually have to be employed.

ERYSIPELAS

This is an *acute, rapidly spreading, non-suppurative* infection of the skin caused by the haemolytic streptococcus. The organism gains access through any minute wound or abrasion

and spreading through the lymphatic channels in the dermis causes a hot, tender and fiery red discoloration of the skin. The advancing margin of this area has a slightly raised edge. Small vesicles may appear within the area of discoloration and when ruptured they exude a thin serous fluid teeming with streptococci. The disease now fortunately uncommon may be spread either by contagion or by infected dust and in the pre-Listerian days of surgery, before the significance of organisms as a cause of disease was recognized, it was partly responsible for the very high incidence of cross-infection in surgical wards. Although it may occur anywhere on the skin's surface it more commonly affects the face and scalp.

Treatment

Large frequent doses of aqueous penicillin by intra-muscular injection have a rapid curative effect but during treatment it is essential that the patient is nursed in strict isolation. All dressings and bed linen must be dumped into a covered receiver *before* they are removed from the cubicle. Immediate incineration of these dressings either in the ward or hospital incinerator should then be carried out. Following this the container should be soaked in a 1 : 20 solution of carbolic acid for half an hour after which it should be scrubbed under running water and then boiled for twenty minutes. When the child has been discharged the bed mattress must be baked, the cot thoroughly washed in disinfectant and the cubicle fumigated.

CELLULITIS

This is an *acute, spreading, suppurative* infection of the subcutaneous tissues caused either by the staphylococcus aureus or the haemolytic streptococcus. The infection is usually of sudden onset and because of the rapid spread is often attended by a severe toxaemia. Suppuration is a late feature and may be associated with extensive tissue destruction. The skin over the area becomes red, brawny, tense and acutely tender. The lymphatic vessels draining the infected area may also become acutely inflamed (*lymphangitis*) and become recognizable as bright red streaks running from the inflamed area towards the regional lymph nodes which themselves become enlarged and tender (*lymphadenitis*).

Treatment

Before suppuration has occurred treatment consists of rest of the affected part, local applications of heat and the systemic administration of large doses of penicillin. These measures will usually cause early resolution. Once suppuration has occurred, however, the pus can only be released by surgical incision into the affected area. The copious discharge of pus which follows this procedure is usually followed during the next few days by the extrusion of dirty grey sloughs through the wound. The evacuation of the pus produces a marked degree of improvement in the general condition of the child. The temperature and pulse return to normal, the child ceases to be perpetually fretful and begins to take an interest in his food and surroundings. Once the slough has been discharged healing of the wound is rapid.

Cellulitis occurring in a deeper plane than the subcutaneous tissues is of particular importance and this is especially so in the deeper layers of the neck. Whereas in cellulitis of the subcutaneous tissues the skin over the area is rapidly involved by the inflammatory reaction and becomes hot, red, swollen and tender, in a cellulitis beneath the deep fascia of the neck (a *deep cellulitis*) extensive suppuration may have occurred before the skin shows any change in its appearance. Thus the likelihood of pus extending along the deep tissue planes of the neck before skin involvement makes the diagnosis obvious renders deep cellulitis a very much more dangerous condition than the subcutaneous type. The clinical appearances of this condition and its treatment will be dealt with in Chapter V.

TETANUS

The infections which we have considered so far have all been caused by organisms which are dependent upon the presence of oxygen for their existence and multiplication (*aerobic organisms*). The organism of tetanus belongs to a group of organisms (the *clostridia*) which thrive in the *absence* of oxygen (*anaerobic organisms*). In addition, the clostridia have the property of turning themselves into *spores* once conditions become unsuited for their existence. These spores are exceptionally resistant both to chemical disinfection and to

extremes of heat and cold. For example, tetanus spores must be subjected to a steam pressure of 30 lb. per square inch (producing a temperature of 260° F.) for thirty minutes before they are destroyed.

The tetanus bacillus normally lives in the intestines of grass-eating agricultural animals and its spores are therefore commonly found in soil and in street dust. They may also be present in coarse woven woollen materials such as blankets and thick flannel. For these reasons any wound which is contaminated by dust, dirt or cloth, especially deep wounds containing devitalized tissue and blood clot, may well be the starting point of a tetanus infection. After an incubation period varying from between two and twenty-one days the tetanus bacillus produces a most virulent toxin which has a specific effect on the nervous system. This toxin reaches the nervous system both by the blood stream and also by passing along nerve trunks, and its effect is to cause a greatly increased reflex excitability of the motor nerve cells. This causes sudden spasms of whole groups of muscles which may either occur spontaneously or may follow the slightest sensory impulse. Inability to open the mouth due to spasm of the masseter muscles (*trismus*), neck rigidity and difficulty in swallowing are usually the first signs of the disease. Later the muscles of the chest, abdomen and spine may become involved causing severe respiratory embarrassment. Death, which may be preceded by hyper-pyrexia (temperatures of 108°-110° F.), is usually due to exhaustion and respiratory failure.

Local tetanus, which is a less serious condition, occurs when the production of toxin is very slight and the only motor nerves involved are those supplying the muscles around the site of the infection.

Tetanus neonatorum is a rare form of the disease in which the infection gains access through the umbilicus during the first day or so of life. Healing of the umbilicus itself may appear to be normal. The first symptom appears at the end of the second week of life and takes the form of trismus which causes difficulty in feeding. Spasmodic contraction of muscles usually follow and may proceed to generalized convulsions.

Never has the old saying ' Prevention is better than cure ' been more true than it is in the case of tetanus. The disease itself carries a mortality of approximately 50 per cent, and as

treatment of the established condition is both difficult and in many ways unsatisfactory, prophylactic (preventive) immunization against the disease, which will prevent the onset of the condition or at least attenuate its severity, is infinitely the wisest course.

IMMUNIZATION

Immunization against tetanus may be either:
         (1) active, or
         (2) passive.

Active Immunization

This is produced by injecting into the body a solution of tetanus toxin which has been treated with formalin (tetanus toxoid) in order to render it incapable of causing the disease. Two intra-muscular injections of 0·5 cc. of tetanus toxoid are given with an interval of six weeks between them. The anti-toxin produced in response to these injections confers an immunity in the body against the action of the tetanus toxin should such an infection subsequently occur. This form of immunity usually lasts between one and two years and if it is to be sustained it requires a ' booster ' injection of 0·5 cc. of tetanus toxoid at yearly intervals. Active immunization is most commonly used to protect members of the armed services against infection by tetanus bacilli of wounds received in battle, but some authorities consider there is a good case for its use in children.

Passive Immunization

Whereas active immunization takes several weeks to produce an immunity, passive immunization is a method of conferring a temporary but immediate protection against the disease. Anti-tetanus serum (A.T.S.) is extracted from horses in which active immunity has previously been produced. It has, however, one serious drawback. The horse's serum in which the anti-toxin is contained may produce a state of sensitivity in the patient's body. Thus the patient who has had one injection of A.T.S. and who, months or even years later receives a further injection of it, may suffer various forms of reaction. Such reactions may consist of a feeling of giddiness, of sickness or of fainting, tightness of breath, skin rashes or oedema

of the face and hands. In its severest form, sudden collapse and even death may follow the injection. *Serum sickness* is a *delayed* form of reaction in which local or generalized patches of oedema of the skin, associated with a pyrexia, may appear up to two weeks after the injection. Occasionally these reactions may occur in patients who have *not* previously been sensitized to horse serum. It is for these reasons that intra-muscular injections of prophylactic A.T.S. are preceded by a small *intra-dermal* injection. If after about twenty minutes a red weal appears at the site of this injection it indicates that the patient is already sensitive to A.T.S. In such an instance the normal dose of 1,500 units of A.T.S. should be given minim by minim over a period of several hours and discontinued at the first sign of any of the symptoms mentioned above. If a reaction should occur, an intra-muscular injection of adrenalin (1 : 10,000 solution) should be given to the child without delay. Very young children should not receive more than 2 minims of adrenalin, but children over ten years of age may receive up to 9 minims. If the reaction is *severe* and there is no improvement following the first dose of adrenalin, the dose should be repeated at two-minute intervals until recovery takes place.

All cases of wounds likely to have been contaminated by tetanus spores should receive a prophylactic dose of A.T.S. *before* the wound is dealt with. This allows the circulation of the anti-toxin throughout the body before the risk of spread of the organisms by surgical interference occurs.

It is important for you to remember that neither active nor passive immunization is an *absolute* guarantee against tetanus. Should tetanus supervene following immunization, however, the disease takes a very much less severe course than it would otherwise have done. Finally, you must realize that both forms of immunization may substantially increase the incubation period of the disease, even up to three or four months. As a general working rule it may be said that the longer the disease takes to appear following infection, the less serious it is likely to be.

Treatment of Tetanus

In an established case of tetanus 50-100,000 units of A.T.S. are at once administered by intra-muscular injection and some authorities advise that this dose should be repeated each day.

On no account, however, should the wound be touched until this therapeutic dose of A.T.S. has been given, for in this way there will always be a circulating anti-toxin in the blood should dissemination of the infection occur when dealing with the wound. In addition to the above dose some authorities also advocate giving a daily dose of 10,000 units of A.T.S. into the spinal theca. The wound itself is inspected and all particulate matter and old blood clot removed. As it is essential that the wound should be disturbed as little as possible, it is left open and a light gauze dressing soaked in 10 volume hydrogen peroxide applied to it. Frequently the wound is also infected with *pyogenic* (pus producing) organisms and in this event penicillin powder should be dusted into the wound and aqueous penicillin given in large doses intra-muscularly.

The child is nursed in a quiet and darkened room in order to protect him as far as possible from any external stimuli which may precipitate muscle contractions. Sedation is employed to abort these muscle spasms and so prevent the child from suffering unnecessary exhaustion. Pentobarbitone ($\frac{1}{2}$ grain per stone body-weight) by mouth or paraldehyde (60-180 minims) per rectum are valuable in this respect, but if the contractions are unduly frequent and severe, muscle relaxants such as 0·25 cc. of tubocurarine in oil may have to be given by intra-muscular injection, and in the event of respiratory embarrassment tracheotomy may have to be performed in order to ensure a clear airway. Feeding should be in the form of a high calorie, fluid diet and while trismus is present it will have to be administered through a nasal catheter.

GAS GANGRENE

Gas gangrene is a rare but exceptionally dangerous form of wound infection which primarily affects muscle tissue. It is caused by a group of anaerobic spore-forming bacilli of the clostridium family which normally inhabit the large gut of humans and animals. When introduced into the tissues they produce powerful toxins which attack and destroy the sugar and protein content of the muscles. It is this decomposition of the muscles which results in the local production of *gas*. Deep wounds which contain devitalized tissue, blood clot or clothing soiled with faeces, or wounds which are contaminated

by soil or manure are most likely to produce this disease. The incubation period is usually between twenty-four to forty-eight hours. The first sign of the disease is a loss of the power of contraction of the muscles in the vicinity of the wound and there may also be a thin blood-stained discharge from the wound itself. The surrounding tissues become increasingly tense and a crackling sensation due to the gas may be felt beneath the skin. At this stage an X-ray of the wound area will show the presence of gas bubbles in the tissues. As the disease progresses the surrounding skin quickly becomes mottled with greenish-yellow patches and offensive-smelling gas bubbles out of the wound. The child, though mentally alert, becomes increasingly pale, the temperature rises to the level of 104°-105° F., the pulse becomes rapid and thready, and vomiting and intense thirst are common. In the severest form of the disease (a *fulminating infection*) the intense toxaemia may result in death even before much gas has been formed. More usually, however, the infection remains localized for a short time in the particular group of muscles which surround the wound (a *group infection*).

As there are three principal organisms which are capable of causing gas gangrene a mixed anti-serum has been prepared which contains the specific anti-sera against each organism. A prophylactic dose of 30,000 units of this mixed anti-gas gangrene serum should be given (with exactly the same precautions as those used in administering A.T.S.) to all cases in which the wound is likely to have been inoculated with the organisms of gas gangrene. In an established case of the disease not less than 100,000 units of the mixed serum should be given by intra-muscular injection and repeated twice a day. Penicillin in doses of 2 million units a day should also be given. As soon as the first dose of anti-serum has been given no time is lost in performing an extensive surgical incision into the infected area and removing the dead and decomposing muscle. Only the lightest gauze dressings are applied so that the toxins may find their way to the surface rather than be absorbed into the blood-stream. Post-operatively a very close watch indeed must be kept for fear of extension of the infection to other muscle groups. In the event of rapid spread, amputation of the limb well above the infected area may be unavoidable.

SEPTICAEMIA AND PYAEMIA

In *septicaemia*, pyogenic bacteria invade the blood-stream, multiply and produce a severe bodily upset. The organisms responsible are usually the haemolytic streptococcus, the staphylococcus or the pneumococcus. A *streptococcal* septicaemia produces a high temperature (105°-106° F.), a rapid pulse, a raised respiratory rate, attacks of sweating, restlessness and even delirium. Skin rashes and purpuric haemorrhages are common and widespread abscess formation may occur. If not treated it runs a quick and frequently fatal course. *Staphylococcal* septicaemia although not usually so severe as the streptococcal variety runs a similar course. It may arise as a result of the introduction of staphylococci into the blood-stream from a boil, an infected wound or in osteomyelitis (see Chapter XIII). When occurring in the newborn, the portal of entry is usually an infected umbilical stump or scar. The condition characteristically produces multiple staphylococcal abscesses which may occur in the lungs, the bones or the subcutaneous tissues.

It is essential in treating a suspected case of septicaemia that a *blood culture* should be performed before commencing treatment. This procedure will tell you firstly the organism that is responsible, and secondly its sensitivity to the various antibiotic drugs. As soon as the blood has been withdrawn for culture the child is placed upon large doses of penicillin without delay and if the subsequent sensitivity tests show the organism to be insensitive to penicillin the appropriate antibiotic is substituted in its place.

Pyaemia is a condition in which clumps of organisms or infected blood clots gain access into the blood-stream. It is usually a sequel to a focus of inflammation where pus is under tension and may occur in osteomyelitis or infections of the middle ear. The infected clots set free from these foci of infection become lodged in the lungs where they form small abscesses from which secondary clumps of organisms may be cast off and disseminated through the arterial system. Treatment of pyaemia is directed to relief of the tension of pus in the primary focus of infection by surgical incision, the administration of large doses of penicillin, and incision and drainage of secondary abscess whenever and wherever possible.

CHAPTER III

THE EFFECTS OF TRAUMA

INJURIES AND WOUNDS

WOUNDS of the body caused by injury may be classified as either *open* or *closed*, depending on whether or not the skin remains intact.

CLOSED WOUNDS

There are two principal varieties of closed wounds:

(1) Haematoma.   (2) Abrasion.

(1) HAEMATOMA.—An haematoma is a collection of blood in the tissue spaces consequent upon the rupture of small blood-vessels beneath the skin, and it is usually slowly absorbed without incident. An haematoma should be treated conservatively for the first day or so, but if severe pain persists it may be aspirated through a wide bore needle. As it is an excellent medium for bacterial growth an haematoma may occasionally become infected, and in this event surgical incision of the infected area should be performed, and the blood and the pus evacuated.

(2) ABRASION.—This is the commonest form of injury you will ever see and it is popularly referred to as a graze. As the superficial layers of the skin have been scraped away, minute nerve endings are laid bare and it is for this reason that an abrasion is a much more painful injury than an haematoma. Sometimes, especially in road accidents, minute particles of grit are forced into the skin and may produce a permanent ' tattooing ' of the area. This is seldom of undue importance, except when it occurs on the face. In such an instance the facial abrasion should be thoroughly cleansed with soap and water or cetavlon and then, under a general anaesthetic, gently scrubbed with a sterile nail brush until all the minute particles are removed. The wound should then be dressed with tulle gras and covered with a light dressing.

OPEN WOUNDS

Open wounds may be:
(1) Incised;
(2) Penetrating;
(3) Lacerated,

and it is most important that before any of them are dealt with by surgical means, the child should *always* receive a prophylactic dose of anti-tetanus serum.

(1) INCISED WOUNDS.—This type of wound is most commonly caused by the surgeon's knife. It may also occur as a result of accidental wounding by glass or any form of cutting instrument. The edges of the wound are invariably cleanly cut and can easily be brought into complete apposition. If produced accidentally, the wound edges and the surrounding skin should be thoroughly cleansed and then the depths of the wound should be explored and all blood clot and any foreign material removed. The edges should then be brought together with non-absorbable sutures.

(2) PENETRATING WOUNDS.—These wounds are much deeper than they are long, and their chief risk lies in the penetration of deeper organs and the possibility of infected foreign material being carried to their depth. They may be caused by stabs, by penetration of the skin in the course of a too-realistic game of bows and arrows, or they may be caused by a fall on to a sharp object such as a spike of 'area' railings. In such injuries the wound and its immediate vicinity should be X-rayed in order to demonstrate any radio opaque foreign bodies that may have been introduced. The skin wound should then be excised, explored and, if small, left open. Penicillin in doses of 1,000,000 units per day should be commenced, the part put at rest, and a close watch for the appearance of infection maintained. Penetrating wounds occurring as a result of street accidents, or those in which there is a likelihood of woollen clothing having been carried into the wound, should as we have already mentioned, *all* receive a prophylactic dose of anti-tetanus serum.

(3) LACERATED WOUNDS.—These are ragged and irregular wounds, in which there is usually some degree of bruising of the wound edges. After thorough cleansing and sterilization of the skin, the wound edges should be cleanly excised, the

depths of the wound explored, and all blood clot and foreign material removed. The wound edges should be approximated with non-absorbable sutures. In the face, as all the muscles are attached to the skin, once the skin has been cut these muscles produce a wide retraction of the wound edges. Such wounds may therefore look very much worse than they are, but due to the abundant blood supply of the skin of the face they invariably heal without incident.

Open wounds which are first seen more than twelve or twenty-four hours following the injury present a slightly different problem. There is always the possibility that infection may already be established but not yet in evidence. In such an instance the skin in the vicinity of the wound should be thoroughly cleansed but the wound itself merely covered with tulle gras and a light dressing. Intramuscular penicillin should be commenced and the part put at rest. After an interval of a day or so the wound is again inspected and if there is no evidence of an established infection then excision of the wound edges and closure of the wound may be carried out. This is called *delayed primary suture* and is employed in order to avoid the possibility of closing the skin over a potentially infected wound.

INJURIES AND WOUNDS IN SPECIAL SITES

With the exception of injuries to the eye and to the tendons we shall consider all other sites of injury in the appropriate chapters.

Injuries and Wounds of the Eye

THE CONJUNCTIVA.—Small vessels lying beneath the conjunctiva may be ruptured as the result of a blow to the closed eye. The resulting *sub-conjunctival haemorrhage* appears as a red discoloration over the ' white ' of the eye and needs no specific treatment as it is slowly absorbed in the course of a week or so.

BURNS OF THE CONJUNCTIVA.—These most commonly occur as the result of household acids and alkalis (such as are found in various cleaning preparations) being splashed into the eye. Immediate and profuse irrigation of the conjunctiva with large quantities of either warm water or saline should be

carried out. If the burning agent is known to be an acid then a tablespoonful of sodium bicarbonate should be added to the pint of irrigating fluid and if it is known to be an alkali then an ounce of vinegar or a tablespoonful of boracic powder should be added instead. In severe burns of this nature adhesions between the inside of the eyelid and the front of the eyeball (*the cornea*) may subsequently develop and if they occur they should be gently separated by a smooth glass rod well lubricated in sterile vaseline.

THE CORNEA.—The most common injuries sustained both by the conjunctiva and the cornea are caused by foreign bodies, such as small pieces of grit. The foreign body may be stuck on the front of the cornea or on the inner surface of the upper lid and in both these instances acute pain is experienced when the child blinks. When the foreign body is beneath the upper lid the lid should be gently everted and the foreign body wiped off the conjunctival surface either by the corner of a clean gauze swab or by a wisp of cotton wool wrapped round an orange stick. When embedded in the cornea the same procedure should be carried out, but if this is unsuccessful it may have to be ' dug out ' with a special metal instrument known as a *spud*. If this procedure causes undue pain to the child then the front of the eye may be anaesthetized by the instillation of a few drops of $\frac{1}{2}$ per cent cocaine. Abrasions of the cornea which are not visible to the naked eye may be revealed by the instillation of a 2 per cent solution of fluorescein which colours the abraided surface of the cornea a brilliant green. In foreign body wounds of the cornea and in simple abrasions, it is most important that the surface of the wound should be prevented from becoming infected and a few drops of 2 per cent Sulph-acetamine or 5 per cent chloromycetin eye-drops should be instilled twice daily for three or four days. The need for the ' careful checking ' of eye drops before use cannot be repeated too frequently. Damage to the eye resulting from the instillation of drops other than those prescribed is both calamitous and unforgivable.

Wounds of Tendons

Tendons may be injured in incised wounds, especially in the vicinity of joints. If the wound is cleanly incised, then, under a general anaesthetic once the wound has been cleansed in the

manner we have previously mentioned, the two ends of the tendon may be united by sutures. If, however, the wound is the slightest bit dirty the cut ends of the tendon should be left as they are and the wound edges united. A week or so later when it has become obvious that the wound is not infected it may then be re-opened and the two cut ends of the tendon united as before. Post-operatively the limb should be immobilized in plaster of Paris in such a position that the muscle and its sutured tendon are placed in the most relaxed position. This form of immobilization should be maintained for three weeks and following its removal active movements of the affected muscle and tendon should be encouraged under the supervision of a physiotherapist.

SHOCK

Shock is one of the most real yet indefinable clinical entities that exist. Its true cause is as yet unknown but the clinical appearances are easily recognized. It may conveniently be divided into two widely differing types:

    1. Primary or neurogenic shock.
    2. Secondary or traumatic shock.

PRIMARY SHOCK

Primary shock is a state of sudden vasomotor collapse which immediately follows an exceptionally painful injury. The blood-pressure falls dramatically and a temporary state of either dizziness or unconsciousness may ensue, but recovery always occurs within a few minutes. This form of shock is thought to be due to a 'bombardment' of the brain with a barrage of sensory impulses arriving from the painful area, which cause a sudden but only temporary paralysis of the cardiac and vasomotor centres.

SECONDARY SHOCK

Whereas primary shock is an *immediate* but *temporary* happening, secondary shock is characterized by a *delayed onset* and a *progressive increase* in the severity of the condition. Secondary shock occurs as a result of severe and usually

4

extensive tissue injury with or without varying degrees of haemorrhage. Although *all* the processes contributing to the production of secondary shock have yet to be discovered, it is known that certain abnormal substances liberated from the injured tissue may gain access into the blood-stream. These substances are called *depressor* substances and have the effect of causing widespread dilation of the arterioles and capillaries in the body (*vasodilatation*).

In the normal state, not all of the vast multitude of capillary vessels in the body are in use. Some are fully open, some only half open and some are closed and thus they offer a resistance to the passage of blood through the tissues. This resistance, against which the heart is having to pump, is largely responsible for the pressure of the blood in the arteries (*the blood-pressure*). You will find this easier to understand by considering the pressure of water in an ordinary garden hosepipe. The bore of the pipe is uniform throughout but is considerably narrowed at the nozzle. When the tap is turned on, the narrowing at the nozzle tip causes the pressure in the pipe to rise so that the water issues from the nozzle as a forceful jet. If now the nozzle (i.e. the resistance to the water flow) is removed, the water merely flows out of the end of the pipe in a lazy and useless manner. Thus, in the case of the arteries, when a much larger number of capillaries than normal is suddenly opened up, the resistance to the blood-flow will be removed and the blood-pressure will consequently *fall*. This is precisely what occurs in secondary shock and is in part due to the vasodilator effect of the depressor substances. As a result of the vasodilatation of large numbers of capillaries, much more blood than usual is circulating through the capillary bed and this fact, combined with the low blood-pressure, produces a sluggish blood-flow through the tissues and thus reduces the rate at which blood is returned to the heart through the veins (*the venous return*). A decrease in the venous return will automatically reduce the amount of blood the heart can pump out with each beat (*the cardiac output*), and for this reason the blood-pressure will fall even further. In this way a vicious circle is set up which, if unbroken, will cause a *progressive* lowering of the blood-pressure and may well terminate in a fatal outcome.

In addition to their vasodilator effect, these depressor substances also cause an increase in the permeability of the

capillary wall. This allows the passage of plasma through the capillary wall into the tissue spaces, with the result that the blood left behind in the vessels becomes more viscous and concentrated than normal (*haemoconcentration*). The degree of haemoconcentration varies not only with the severity of the injury but also with the nature of the injuring agent and is of particular importance in burns, when it may be extensive. This increased viscosity of the blood reduces the rate of the

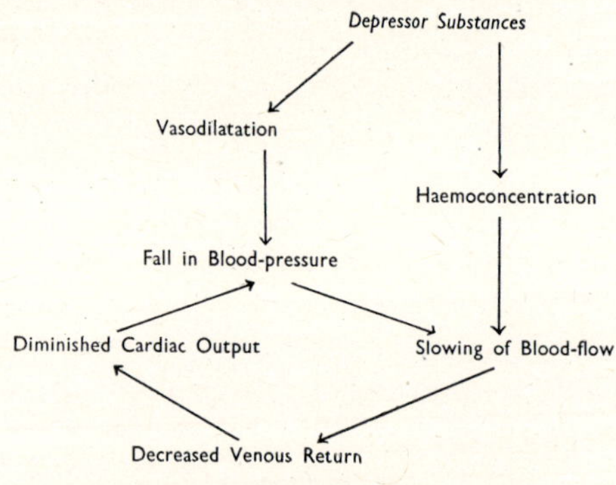

FIG. 13

The vicious circle established in Secondary Shock, showing the contributions subscribed by the depressor substances.

blood-flow through the capillaries still more and thus contributes to a further decrease in the venous return to the heart. This sequence of events is summarized in Fig. 13.

The response of the body to the state of affairs we have just described, is to attempt to raise the blood-pressure in order to ensure an adequate blood supply to vital organs such as the brain. The body does this in two ways. Firstly, it increases the pulse rate so that more blood is pumped out of the heart per minute, and secondly, it attempts to constrict the arterioles and the capillaries in order to restore the peripheral resistance. The clinical course of a patient suffering from secondary shock is largely dependent upon the ability of the body to institute and maintain these compensatory measures and it is to *assist* them that all treatment is directed.

Clinical Appearances

Typically the symptoms and signs of secondary shock begin to appear within an hour or so of injury. The child becomes

noticeably listless, increasingly pale, and may complain of dizziness and faintness. The temperature falls, the pulse begins to increase in rate and in severe degrees of shock a cold sweat may appear on the forehead and the palms of the hands. As a result of the slowing of the circulation and the increased number of dilated capillaries, the blood in these vessels becomes more de-oxygenated than usual and the local tissue anoxia resulting from this is revealed by a bluish tinge in the skin of the feet and hands and the lobes of the ears. Minor degrees of *cerebral* anoxia are evidenced by increasing restlessness and even delirious behaviour. As the state of shock proceeds, so all these signs increase in severity and not only does the pulse rate continue to rise, but the pulse volume begins to fall, giving it a weak and thready feel. This increasing feebleness of the pulse is a sign of critical importance, for it indicates the failure of the compensatory mechanisms of the body to overcome the state of shock. It is upon the nurse's constant and accurate observation of these symptoms and signs that the surgeon must always be able to depend. It is the nurse who has the first opportunity to observe any change in the condition of the child and it is the efficiency with which she discharges this responsibility and the promptitude with which she informs the correct authority that may be the deciding factors in the survival of her patient.

Treatment

It cannot be emphasized too strongly that the compensatory mechanisms against shock in a child's body are not so effective, neither are they capable of being sustained for such a long period, as they are in the adult. It is, therefore, of paramount importance in children's surgery that the first signs of shock should be recognized for the omens that they may be and no time should be lost in instituting treatment.

REST.—As in all acute conditions affecting the human body, rest is the first and one of the most important measures. The child should be nursed in a quiet room and subjected to the minimum amount of disturbance, for in this way none of the child's energy will be needlessly wasted. The foot of the bed should be raised about six inches from the floor in order to assist the return of venous blood back to the heart from the

lower limbs and the abdomen. If restlessness due to pain is a prominent feature, an intramuscular injection of Papaveretum or Nepenthe should be administered.

WARMTH.—It is important to stress that warmth is desirable only to *restore* the body temperature, not to increase it. The effect of heat when applied to the skin is to cause *vasodilatation* and *sweating*. As we have already said, one of the principal ways in which the body is trying to combat the effects of secondary shock is by producing a *vasoconstriction* in the capillary bed. If this compensatory vasoconstriction is interfered with by an over-zealous application of heat, then the vasodilatation and the increased fluid loss (due to sweating) that this procedure produces, will result in the state of shock *increasing* rather than *decreasing* in severity. A very careful watch should therefore be kept, so that over-heating does not occur. Hot water-bottles placed between the blankets is the time-honoured and usually the most successful method of keeping the body warm. Electric blankets and heat cradles always incur the risk of over-heating and if they are employed then constant attention and regulation must be observed.

FLUID ADMINISTRATION.—This aspect of treatment is directed to restoring the circulating blood-volume and decreasing any haemoconcentration that is present. In minor degrees of shock (other than those caused by penetrating abdominal injuries) the administration of oral fluids in the form of glucose water is usually sufficient. In more severe degrees of shock an intravenous infusion of fluid will have to be employed. The most readily available intravenous fluid in any hospital is 4·5 per cent dextrose and N/5 saline solution, and an intravenous infusion of this fluid should be instituted at once. This solution has, however, a serious drawback in that it rapidly passes through the now more permeable capillary walls. Its action, therefore, though immediately beneficial is only temporary in effect. The intravenous administration of *plasma*, on the other hand, confers a more permanent effect, as it does not diffuse through the capillary walls so rapidly as dextrose saline solution.

It goes without saying that shock associated with severe blood loss can only be treated satisfactorily by the replacement of whole blood.

THE CRUSH SYNDROME

This clinical syndrome is not common in childhood, but it may sometimes follow severe crushing injuries of the limbs. It may also occur as a tragic sequel to a tourniquet having remained, by mistake, in place for a number of hours. The limb becomes firm and tense and may show blistering of the skin. After an interval varying between two and six days the urinary output of the child suddenly begins to fall (*oliguria*). This usually proceeds to complete cessation of the secretion of urine (*anuria*), and the blood urea values begin to increase and may reach as high as 300 or 400 mg. per cent. If the secretion of urine is not re-established the blood urea continues to rise until the child passes into the coma of uraemia and shortly dies. On the other hand, the secretion of urine may quite suddenly become re-established with rapid improvement in the child's clinical condition and a return of the blood urea values to normal.

The precise nature of this condition is still a matter of controversy, but it is thought that crystals of altered blood in the crushed area may find their way to the kidneys where they produce either a temporary or permanent blockage of the renal tubules. Treatment is most unsatisfactory, but should consist of the rapid and profuse administration of intravenous N/5 saline as soon as the oliguria is revealed.

HAEMORRHAGE

The effects of severe blood loss on the body are almost indistinguishable from the state of shock that we have just described—in other words, severe blood loss, even unassociated with severe tissue injury, can itself be the cause of a profound degree of shock. Thus, with the exception of replacing the blood by transfusion, the management and treatment of haemorrhage does not differ from that already described for secondary shock. The sequence of events in the two conditions is much the same. As a result of the haemorrhage there is a sudden decrease in the circulating blood-volume. This in turn causes a decreased venous return to the heart, which in its turn is responsible for a decrease in the cardiac output and as a result of this the *blood-pressure falls*. To this state of affairs

the body applies its compensatory mechanisms—firstly, of increasing the pulse rate (to increase the cardiac output), and secondly, of reflex vasoconstriction (to shut down all the unwanted arterioles and capillaries in an attempt to raise the blood-pressure).

Thus, the clinical appearance of haemorrhage is a pallid listless child with a subnormal temperature, a pulse which is raised in rate and decreased in volume, and a blood-pressure that is below the normal level.   Added to this there may be, in cases of severe haemorrhage, the phenomenon of *air hunger*. When this is present the child appears to be gulping air down in an effort to fill its lungs.   It is a sign of critical importance and indicates a most severe degree of blood loss.   It is important to emphasize again that children cannot stand a rapid blood loss, and once the compensatory mechanisms begin to fail their decline is far more rapid than in the adult.

TYPES OF HAEMORRHAGE

Haemorrhage may be classified as being principally:

1. Arterial.
2. Venous.
3. Capillary.

1. Arterial Haemorrhage

Arterial haemorrhage may be either:

(*a*) Primary.
(*b*) Reactionary.
(*c*) Secondary.

(*a*) PRIMARY ARTERIAL HAEMORRHAGE.—This type of haemorrhage is most commonly encountered during the course of a surgical operation.   The bleeding vessel is clamped in a haemostat and subsequently ligatured with a piece of catgut. Occasionally you will come across street or domestic accidents in which primary arterial haemorrhage is a predominant feature.   By far the most effective first-aid treatment is to apply a dressing and firm bandage to the wound, and this is invariably sufficient to control the haemorrhage until formal surgical arrest of the bleeding may be performed.   In the rare instance when bleeding continues in spite of this treatment a tourniquet

must be applied above the wound in order to compress the main arterial vessels supplying the wound area. You must remember that the *whole* limb distal to the tourniquet is being deprived of its blood-supply, and unless the tourniquet is removed every fifteen to twenty minutes in order to allow arterial blood to enter the deprived area, the limb beyond the tourniquet may suffer irreparable changes. It is essential to emphasize that a tourniquet is a potentially dangerous instrument and should only be applied in the direst emergency.

(*b*) REACTIONARY HAEMORRHAGE.—This term refers to haemorrhage which *recommences* in a wound (operation or otherwise) up to forty-eight hours after the primary arterial haemorrhage has been arrested. It is invariably due to a ligature around an artery slipping off and if the haemorrhage cannot be controlled by a pressure dressing, then the wound should be reopened, the bleeding vessel located and religatured. Reactionary haemorrhage may also occur consequent upon a state of shock, as the low blood-pressure may fail to cause bleeding from some of the smaller arterial vessels in a wound. Once recovery from the shock occurs, however, then the restoration of the blood-pressure to normal may cause a resumption of bleeding.

(*c*) SECONDARY HAEMORRHAGE.—This is a haemorrhage commencing between seven to ten days after wounding or after operation and is due to a low-grade infection which has involved the wall of an artery. As a result of the infection the arterial wall may give way and bleeding ensue.

2. Venous Haemorrhage

This most commonly occurs during the course of surgical operations. Both ends of the cut vein should be ligated with catgut. Very occasionally cuts of the forearm may result in venous haemorrhage. A dressing and firm bandage should be applied until such time as formal ligation may be performed.

3. Capillary Haemorrhage

This is of far less importance than arterial or venous haemorrhage and it invariably stops of its own accord. If it should prove to be troublesome, then a firm dressing is sufficient to control it.

CONCEALED HAEMORRHAGE

A concealed haemorrhage is one in which the bleeding is not revealed by an issue of blood on the surface of the body. Thus it may result from rupture of an intra-abdominal organ or blood-vessel consequent upon an injury, or it may be due to an intra-abdominal or intra-thoracic reactionary haemorrhage. As the bleeding is *concealed* in nature the diagnosis rests upon the observation of the general symptoms and signs of haemorrhage that we have already discussed, and it is for this reason that such a close record of the pulse, the colour and of the appearance of a child must be kept for at least twenty-four hours after either an abdominal injury or operation. We shall discuss the subject of intra-abdominal injuries and their treatment in Chapter X.

BURNS

A burn is one of the most painful injuries that a child can suffer, and may be caused by a wide variety of agents. The commonest forms of burns in children occur as a result of domestic accidents, and it is important to realize that even an ordinary cup of tea, which when spilt over the adult skin may produce little more than a local reddening, may produce quite severe blistering in the child. The first consideration in all cases of burning is to assess the degree of shock resulting from the injury. Roughly speaking, burns involving less than 10 per cent of the body surface do not cause a significant degree of shock, and so the burn itself may be treated without delay. In more extensive burns (i.e. over 10 per cent of the body surface) it is the *shock* that must first be treated and the burn itself attended to when the child has been sufficiently resuscitated to withstand further treatment.

Burns, irrespective of the agent that caused them, may be classified into either *superficial* or *deep*. The term *superficial* refers to a burn which involves only a partial thickness of the skin, whereas *deep* indicates a burn in which the full thickness of the skin has been destroyed and deeper structures laid bare. Some authorities prefer to classify burns in six degrees:

First degree—a burn producing no more than a local reddening (*erythema*) of the skin.

> Second degree—in which the superficial layers of the skin
> have been destroyed and are lifted off the deeper layers
> of the skin by an exudate of plasma (i.e. *a blister*).
> Third degree—a burn in which the full thickness of the skin
> has been destroyed.
> Fourth degree—burns involving subcutaneous tissue.
> Fifth degree—burns involving muscle.
> Sixth degree—burns extending down to bone.

From this you will see that the first two degrees of burning are
superficial, whereas the latter four degrees are *deep*. It is
occasionally difficult to assess whether a burn is of a second
or third degree, and an interval of four or five days may be
necessary before it can be estimated whether or not the whole
thickness of the skin has, in fact, been destroyed.

The Effects of Burning

The effects of burns may be divided into *local* effects and
general effects.

Local Effects

The capillary vessels in a burned area become very much
more permeable than normal and as a result of this there is a
considerable local outpouring of plasma into the tissues. This
is most commonly seen in the formation of an ordinary blister,
but in deep burns plasma loss may be so extensive that a severe
degree of haemoconcentration may result from it. In addition,
the burned area consists of dead and dying tissue and as this
is a most attractive medium for bacterial growth the most
stringent aseptic precautions must be taken in order to prevent
infection.

General Effects

A marked degree of primary shock accompanies practically
every burn. In burns involving more than 10 per cent of the
body surface, primary shock gives way during the course of the
succeeding few hours to a severe degree of secondary shock.
This is due both to the plasma loss at the burned site itself and
also to a generalized increase in capillary permeability throughout the body. The degree of secondary shock following a

severe burn is frequently more profound and more protracted than shock resulting from other forms of injuries, and it is thought that this is due to the absorption into the blood-stream of certain toxic substances which are only liberated in burned tissue.

The Management of Burns

General Management

Fluid loss, both into the tissues and to the exterior through the burned area, has the most devastating effect on the burned child and it is to the correction of this fluid loss that the general management of burns is directed. The precise amount and type of fluid that needs to be replaced is calculated on a mathematical basis according to the weight of the patient and the extent and degree of the burn in question. You will not be called upon to perform this calculation yourself, but you must be aware of the reasons for its administration. (See *Shock—fluid replacement*.) Roughly speaking, all patients with superficial burns amounting to less than 10 per cent of the body surface will only need their fluid to be replaced by the oral route, and this is usually given in the form of glucose drinks. For superficial burns of up to 25 per cent of the body area, intravenous administration of both plasma and saline solution will have to be employed. For deep burns amounting to the same extent and superficial burns amounting to more than 25 per cent, the fluid should be replaced in the first instance as whole blood, followed by plasma and then continued by saline solution. Blood is employed in this last instance due to the fact that severe burns may cause wide destruction of red blood corpuscles and thus a significant loss in the oxygen-carrying power of the blood. The systemic administration of large doses of penicillin should always be instituted at the earliest moment following burning in an attempt to prevent the onset of infection in the devitalized burned tissues.

Should skin grafting ultimately become necessary, the haemoglobin level of the blood should be above 90 per cent, otherwise failure of the graft to 'take' may occur. If the haemoglobin level is below this value, then blood transfusion should be employed in order to raise it.

As the loss of plasma resulting from a burn is a loss of essential body protein, a high protein and high calorie diet should be given to the child once it has recovered from its state of secondary shock.

Local Management

SUPERFICIAL BURNS.—The *first-aid* management of a recent burn is to cover it with a clean or sterile towel and to disturb the burned area as little as possible. No chemical preparations or creams should be applied to the area, and in the case of the face, the area should be left exposed. Once in hospital the burned child should be nursed in an atmosphere of 70°-75° F., and if restlessness due to pain is a prominent feature sedation with intramuscular Papaveretum should be employed. Providing the burn is less than 10 per cent of the total body surface, treatment should be carried out within the course of the next hour or so. The child should be given a light general anaesthetic and, under *full aseptic precautions* in the operating theatre, the whole of the burned area and all the surrounding skin should be gently and carefully cleaned with a 1 per cent solution of cetavlon. Any obviously dead skin should be removed, blisters should be punctured and providing they are clean they may be left *in situ*. Once this has been done the whole area should be gently mopped dry with a soft towel. From this you will see that the whole aim of local treatment is to prevent any form of infection and at the same time to refrain from damaging the burned area any further. Once these measures have been carried out one of two techniques may be followed:

> (1) The dressing technique.
> (2) The exposure technique.

(1) DRESSING TECHNIQUE.—The whole of the burned area should be covered with a single layer of tulle gras from which most of the vaseline has been scraped off. This should be covered by a gauze pack (which some authorities prefer to be moistened in saline solution) and a thick layer of sterile cotton wool. These dressings are then kept in place by a firmly applied crepe bandage. Providing the child does not complain of increasing pain, and providing there is no oedema distal to this dressing and no evidence of infection as might be

revealed by an increase in the temperature, this dressing may be kept in place for up to ten days so that the growth of the new skin is not interrupted. Should any of the complications we have just mentioned appear, the gauze and cotton wool should be removed and the wound inspected through the layer of tulle gras.

(2) EXPOSURE TECHNIQUE.—In this method of treatment no dressings whatsoever are applied to the burned area. The child should be covered by a bed cradle, over which a sterile sheet is draped. During the course of the next two to three days a thick crust forms over the burned areas, and it is essential that this should be prevented from cracking by adequate immobilization. Should cracking of the crusts occur, the ' dressing effect ' that they provide will be destroyed and the treatment will have failed in its purpose. From this you will readily appreciate that it is the ingenuity and constant care that the nurse displays in keeping the limb at rest and the child undismayed upon which the success of this form of treatment largely depends. The crusts begin to separate from the burned area about the tenth day and have usually separated by the fourteenth day following burning. The advantages of this method of treatment are that the wounds may be inspected at all times and the necessity of dressings is obviated. It is not so satisfactory as the dressing technique, however, when the burned area completely encircles the limb, as in such an instance oedema developing beneath the burn may cause the thick crust to act as a tight band.

DEEP BURNS.—Deep (whole thickness) burns of less than 10 per cent of the body surface which have not produced a significant degree of shock should be regarded as a surgical emergency. The wound should be cleansed in the same way as we have already described, the burned area then cleanly excised and a skin graft applied to cover it.

Burns of Special Sites

THE HANDS AND FINGERS.—Exposure technique in burns involving the hands and the fingers is not so satisfactory as the dressing technique as it is essential that movements of the fingers should be practised from the first day after burning in order to prevent stiffening of the joints. When the hand has

been dressed it should be elevated above the level of the head and maintained there for five or six days in order to minimize any oedema that may appear.

THE FACE.—Treatment by exposure is the method of choice in superficial burns of the face, and providing the arms are not burned they should be adequately splinted to prevent the child from touching the wounds. Particular attention should be paid to any nasal discharge running over the burned upper lip. Any such discharge should be removed with moist cotton wool swabs.

THE PERINEUM.—Exposure is again the method of choice in this situation. Soiling of the area by faeces and urine should be swabbed away as soon as it has occurred and if the genitalia are severely burned some authorities advise the use of an indwelling catheter in the bladder. In children up to about two years of age, nursing in Gallows' traction (see p. 271) often secures greater comfort and cleanliness.

THE MOUTH.—Children with burns involving the oral cavity and pharynx, received as a rule from the accidental inhalation of steam, are particularly prone to develop oedema of the glottis and lungs. In this instance the maintenance of a clear airway is of first importance and tracheotomy may have to be employed. Aspiration of the pharynx with a nasal catheter attached to a sucker should be performed regularly. This particular type of burn is additionally dangerous in that oedema of the glottis may take some time to develop. When seen shortly after the accident, the child may appear to be normal and without any form of respiratory embarrassment, but oedema of the glottis may supervene as much as twelve hours later with the likelihood of suffocation and a fatal outcome. For this reason it is most important that children who have suffered such accidents should be admitted to hospital for observation, irrespective of how well they seem to be at the time.

SPECIAL TYPES OF BURNS

Electrical Burns

Electrical burns merit special consideration as, although seldom extensive, locally they are invariably severe. Contact with a live electric wire may produce at the site of contact an

apparently small and insignificant amount of charring. Over the few weeks following the burn, it becomes apparent that the depth of the burn has become much greater than was at first thought. Electrical burns are characterized by continued sloughing of the wound edges and gradual extension of the burn until what was once a small point of charring later becomes a wide, sloughing, necrotic area. After a few weeks the burned area ceases to extend and the sloughs separate from its base. Once the wound has been proven bacteriologically sterile, repair of the area by the application of split skin grafts is then undertaken.

X-ray and Radium Burns

Both these agencies are used in the treatment of malignant disease by virtue of the power of their rays to penetrate the skin and thus produce their effect at any depth beneath the skin's surface. The skin as well as the tumour will necessarily be irradiated and should this exceed a certain value which is known as the *skin tolerance dose* then burning of the skin will occur. Such burns are now fortunately very rare, for their main characteristics are the slow and gradual extension of the skin loss together with a remarkable reluctance to heal. Skin grafts applied to radium burns, even as much as two or three months after burning has become apparent, invariably fail to ' take ' and even later on, when skin grafting *is* successful, a breakdown in the healed area is always liable to occur.

Before leaving the subject of burns you must remember that for the first few days after burning you are not only dealing with a sick child but you are also nursing a *frightened* one. The memory both of the accident which caused the burn and the pain which followed it are still fresh in the child's mind and any simple nursing procedure that you are about to carry out may be interpreted by the child as a ' portent of pain to come '. Failure to appreciate this natural fear will only add to the child's distress and delay recovery. Only infinite patience and gentleness will succeed in assuring the child of your good intentions and only a real sympathy will afford true comfort.

CHAPTER IV

THE FACE AND THE MOUTH

CLEFT LIP AND CLEFT PALATE

THIS subject invariably causes the student nurse an unnecessary amount of difficulty. In order to understand it properly it is essential that we first consider how the face is normally formed. Once we have done this the anatomical and functional errors of development will be more readily appreciated and the aims of treatment will become apparent. The details of the operations designed to correct these conditions are not in your province. Remember that it is what the surgeon is trying to do and not the way in which he does it that is your primary concern.

THE DEVELOPMENT OF THE FACE AND THE PALATE

The face of the embryo is developed from five principal components. Two of these, the *mandibular* processes, grow inwards towards the mid-line, each fusing with its opposite number to form the flesh and bone of the *lower jaw*. Failure in fusion between these two processes is known as a median cleft of the lower jaw and as it is exceptionally rare it need concern us no more.

The face and upper jaw are formed by three main processes:

(1) The fronto-nasal process.
(2) Two maxillary processes.

The *fronto-nasal process* (the dotted portion in Figs. 14 and 15) grows downwards in the mid-line to form:

(*a*) The nose and nostrils (Fig. 14).
(*b*) The mid-portion of the upper-lip (the *philtrum*) (Fig. 14).
(*c*) The front portion of the hard palate (the *pre-maxilla*) (Fig. 15).

The two *maxillary processes* (the shaded portion in Figs. 14 and 15 grow inwards toward the mid-line to form:

(*a*) The Cheek (Fig. 14).
(*b*) The upper lip on either side of the philtrum (Fig. 14).
(*c*) The two halves of the hard and soft palate behind the
    pre-maxilla (Fig. 15).

All the components of these three processes finally fuse together to form the normal face and palate, and whereas the lines of fusion do not remain visible on the face itself, they remain in the skeleton of the hard palate as a Y-shaped suture line joining the pre-maxilla and the two halves of the hard

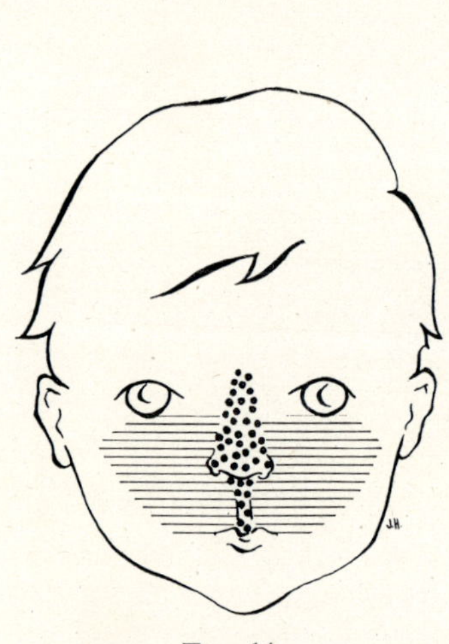

FIG. 14

To show the contribution of the fronto-nasal process and the two maxillary processes in the formation of the face.

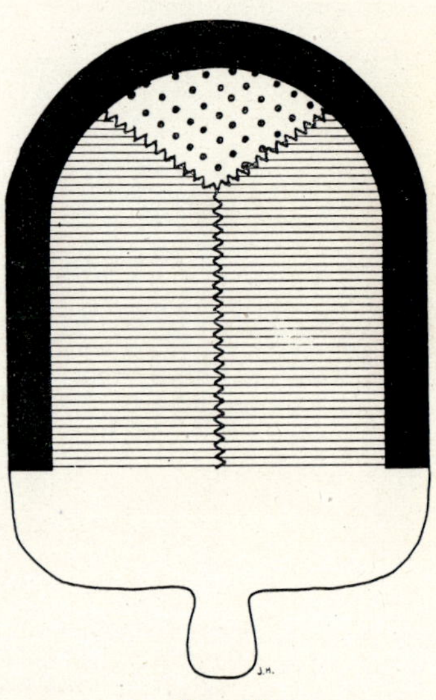

FIG. 15

To show the contribution of the fronto-nasal process and the two palatal processes (of the maxillary processes) in the formation of the hard palate. The thick black line represents the gum margin.

palate (Fig. 15). From this account you will see that failures in fusion between the components of the fronto-nasal process and the maxillary processes will result in a variety of deformities.

CLEFT LIP

A cleft lip occurs at the site where the upper lip would normally join the philtrum. The cleft involves the full thickness of the lip and usually extends up into the floor of the

5

nostril. You will notice in Fig. 16 that the nostril itself is flattened and widened, and this splaying of the nostril is a constant associated deformity. Cleft lip may be:

(1) Unilateral, (2) Bilateral,

and each of these varieties may or may not be associated with clefts in the palate.

Unilateral Cleft Lip

The obvious disfigurement of this condition is at once apparent. Opinions differ on the best age at which to perform

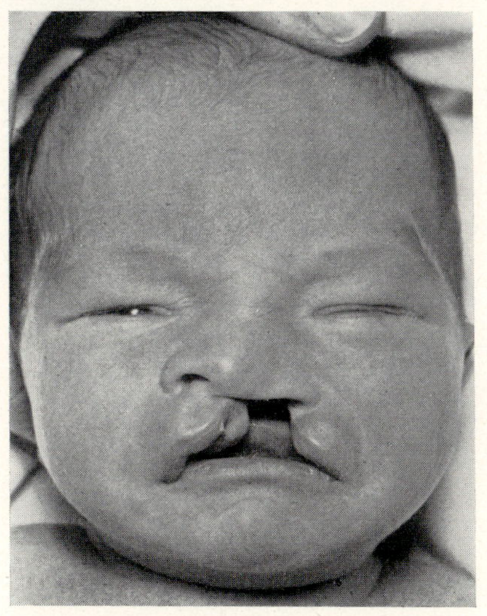

FIG. 16
Complete unilateral cleft lip and palate.
Note the splaying of the nostril and the
deviation of the philtrum.

operative correction of the deformity and you will no doubt see cleft lips repaired at ages varying between the first day of life and three or four weeks of age. A good working rule, however, is to operate on or about the tenth day of life. At this time the baby has regained its birth-weight and has thus become a better operative risk. A further convenience is that the mother is up and about by the tenth day and can either be admitted to hospital with the baby, or visit it regularly in order to express her milk so that breast feeding is *not* discontinued.

Pre-operative Management.—A few spoonfuls of sterile

water are given following each feed and the cleft and gum are then cleaned with sterile water to remove all remaining traces of milk. Intra-muscular injections of aqueous penicillin in doses of 6,000 units per pound body-weight three times a day are commenced two days before operation and continued until the fifth post-operative day.

Operation.—The aims of the operation are to restore the continuity of the mucous membrane on the back of the lip, to unite the orbicularis oris muscle which normally surrounds the whole mouth and to bring the skin margins together as inconspicuously as possible. Under a general anaesthetic administered through an endo-tracheal tube the cleft margins are 'pared' with a scalpel. The mucous membrane on the back of the lip is then united with catgut sutures; the muscle is firmly sewn together with cat-gut and finally the skin edges are united with very fine silk stitches. Particular attention is paid to re-forming the normal 'cupid's bow' appearance of the red margin of the lip. At the close of the operation the skin wound is lightly dusted with penicillin powder. Some-times you will see a *Logan's bow*

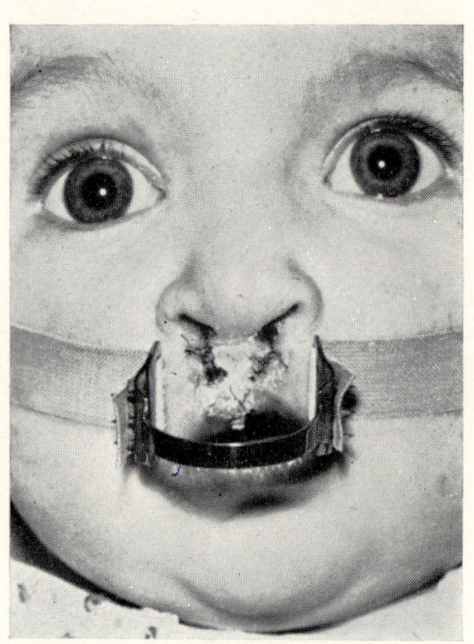

FIG. 17

A Logan's Bow in position following repair of a bilateral cleft lip.

applied to the face when the operation has been completed. This appliance consists of a metal bow which is fitted over the nose and kept in place by a length of strapping applied to each cheek (Fig. 17). It is designed to relieve any tension on the stitches closing the cleft and is worn until the seventh or tenth post-operative day.

Post-operative Management.—On return to the ward both the child's arms are splinted to prevent him disturbing the operation area. Spoon-feeding is commenced four hours after operation and continued for five days. Alternate stitches in the white portion of the lip are removed on the second day and the remainder on either the fourth or fifth days. Following

this the child is put to the breast and providing there is no cleft in the palate subsequent feeding is in no way different from the normal.

Incomplete Cleft Lip

This is a condition in which the cleft only involves a small portion of the lip and does not extend up into the floor of the

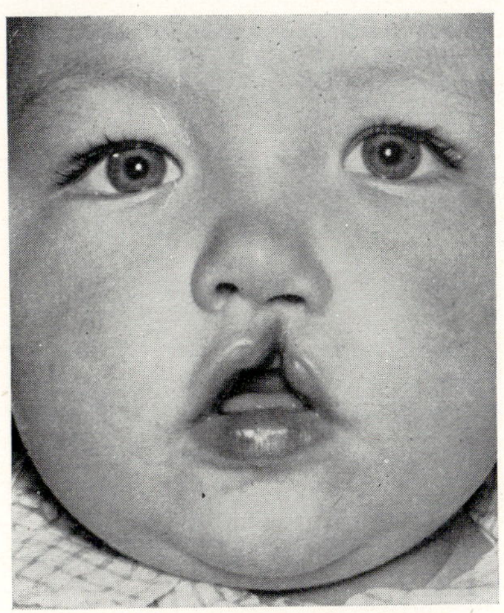

FIG. 18
An incomplete cleft lip.

nostril (Fig. 18). As the gap between the margins of the cleft is always small, operation is usually delayed until about three months of age.

Bilateral Cleft Lip

This condition which is fortunately less common than the unilateral variety is very much more difficult to treat. When associated with a bilateral cleft palate in which the pre-maxilla is completely separated from the other two components of the hard palate, the philtrum and the pre-maxilla jut forward from the rest of the face producing a gross degree of disfigurement (Fig. 19). Treatment of this condition is usually deferred until the child is three months of age as it is an extensive procedure and sometimes may have to be performed in stages. At operation the pre-maxilla and philtrum are pushed back so that they fall into line with the rest of the upper lip and an attempt

is made to unite the pre-maxilla with the maxillary processes. Following this the two clefts in the lip are repaired in the usual fashion. The pre- and post-operative management do not differ from that already described.

CLEFT PALATE

As we have already seen, the hard palate is formed by fusion of the pre-maxilla (the palatal portion of the fronto-nasal process) and the two palatal portions of the maxillary processes. Following this union the posterior lip of the hard palate grows

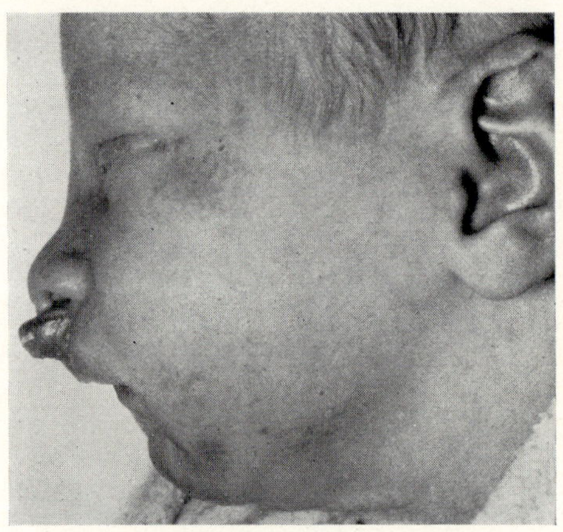

FIG. 19

To show the pre-maxilla jutting forward in a
case of bilateral cleft lip and palate.

downwards and backwards to form the soft palate. The soft palate, which contains no bony tissue, is best regarded as a muscular flap which can be raised or lowered.

Although the abnormalities resulting from failure in this normal formation of the palate may be both wide and varied, there are three *principal* types:

(1) A simple cleft between the two halves of the hard and soft palate. (An *incomplete* cleft palate or *inter-maxillary* cleft) (Fig. 20).

(2) A cleft of the hard and soft palate extending between the palatal portion of the maxillary process on one side and the fused pre-maxilla and palatal processes on the other side (a *complete unilateral* cleft palate) (Fig. 21).

(3) A cleft between both halves of the palate which extends forwards on *either* side of the pre-maxilla (a *bilateral* cleft palate) (Fig. 22). (See also Fig. 19.)

In order to understand the significance of these abnormalities and the disabilities that they produce, we must first study the mechanism of normal speech.

NORMAL SPEECH.—During quiet breathing with the mouth closed, the muscles of the soft palate are relaxed. This allows the inspired and expired air to enter and leave the respiratory system through the space between the free edge of

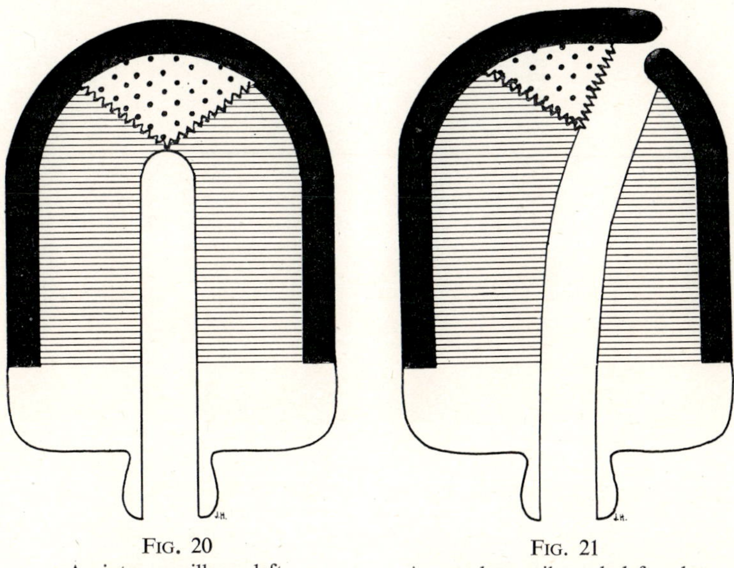

<table>
<tr><td>FIG. 20
An inter-maxillary cleft.</td><td>FIG. 21
A complete unilateral cleft palate.</td></tr>
</table>

the soft palate and the posterior pharyngeal wall (Fig. 23 A). During speech, however, the muscles of the soft palate contract and lift it up against the posterior pharyngeal wall, thus separating the nasal cavity from the oral cavity. In this way the sound waves produced by the vibration of the vocal cords make their exit through the mouth (Fig. 23 B). The only exceptions to this mechanism are the sounds MN, NM and NG in which the *oral* cavity is occluded by the lips or the tongue and the sound waves must therefore make their exit through the *nasal* cavity. You can easily verify this for yourself by placing a pocket mirror just beneath the nostrils while pro-

nouncing these sounds, and you will notice that the glass of the mirror becomes blurred with the breath issuing from the nasal cavity. You will also notice that the pronunciation of words *not* containing these combinations leaves the mirror quite clear thus demonstrating the fact that the nasal cavity is no longer in communication with the pharynx. All other sounds in speaking are produced by an infinite variety in the positions of

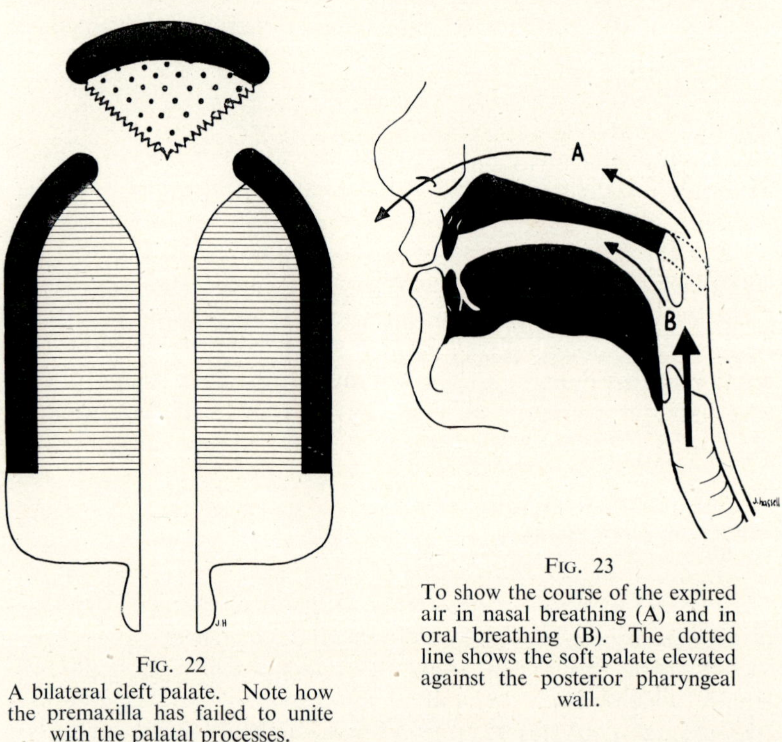

FIG. 22

A bilateral cleft palate. Note how the premaxilla has failed to unite with the palatal processes.

FIG. 23

To show the course of the expired air in nasal breathing (A) and in oral breathing (B). The dotted line shows the soft palate elevated against the posterior pharyngeal wall.

the lips, cheeks and tongue which combine to mould the sound waves into the multitude of successive noises that we recognize as speech. For instance, vowel sounds are produced by passing the sound waves over varying positions of the tongue and then allowing them to issue through differently shaped apertures formed by the lips. On the other hand a consonant such as T is produced in an entirely different way. The soft palate is elevated in order to close off the nasal cavity; the tip of the tongue is placed against the back of the upper incisor teeth; a

pressure of breath is raised behind this junction and is then allowed to escape by withdrawing the tip of the tongue. In this way you will see that the oral cavity has been converted into an ' explosion chamber '. Consonants such as B, D, G, K, P and Q are produced in a similar manner, the mechanism differing only in so far as the site of occlusion in the mouth is concerned. These consonants are therefore most suitably referred to as *explosive* consonants, and it is the inability to produce them that is the chief characteristic of cleft palate speech.

CLEFT PALATE SPEECH.—When a cleft is present in the palate, no amount of contortion of the lips and tongue or elevation of the soft palate will prevent the sound waves from entering into the *nasal* cavity. This sharing of the sound waves by both nasal and oral cavities is known as *nasal escape* and as a result of it, the ability to produce explosive consonants is completely lost. Sounds such as ' tee ' and ' kay ' become ' hee ' and ' hay '. It is primarily for this reason that the repair of cleft palate is undertaken, and you will readily appreciate that this must be performed before the child has got into the habit of speaking through the cleft in its palate. Thus operation is generally performed at or about the tenth month of life.

Inter-Maxillary Cleft

In addition to the requisites of speech, the act of swallowing also demands complete separation of the oral and nasal cavities otherwise regurgitation of food through the nasal cavity will occur. For this reason the infant is fed with a cleft palate spoon which allows the milk to be deposited on the back of the tongue, and thus regurgitation through the nasal cavity is reduced to a minimum.

Pre-operative Management.—For four days before operation the child is nursed in strict isolation in a cubicle in order to prevent contact with any intercurrent upper respiratory infections. Throat and nasal swabs are taken each day to determine whether the child is harbouring any patho-genic bacteria, and providing these swabs are reported as sterile, intra-muscular injections of penicillin are com-menced on the third day before operation. Particular atten-tion is paid to the toilette of the cleft itself after feeding.

A few spoonfuls of sterile water are given after each feed in order to 'rinse' the mouth of milk, and if necessary the margins of the cleft may be gently swabbed clean with sterile water.

Operation.—The details of these complicated operations do not concern you. It is only the principle of the operation, namely the closure of the cleft, which you are required to understand. The anaesthetic is administered through an endotracheal tube and a small gauze pack is placed around this tube in the pharynx to prevent the aspiration of blood into the lungs. The aim of the operation is to shift the muco-periosteum covering each half of the hard palate inwards to the mid-line. To facilitate this, long incisions are made into the lateral margins of the muco-periosteum just where it joins the gum. These incisions are called relaxing incisions and allow the muco-periosteum to be lifted off the underlying hard palate and brought to the mid-line without tension. The margins of the cleft itself are pared with a scalpel and then united together with stitches. Particular attention is paid to the union of the muscle tissue in each half of the soft palate.

Post-operative Management.—The child is returned to the cubicle and remains there for a further ten days. During this time the administration of penicillin and the feeding of the child are continued as in the immediate pre-operative management. The arms are both splinted to prevent the child from thumb sucking and thus running the risk of interference with the wound and the introduction of infection into the mouth. It is an advantage to institute splinting of the arms two days before operation in order to allow the child to get used to them. As far as possible crying is prevented both by 'petting' and by the administration of chloral (2 grains by mouth) when necessary.

Complete Unilateral and Bilateral Cleft Palate

The pre-operative and post-operative management in both these conditions do not differ in any way from that employed in inter-maxillary cleft. The operation differs only in the extent of the cleft to be closed, and in the case of bilateral cleft palate the added difficulty of bringing the gum margins into line with each other.

AFTER CARE

When the child begins to speak it is encouraged to play 'blowing games' such as 'blowing bubbles' and 'blow football' in order to exercise the soft palate as much as possible. Instruction in these games is given to the mother by a speech therapist and from then on they should be practised at home. If by the age of three years there is still some degree of nasal escape, further more complicated exercises and training should be carried out under the direct supervision of the speech therapist. Should nasal escape continue in spite of these measures, further surgical operations designed to lengthen the soft palate may have to be performed.

Orthodontic Treatment

This is not as yet an established method of treating cleft palates nor is it of use in all forms of the condition, but it is of interest to consider it at this point. The treatment is based upon the fact that the edges of a cleft in the *hard* palate when subjected to constant stimulation are capable of growing inwards towards the mid-line. In order to subject the margins of the cleft to constant mechanical stimulation, a 'plate' is moulded to fit the gap. On the oral aspect of this plate is fitted a small contrivance which is constantly moved by the tongue during the course of speech and this has the effect of subjecting the margins of the cleft to a mechanical 'rubbing' stimulation. As the cleft margins begin to grow towards the mid-line so new plates are fashioned to fit the decreasing size of the gap, and it is reported that small clefts in the hard palate have been closed by this method in as short a time as seven months. As this form of closure is as yet largely experimental it remains to be seen what part it will eventually play in the treatment of this condition.

DERMOID CYSTS OF THE FACE

A dermoid cyst on the face is unusual in that it is situated just above the outer angle of the eye. In this situation it is referred to as an *external angular dermoid*. The cyst itself lies deep to a wide circular band of muscle (the orbicularis oculis)

which completely surrounds the eye. You can easily demonstrate this fact to yourself by placing a finger on the cyst and then asking the child to ' screw his eyes up '. When he does so you will notice that the cyst disappears as the contraction of the orbicularis oculis renders it impalpable. Treatment consists of removal, and in order to conceal the subsequent scar the incision is usually made in the eyebrow. Dermoid cysts may occasionally occur in the mid-line of the face immediately between the eyes. This is a very much less common situation than the external angular variety and is treated by surgical excision.

CONGENITAL ABNORMALITIES OF THE PINNA

The portion of the external ear known as the pinna or auricle is developed in embryological life from a series of small

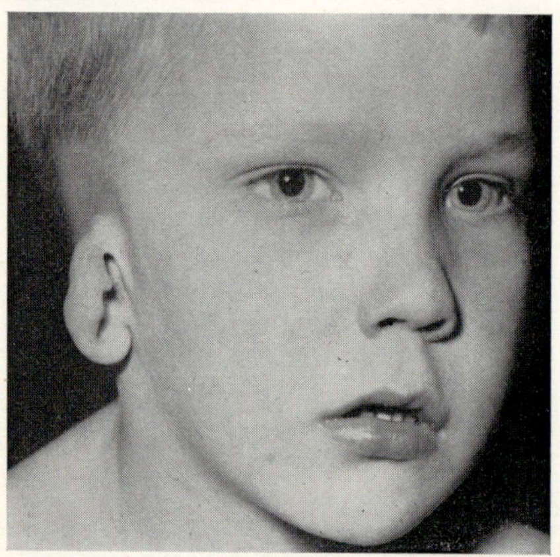

Fig. 24
Congenital deformity of the right pinna.

eminences which appear around the external auditory meatus. Ultimately these eminences fuse together to form the skin and cartilage of the external ear, and errors in this development may result in a wide variety of abnormal shapes and sizes of the pinna (Fig. 24). There may be complete absence of the auricle altogether or it may consist solely of a small lump of skin and cartilage which bears little or no resemblance to the

normal appearance (a rudimentary auricle). Deafness seldom occurs with either of these conditions as the external auditory meatus is invariably patent.

ACCESSORY AURICLE.—In this condition there is a small lump of skin and cartilage just in front of the root of the ear (Fig. 25). It seldom if ever causes any trouble, and can be removed without difficulty in order to improve the cosmetic appearance.

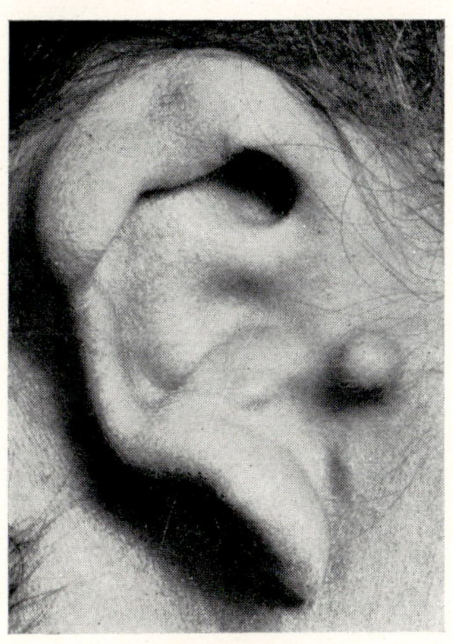

FIG. 25
An accessory auricle.

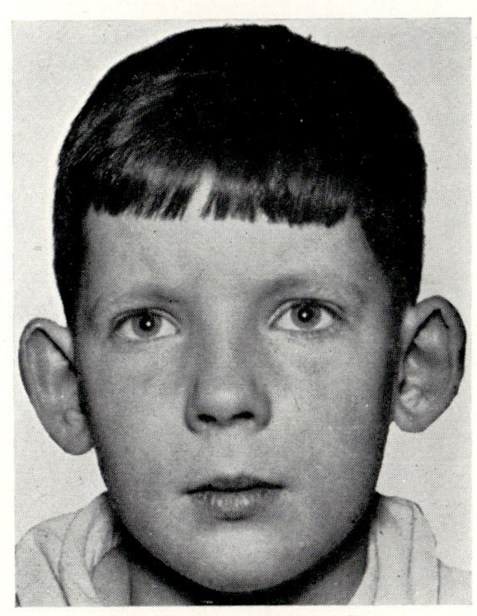

FIG. 26
Bat ears.

PRE-AURICULAR SINUS.—A pre-auricular sinus is situated just in front of the external auditory meatus and consists of a minute opening in the skin which leads down into a small blind pit. Frequently the sinus becomes inflamed and if the opening to the surface becomes blocked, a small abscess may develop. It is for this reason, rather than for cosmetic improvement, that excision of the sinus is advisable.

BAT EARS.—This somewhat unacademic term refers to ears which stick out almost at right angles from the side of the head (Fig. 26). The condition may be unilateral or bilateral. It is doubtful if there is a true surgical indication for operating upon them, but occasionally you will come across children or their parents who are genuinely distressed by the appearance that this condition produces. Operative reconstruction entails removal of an ellipse of skin from the back of the ear and the

adjacent scalp. In addition, a wedge of the auricular cartilage is sometimes then removed, the ear folded back on itself and the raw edges of the skin united by sutures. A crepe bandage is applied to keep both ears back in position and should be worn until the stitches are removed on the tenth post-operative day.

THE MOUTH

Ranula

A ranula is a blue-coloured cystic swelling of the floor of the mouth and is always situated to one or other side of the mid-line. When large, it causes displacement of the same side of the tongue, yet it seldom produces difficulty in either swallowing or in speech. Surgical excision may prove to be exceptionally difficult due to the fragile walls of the cyst and because of this, treatment is usually confined to excising only the accessible portion of the swelling and leaving the floor of the cyst *in situ*.

Dermoid Cyst

Unlike a ranula, a dermoid cyst is a bright yellow swelling which is always situated in the mid-line of the floor of the mouth. As it increases in size it displaces the whole of the tongue upwards. Surgical excision is comparatively easy as the capsule is firmer and tougher than in the case of a ranula. The cyst is approached through the mouth and, following excision, the floor of the mouth is repaired with catgut sutures. These sutures do not need to be removed as they are absorbed by about the eighth post-operative day. After operation the child is fed on sterile milk for five days and after each feed the mouth is irrigated with a mild antiseptic mouthwash. If the child is a 'thumb-sucker' the arms should be splinted to prevent the introduction of infection into the mouth. Normal feeding is resumed on the sixth post-operative day.

Tongue Tie

In this condition the normal degree of protrusion of the tongue is prevented by an unusually short frenulum linguae. It frequently causes concern to the mother of the child as she naturally feels that the child's speech will be abnormal, but it

has been found in the majority of cases that once the child begins to speak the frenulum becomes sufficiently stretched to allow normal mobility of the tongue. If, however, the frenulum is so tight that the tip of the tongue is tethered by it to the floor of the mouth, then surgical division of the frenulum should be undertaken. It is most important that this operation should be performed on the child as an in-patient, for if the degree of division is too extensive, serious and even dangerous haemorrhage may ensue. Normally, however, there should be little or no bleeding at all.

Lymphangioma

In this condition the under surface of the *anterior two-thirds* of the tongue is occupied by a mass of minute lymphatic cysts (a capillary lymphangioma). As a result the tongue is displaced upwards and forwards and can hardly be accommodated inside the oral cavity. As a result of this, the mouth is perpetually held open and saliva continually dribbles over the lower lip. Infection within the lymphangioma is a common and frequent occurrence and may produce an alarming increase in its size, but as this condition is always limited to the anterior two-thirds of the tongue, interference with the pharyngeal airway does not occur. Feeding, however, may become increasingly difficult and may have to be limited to fluids whilst the infection is still present. Irrigation of the oral cavity with three-volume hydrogen peroxide solution assists in cleaning up the surface of the lymphangioma, and if this is not sufficient to deal with the infection antibiotic therapy should be employed. Alarming though these episodes of infection may be they are, in fact, beneficial as fibrous tissue replacement within the lymphangioma follows each attack. Over a period of years these attacks of infection produce quite a marked degree of shrinkage and reduction in size of the lymphangioma.

Phagedena (cancrum oris)

This is a very severe gangrenous infection involving the oral cavity and the cheek. It is now fortunately very rare but when it does occur it produces a wide, sloughing, offensively-smelling area of gangrene in the cheek and is invariably fatal in its outcome.

Salivary Calculus and Sialoadenitis

Stones (calculi) and infections (sialoadenitis) of the salivary glands are uncommon conditions in childhood and are invariably confined in their incidence to the submandibular gland. A salivary calculus (which is composed of a mixture of calcium phosphate and calcium carbonate and which is formed within the substance of the submandibular gland) seldom causes any symptoms until it has entered and becomes stuck (impacted) in the submandibular duct. This produces

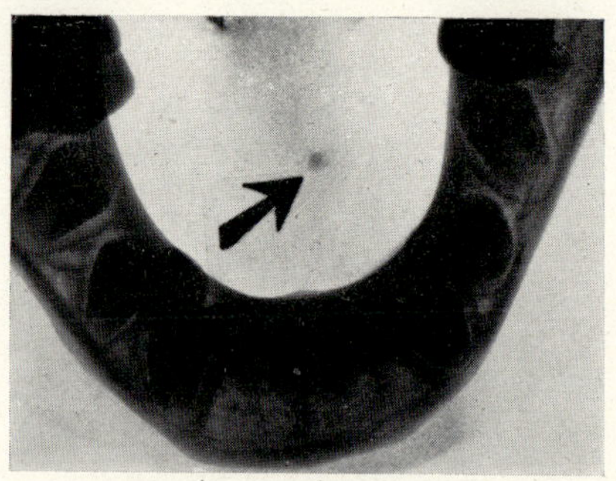

FIG. 27

An X-ray of a small salivary calculus impacted in the opening of the left submandibular duct.

an obstruction to the outflow of saliva which in turn causes distension and pain in the submandibular gland. The pain is aching in character and always appears when the secretion of saliva is greatest, that is to say, either in anticipation of a meal or during the eating of it. Enlargement of the gland during the episodes of pain is frequently present and serves to differentiate this form of pain from other causes such as toothache. The situation of the stone may be discovered by feeling it in the duct as it crosses the floor of the mouth, and also by X-ray examination (Fig. 27). Under either a general or a local anaesthetic, a small incision should be made into the duct immediately over the stone, and the stone then removed. No repair to the duct is necessary as the opening which has been made into the duct forms a new but perfectly satisfactory site for the outflow of saliva.

Infection of the submandibular gland usually results from the effects of a long standing partial obstruction in the

submandibular duct.   Attacks of acute infection are revealed by a continuous pain in the gland and a reddening of the skin over it.   Hot mouth washes, hot fomentations to the neck and intensive penicillin therapy are usually sufficient to bring about a temporary improvement but a chronic state of infection invariably remains behind.   Children who continue to suffer from such recurrent infections after the obstruction has been relieved should have the affected submandibular gland removed.

CHAPTER V

THE NOSE, THROAT AND EARS

THE NOSE

Injuries

INJURIES to the nose always result from direct violence and they are invariably followed by a considerable degree of soft tissue swelling which is usually sufficient to mask any underlying deformity that may be present due to fracture of the nasal bones. Unless X-ray examination reveals gross displacement of such a fracture the most satisfactory course to follow is to withhold treatment for a week until all the swelling has subsided, and if at the end of this time there is any residual deformity reduction should then be carried out. Under a general anaesthetic the nasal bones should be manipulated into the correct position, following which both nostrils should be packed with vaseline gauze for twenty-four to forty-eight hours in order to maintain the reduction. It is important for you to realize that as the nasal cavity is potentially an infected area, the pack should be removed as soon as possible, and for this reason if the surgeon requires it to be left *in situ* for more than twenty-four hours he will give definite instructions to that effect. Irrespective of whether the injury is complicated by fracture, the nasal septum should always be closely inspected for the presence of a haematoma. If present it should always be opened and the blood clot evacuated, for should a septal haematoma become infected it will proceed to abscess formation and subsequent perforation of the nasal septum.

Foreign Bodies

Quite frequently young children for reasons best known to themselves, introduce foreign bodies such as small beads, peas and bits of rolled up paper into the nostrils. Sometimes these foreign bodies may become irretrievable and the child, rather than disclose the fact to his or her parent, may prefer to forget the incident altogether. In such cases the foreign body sets up a state of inflammation around itself which is revealed some

days later by a mucoid or purulent discharge from the blocked-up nostril. If radio-opaque the foreign body will be revealed by X-ray examination and if it is situated far back in the nasal cavity it is usually safest to remove it under a general anaesthetic, in order to prevent the possibility of its aspiration into the trachea. When situated just inside the nostrils foreign bodies are usually quite easily removed with a pair of forceps or better still a blunt hook, but even so they often have the disconcerting habit of slipping further and further back into the nasal cavity with each successive attempt at removal.

Epistaxis

Bleeding from the nose is a very common happening in children and is most frequently due to rupture of a small vein just inside the nostril. It is most important for you to realize, however, that epistaxis may be the first sign of far more serious conditions such as leukaemia, purpura and haemophilia. Simple epistaxis may not always be revealed by an issue of blood from the nostrils for if the site of bleeding is at the back of the nasal cavity, the child may swallow the blood and the epistaxis only be revealed after the child has vomited digested blood. Simple epistaxis should be treated by gentle compression of the nostrils by the finger and thumb but if this is insufficient to control the haemorrhage, the nostrils should be packed with ribbon gauze soaked in 5 minims of 1 : 1000 adrenaline solution.

Congenital Syphilis

This condition, which is fortunately becoming increasingly rare, may be present at birth or become apparent later in childhood. The nasal mucous membrane and the muco-periosteum are infected with the spirochaeta pallida which produces a highly infectious nasal discharge of mucopus (on account of which the condition is sometimes called ' the snuffles '). The skin around the nostrils becomes excoriated and sore and the nurse must observe the most rigid precautions in order to prevent her skin from becoming contaminated by the discharge. If left untreated the nasal septum may be destroyed and leave a ' saddle-backed ' deformity of the nose. Modern treatment favours intra-muscular injections of penicillin

(40,000 units per kg. of body-weight every six hours) in preference to the use of arsenical compounds and Bismuth.

New Growths

The only new growth that occurs in the nose in childhood is a particular form of fibroma. It occurs in the periosteum of the roof of the nose and although locally invasive it does not metastasize to other parts of the body. It is fortunately extremely sensitive to irradiation.

THE PARANASAL AIR SINUSES

ANATOMY.—The paranasal air sinuses are cavities within the bones of the facial skeleton which are in communication with the nasal cavity. The cells which make up the lining of these sinuses are known as ciliated epithelial cells for they are furnished with numerous microscopic hair-like projections whose function it is to waft any invading particles of foreign material back towards the nasal cavity. In all there are six paranasal air sinuses, arranged in three groups of two.

1. **The Maxillary Antra.**—These are situated within the bone of the maxilla, one on either side of the nose and each one communicates with the nasal cavity through a small hole high up on the medial wall of the antrum (Fig. 28).

2. **The Ethmoid Air Sinuses.**—These are a number of irregular spaces in the bone, disposed in two principle groups on either side of the roof of the nasal cavity with which they communicate through a series of small holes. Each group of ethmoid air sinuses is bounded on its outer aspect by the medial wall of the orbit (Fig. 28).

3. **The Frontal Air Sinuses.**—Unlike the maxillary antra and the ethmoid air sinuses, the frontal group are not present at birth and do not usually appear until about five to seven years of age (and sometimes indeed they may fail to appear altogether). They develop as large spaces within the frontal bone and are situated just above the bridge of the nose. They communicate with the nose through narrow canals, each of which open low down on the lateral wall of the nasal cavity.

Before considering the appearances and the effects of infections of either the nose, the paranasal air sinuses, the throat or the ears, it is most important for you to realize that although an infection may appear to predominate in any one of them, they are all in communication with each other and thus are usually all involved to a greater or lesser degree.

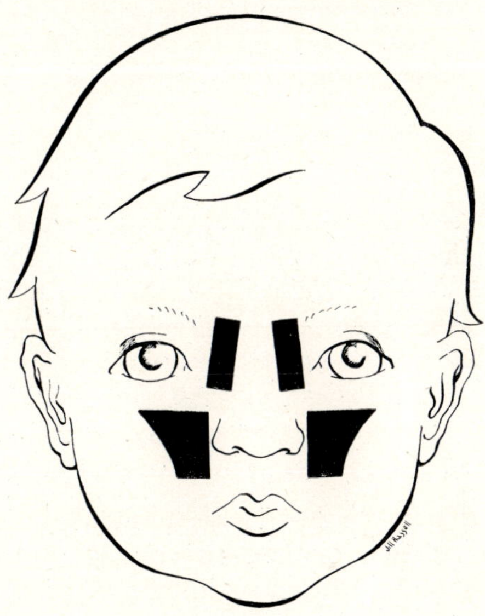

FIG. 28

The surface markings of the Maxillary Antra
and the Ethmoid air cells.

Acute Ethmoiditis

Acute inflammation of the ethmoid air cells occurs most commonly in young infants. Swelling and redness of the skin on either side of the nose is usually present and the oedema may even extend into the skin of the orbit and the eyelids. Constitutional signs are usually severe. The temperature is raised to 103°-104° F. and symptomatic vomiting and even diarrhoea may also be present. Treatment of the condition is by the oral administration of sulphonamides or by systemic penicillin and also by spraying the roof of the nasal cavity with a solution of $\frac{1}{2}$ per cent ephedrine in an attempt to shrink the epithelium and thus assist the drainage of pus from the ethmoid air cells. As in all acute pyogenic infections in infants, fluid administration

must be carefully watched in order to prevent the onset of dehydration.

Infections of the Maxillary Antra

Acute infections of the maxillary antra are uncommon in infants and occur more frequently in older children. Minor involvement of both antra always occurs with a severe 'cold' but as a rule the inflammation within the antra subsides together with that in the nasal cavity. Sometimes, however, the inflammatory oedema around the communicating hole between the nose and the antrum may be sufficient to occlude it and in

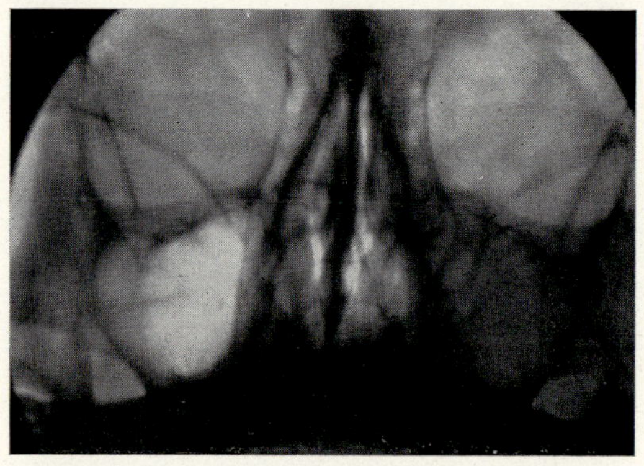

FIG. 29

An infection of the left maxillary antrum. Note that the infected antrum is more opaque than the normal one on the other side. (The ethmoid air cells are also visible between the nasal cavity and the medial wall of the orbit.)

this event drainage from the antrum is prevented, and pain, tenderness and swelling of the skin over the affected antrum shortly make their appearance. Oral administration of sulphonamides should be commenced and the lateral walls of the nasal cavity sprayed with $\frac{1}{2}$ per cent ephedrine solution in order to shrink the nasal mucosa and re-establish drainage from the blocked antrum. If the child is old enough to co-operate, inhalations of menthol vapour will assist this process.

Chronic infection of the antra may follow the unsuccessful treatment of an acute attack, or it may arise for no apparent cause. In the latter instance chronic enlargement of the adenoids and of the tonsils is a common associated finding.

There is a constant mucoid or mucopurulent discharge from the nostrils and X-ray examination shows an opacity in the affected antrum denoting the presence of inflammatory fluid (Fig. 29). Treatment of this chronic condition consists firstly of regular ephedrine spraying of the nostrils and menthol inhalations, and secondly in treating any dietary deficiencies

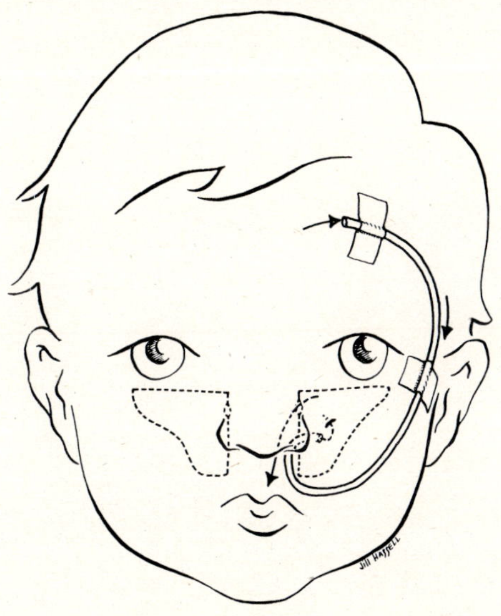

FIG. 30

Polythene tubing in position for daily irrigation of the left antrum. The arrows denote the direction and the course of the injected saline solution.

that may be present. If possible the child should be sent to a convalescent home for at least a month, and these measures are frequently sufficient to secure an improvement in the condition. If the tonsils and adenoids remain enlarged they should be removed. If, as all too frequently occurs, the condition fails to improve, then puncture and irrigation of the offending antrum should be carried out. Under a general anaesthetic a wide bore needle is introduced into the cavity of the antrum through the lateral wall of the nasal cavity (antral puncture); sterile normal saline solution is then introduced through this needle and having filled up the antrum overflows through the communicating aperture into the nasal cavity, from where it is removed by a sucker. In this way the antrum

is thoroughly cleared out and some authorities advocate leaving *in situ* a length of polythene tubing through the needle hole in order to connect the antrum with the exterior so that irrigation of the antrum with saline solution may be repeated daily for seven to fourteen days. The outside end of the polythene tubing is secured to the cheek and forehead (Fig. 30), and when the antra are irrigated the child should bend forward over a bowl so that the issue of saline from the nasal cavity does not enter the naso-pharynx. The procedure causes the child no discomfort whatsoever.

THE THROAT

THE PHARYNX

The function of the two faucial tonsils is to provide an immediate defence against pathogenic bacteria in the throat, and in performing this duty they frequently become acutely inflamed. The tonsils become greatly enlarged and bright red in colour, the child experiences difficulty in swallowing and secondary enlargement of the cervical lymph nodes usually follows in a day or so. The temperature is elevated to 103°-104° F. and anorexia and symptomatic vomiting are often present. In addition to the above symptoms and signs, the child not infrequently complains of a generalized abdominal pain. The precise reason for this is obscure but it is generally assumed to be due to a ' sympathetic enlargement ' of some of the lymph glands within the abdomen and in some cases the pain may be so pronounced that it closely simulates the early phase of acute appendicitis.

The treatment of acute tonsillitis has been revolutionized since the advent of penicillin. A throat swab should always be taken in order to discover the identity and sensitivity of the causative organism and then systemic penicillin should be commenced at once. Copious amounts of oral fluid should be administered and, because of a natural reluctance to swallow, there is often some difficulty in persuading the child to take them. Careful attention should be paid to the regular opening of the bowels, as constipation is a common associated finding in acute tonsillitis. The use of gargles is of doubtful value. Only a few children seem to be able to gargle at all and those

who can, invariably do so in an explosive and ineffective manner and for these reasons gargling is regarded as being of little or no use.   Penicillin therapy should be continued for a minimum period of five days and during this time a close watch should be kept for the onset of secondary infection of the middle ear or suppuration in the cervical lymph nodes (see below).

Peritonsillar Abscess (A Quinsy)

This condition is usually consequent upon an attack of acute tonsillitis and is due to an extension of the infection into the tissues surrounding the tonsil.   A large swelling appears in the upper portion of the tonsillar fossa which pushes the tonsil downwards and often displaces the uvula to the opposite side (Fig. 31).   The child experiences increased difficulty in swallowing, the cervical lymph nodes on the same side as the abscess begin to enlarge, and the temperature swings dramatically. Penicillin therapy should be commenced at once, and under a general anaesthetic a pair of sinus forceps should be gently introduced into the most prominent portion of the abscess. As the pus gushes forth it is removed with a sucker in order to prevent it entering the trachea.   Following this procedure systemic penicillin should be continued for a further five days during which time healing of the wound is rapid and uneventful. In older children the use of a general anaesthetic is not always necessary, and the abscess may be punctured simply by thrusting a pair of sinus forceps into the swelling.   In this way the risk of inhalation of pus is reduced to a minimum (as the cough reflex is present) and the child is able to spit out the discharge and co-operate in washing out the mouth.

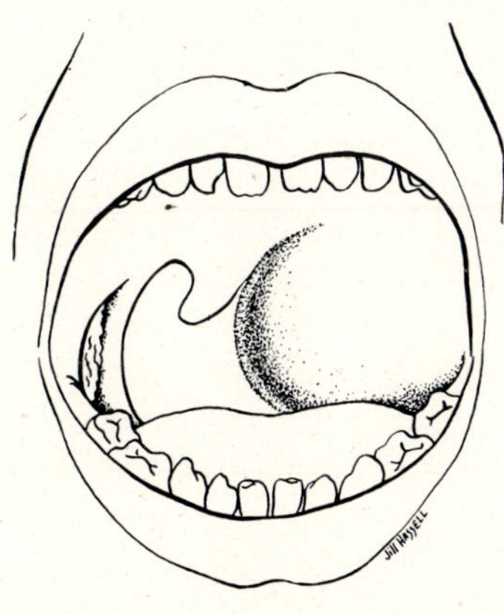

Fig. 31

A large peritonsillar abscess.   Note how it has pushed the uvula towards the opposite side and displaced the tonsil out of sight.

Retropharyngeal Abscess

The lymphatic vessels draining the adenoids pass down-

wards and backwards to a group of small lymph glands lying immediately beneath the posterior pharyngeal wall, and these glands may be the seat of suppuration secondary to a primary infection of the adenoids. The retropharyngeal abscess that results, presents as a tense, fiery red swelling in the mid-line on the posterior pharyngeal wall and it should be treated in precisely the same way as a peritonsillar abscess.

Within two or three months following recovery from either a peritonsillar or a retropharyngeal abscess both the tonsils and the adenoids should be removed as a safeguard against further similar episodes of abscess formation.

Chronic Tonsillitis

Fibrosis within the substance of the tonsil with consequent impairment or loss of its protective function is the usual sequel to repeated attacks of acute tonsillitis. Pathogenic bacteria are harboured in the deep crypts and folds of the tonsillar surface and provide a constant septic focus which may be responsible for episodes of acute otitis media, cervical adenitis or further attacks of acute tonsillitis. The tonsils remain in a state of moderate enlargement and in children who habitually sleep on their backs, the relaxation of the throat muscles during sleep may allow the tonsils to fall downwards and backwards and cause the child to awake with a sudden sense of suffocation. This is not an uncommon cause of ' night terrors ' in children, and involuntary bed-wetting may occur at the same time. Chronic enlargement of the adenoids is an invariable accompaniment of chronic tonsillitis and the obstruction to the nasal airway that this produces results in mouth-breathing and snoring at night. The only satisfactory treatment of chronic enlargement of the tonsils and adenoids is surgical removal, but this should never be performed sooner than one month following recovery from an attack of acute inflammation.

TONSILLECTOMY AND ADENOIDECTOMY.—Nowadays this operation is always performed under an ' umbrella ' of penicillin; that is to say, systemic penicillin is commenced the day before operation and continued for five days afterwards in order to deal with the dissemination of septic material that may be liberated during the course of the operation. The details of the operation are not primarily your concern. Suffice it to say that the tonsils are dissected from their beds and catgut

ligatures are applied to any troublesome bleeding vessels. The adenoids are removed by a curette which scrapes them off the roof and off the back of the nasal cavity. The two principal complications of this operation are firstly, aspiration of blood or blood clot into the trachea or bronchi and secondly, reactionary haemorrhage. It is the prevention of the first of these complications and the speedy recognition of the second that is the nurse's prime responsibility in the immediate post-operative period. When the child leaves the operating theatre he, or she, is laid either prone or on one side over a pillow placed at the level of the armpits, so that the head and neck are in a slightly dependent position. This allows blood to gravitate into the mouth rather than into the lungs. When received into the cot or bed the same position should be maintained; the pillow beneath the chest may be removed and the foot of the bed raised six inches to a foot in order to keep the head at a lower level than the chest. A clean white towel should be placed beneath the head so that the amount of any subsequent bleeding may be roughly estimated by the size of the stain that it produces. There is invariably a slight amount of ' oozing ' of blood from the adenoid bed but this should not amount to a stain larger than half-a-crown. The child's neck should not be allowed to become flexed but should be maintained in a slightly extended position so that the air-way remains clear. (If there is the slightest degree of obstruction to the air-way it causes venous congestion of the head and the liability to haemorrhage from the tonsillar fossae is correspondingly increased.) The pulse should be taken every ten minutes, a record being kept both of the rate and of the volume and the nurse in charge of the patient *should not leave the bedside* until the child has recovered consciousness. When conscious, the child is usually given an intramuscular injection of Papaveretum in order to allay restlessness, and shortly after this the bed may be returned to the horizontal position and an hourly pulse chart commenced. Reactionary haemorrhage is revealed by the efflux of bright red blood from either the nostrils or the mouth and if this occurs ice-packs should at once be applied to the upper cervical region on both sides of the neck. A further small dose of Papaveretum may be given and these measures are usually sufficient to deal with minor bleeding resulting from the dislodgment of a small clot. If the haemorrhage is more

severe, the bleeding persists in spite of the treatment we have mentioned and the pulse rate shows a progressive increase. In this event no time should be lost in returning the child to the operating theatre where ligation of the bleeding vessel is carried out. If, however, it is found that the haemorrhage is occurring in the adenoid bed then ligation is impossible and a pack should be introduced instead. The tapes attached to the pack are led out through the nostrils and secured to the cheek with adhesive plaster in order to prevent it falling downwards into the oropharynx. It should be removed within twenty-four hours, after which there is seldom any further bleeding. Once again we must stress the fact that children, especially young ones, do not tolerate blood loss at all well and the sooner troublesome bleeding is dealt with the better. From what we have said it will be obvious to you that it is the skill of the immediate post-operative nursing, and the prompt recognition of the signs of reactionary haemorrhage, upon which the surgeon depends in order to ensure the successful outcome of the operation.

THE LARYNX

Foreign Bodies

As you already know, young children frequently put almost anything they can lay their hands on into their mouths. A sudden inspiratory effort whilst sucking such objects as sweets, beads and small marbles may carry the foreign body backwards and downwards into the larynx. If complete obstruction to the airway results from this accident the child will make violent inspiratory efforts and exhibit rapidly increasing cyanosis. In this event the promptest measures are called for in order to avert a disaster. The child should be lifted up by the feet and heartily thumped on the back and at the same time a finger should be passed into the mouth in an attempt to hook out the foreign body. In the rare instance when this treatment fails, immediate tracheotomy is the only hope of survival. Quite commonly a small foreign body such as a bead, may enter the larynx but come to rest to one side of the vocal cords and thus cause no interference with the airway. In such a case there are no signs of obstruction and all that is noticed is a constant cough and an increasing hoarseness of the voice; symptoms in fact which would appear to be caused by laryngitis rather than

the presence of a foreign body.   Removal is most satisfactorily carried out by direct laryngoscopy under a general anaesthetic.

Papillomas of the Vocal Cords

Multiple papillomas of the vocal cords is a condition confined entirely to childhood.   Attention is first drawn to their presence by a gradually increasing hoarseness of the voice and they are treated by removal under a general anaesthetic. Unfortunately they show a remarkable tendency to recur and repeated operations for their removal may have to be performed before a final cure is obtained.

THE EARS

(For congenital deformities of the external ear and pinna, see Chapter IV.)

Foreign Bodies in the External Ear

Small foreign bodies seem to find their way into the external auditory meatus as regularly as they are placed into the other natural orifices of the body.   Unless they are just within the meatus it is wisest to remove them under a light general anaesthetic in order to obviate the risk of damage to the ear drum by any struggling on the part of the child.   If for fear of the consequences the child fails to declare what he or she has done the presence of a foreign body may not be suspected until it causes a purulent discharge from the meatus.   In this event authorities differ as to the correct treatment.   Whereas some advise immediate removal others, rather than interfere with it, wait for the foreign body to be pushed out by the discharge that it has caused.

The Anatomy of the Middle Ear

As you will recall, the cavity of the middle ear communicates with the nasopharynx by a short canal called the Eustachian tube, the function of which is to allow the same pressure within the middle ear as is the atmospheric pressure outside, so that the ear drum (the tympanic membrane) is able to vibrate freely. The pharyngeal end of each of these tubes is situated to one side of the mid-line just beneath the adenoids and is surrounded by a collar of lymphatic tissue which itself is liable to be

inflamed during the course of a nasopharyngeal infection. It is not surprising, therefore, that an ascending infection of the middle ear (otitis media) via the Eustachian tube is so frequently associated with a chronic nasopharyngeal infection and particularly with chronically infected adenoids.

Acute Otitis Media

There are two principal forms of acute otitis media, catarrhal and suppurative. The catarrhal form is usually secondary to a generalized catarrhal inflammation of the nasopharynx. Swelling of the collar of lymphatic tissue around the pharyngeal end of the Eustachian tube causes occlusion of its lumen and consequently unequal pressure on either side of the ear drum, and this produces a temporary deafness. This occlusion although complete is not usually sustained for long periods and from time to time the Eustachian tube becomes momentarily patent. When this happens the child is conscious of a ' popping ' in the ear as the pressures on either side of the drum are suddenly equalized. Catarrhal otitis usually runs a mild course and frequently resolves of its own accord. It may, however, proceed to the *suppurative* form. Suppurative otitis media is characterized by a severe earache and a high temperature, but it is not always accompanied by deafness. Inspection of the drum through an auriscope shows it to be acutely inflamed but as the condition progresses and pus is formed within the middle ear, the drum becomes dull white in colour and begins to bulge in an ominous manner. Treatment with large doses of intramuscular penicillin should be commenced as soon as the diagnosis is made, and in a large number of cases resolution of the infection will follow. It is most important, however, that a close watch should be kept on the drum, for if it shows signs of bulging it should be incised under a general anaesthetic (myringotomy) in order to provide free drainage of the pus through a small pre-arranged wound, and thus prevent the considerable damage it would sustain if it were allowed to rupture of its own accord. Following the operation a large pad of warm cotton-wool is usually worn over the ear for a day or so in order to mop up the discharge of pus, and the external auditory meatus should be gently swabbed out at least twice a day. After a few days, a sterile-wool wick is the only dressing necessary and this is worn until examination shows good

healing of the drum.   If the tonsils and adenoids show evidence of chronic enlargement, they should be removed a month or so after the child has recovered from the otitis media.

Acute suppurative otitis media in infants, like so many acute infections in this age-group may occur without any symptoms directly referable to the primary focus. (See Chapter XI, Pyelitis.)   A high temperature (104°-105°F.) is always present and vomiting, diarrhoea and even convulsions are common associated findings.   It is not until the ear drum has been examined that the diagnosis becomes obvious.   The treatment does not differ from that we have already mentioned.

Chronic Otitis Media

This condition is invariably a legacy from an unresolved attack of acute otitis media and it is characterized by a continual painless discharge through an old perforation of the ear drum (otorrhoea).   It is a difficult condition to treat, as apparent improvement is often followed by a relapse.   The external auditory meatus should be swabbed dry at least twice a day and two or three spirit drops instilled into it.   Some authorities advocate a week's course of penicillin.   Chronic infection in the mouth and nasopharynx such as dental sepsis and enlarged tonsils and adenoids should be sought for and dealt with accordingly.   Like all chronic infections of the nose, throat and ears, attention to the child's general health is of great importance.   Dietary errors and deficiencies should be corrected and for town children, a period of convalescence in the country or better still the sea-side, is frequently beneficial.

Acute Mastoiditis

The cavity of the middle ear is in direct communication with the air-cells lying within the mastoid process and acute inflammation of the bone surrounding these air-cells (acute mastoiditis) may result from the extension of a pre-existing infective process within the middle ear.   Although acute mastoiditis may sometimes occur as a complication of acute otitis media it more commonly supervenes during the course of a *chronic* otitis media, in which the drainage of pus from the middle ear has temporarily become blocked.   The child becomes ill quite suddenly.   The temperature is usually of the order of 104°-105° F. and symptomatic vomiting may also be

present. The child complains of acute pain just behind the pinna, there is exquisite tenderness over the mastoid process and narrowing of the external auditory meatus from behind forewards is always present. In cases where there is a rapid extension of the pus to the surface of the mastoid process, a subcutaneous abscess is formed and the pinna is pushed forwards and slightly downwards (Fig. 32). Since the advent of penicillin, opinions as to the advisability of operation are somewhat divided. In the early stages of the condition systemic penicillin or oral aureomycin is often sufficient to produce pronounced clinical improvement within a few days. If, however, no such improvement occurs or if an abscess is formed, then operation should be undertaken at once. The purpose of the operation is to open the mastoid process behind the pinna and gouge out and scoop away all the infected bone. Following this the wound is lightly packed with tulle gras or vaseline gauze and a large cotton-wool dressing is applied over it. The response to this operation is usually dramatic—the temperature falls to normal within a day and the child rapidly begins to take an interest in his food and his surroundings once more. After five days the dressing is changed under a light general anaesthetic and thereafter dressings are done every two to three days without an anaesthetic. The wound is usually healed within two to three weeks. Very occasionally acute mastoiditis is accompanied by the dangerous complications of brain abscess and/or thrombosis of the lateral venous sinus (which lies in close relation to the mastoid process). The former is recognizable by the onset of meningitic symptoms and by a fall in the pulse rate without an accompanying fall in temperature and in the latter complication, septic emboli may be cast off into the general circulation causing secondary

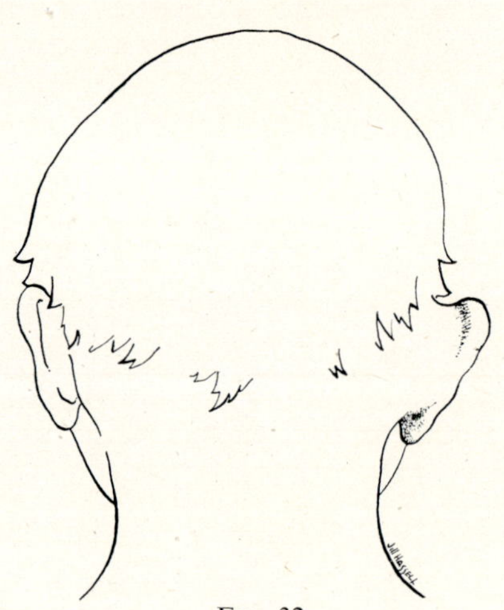

FIG. 32

Acute mastoiditis.   See text.

abscess formation throughout the body. Both these complications are accompanied by a high mortality.

DISEASES OF THE LYMPH GLANDS OF THE NECK

As you will recall the lymphatic system of the body consists of a widely ramifying system of small vessels (the lymphatics) which absorb the tissue fluid and finally empty their contents into the venous system. Along the course of these vessels are groups of lymph glands whose principal function is to filter off any bacteria that the lymph may contain and thus prevent bacterial infection of the bloodstream. Once bacteria have been 'arrested' in a lymph gland they may either be overcome and destroyed then and there, or they may produce a secondary focus of infection within the substance of the gland (*lymphadenitis*) which, like all acute inflammations may either *resolve* or proceed to *suppuration*. Such a focus of infection within the gland may destroy its effectiveness as a filter and in this event bacteria will be conducted onwards to the next group of glands. Thus the succeeding groups of lymph glands into which the lymph drains from any part of the body are best regarded as a series of lines of defence.

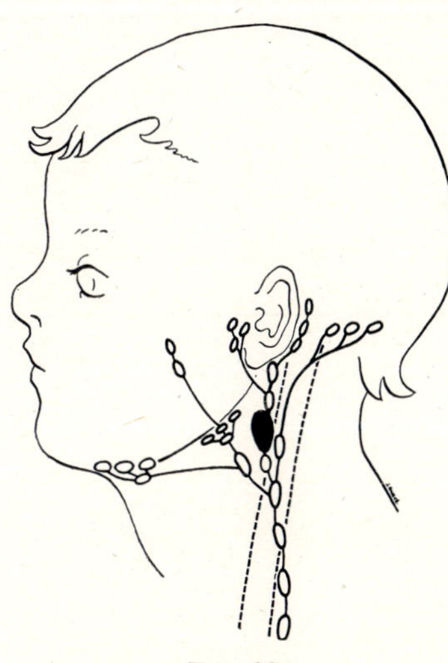

FIG. 33

The lymphatic glands of the neck (the second and third lines of defence). The dotted line indicates the position of the sterno-mastoid muscle and the tonsillar gland is coloured black.

The distribution of the lymphatics and the lymph glands in the neck are arranged in a *three-line defence system*. The first line of defence is formed by the four main aggregations of lymphatic tissue at the back of the nose and throat, the two faucial tonsils, the nasopharyngeal tonsil (the adenoids), and the lingual tonsil (which lies out of sight on the back of the tongue). The second line of defence is in the shape of a ring and consists of a series of glands beneath the chin (the sub-

mental group), beneath the angle of the jaw (the submandibular group), in the cheek and over the parotid gland (the facial and parotid groups), behind the ear (the post-auricular group), and around the occipital region of the head (the occipital group) (see Fig. 33). The third line of defence consists of two vertical chains of glands lying around the carotid artery and the jugular vein (known as the *deep cervical* glands), which terminate at their lower ends in a duct which returns the lymph into the blood-stream at the junction of the subclavian and jugular veins on either side of the neck.

ACUTE LYMPHADENITIS

The onset of acute inflammation in the lymph glands of the head and neck is always consequent upon a primary focus of infection within the area that drains into the affected glands. This primary focus of infection must always be sought for and, if found, should be treated just as energetically as the lymphadenitis that it has caused. Acute lymphadenitis is revealed by the painful enlargement of the gland or glands involved and also by increasing warmth and redness of the overlying skin. The temperature is usually raised one or two degrees and if the deep cervical glands are affected the child frequently holds its head towards the side of the inflammation in order to reduce the tension on the enlarged glands and thus relieve the pain. If there is no evidence of pus within the gland, hot fomentations should be applied to them and intra-muscular penicillin given in large doses. This is often sufficient to cause resolution of the infection but once pus has been formed no conservative treatment is of any use and surgical incision is indicated. Under a general anaesthetic a small incision is made through the skin overlying the most prominent portion of the swelling, a pair of sinus forceps are thrust into the abscess and the pus is allowed to escape. A small, soft rubber or tulle gras drain is introduced into the abscess cavity for twenty-four hours in order to assist the drainage of pus. The wound should be dressed each day until it is healed.

DEEP CELLULITIS OF THE NECK.—Beneath the skin and subcutaneous tissues of the neck there is a collar of tough connective tissue which completely encircles the deeper struc-tures. This is known as the *deep fascia* and the submandibular

and deep cervical glands are situated beneath it. If infection within these glands spreads into the surrounding tissues it will cause an *acute, suppurative, spreading* infection of the tissue planes beneath the deep fascia. This is revealed by a tense, brawny swelling of the neck, a high swinging temperature, anorexia and sometimes vomiting. No time should be lost in carrying out surgical incision into the inflamed area and intensive penicillin therapy should be instituted at the same time. Deep cellulitis of the neck is potentially a most dangerous condition for the pus in tracking along the deep tissue planes of the neck may cause *oedema of the glottis* with the resulting possibility of obstruction to the airway and subsequent suffocation. *Ludwig's angina* is one particular form of deep cellulitis of the neck and is caused by suppuration in the submandibular glands. It commonly results from an infected tooth socket in the lower jaw and may sometimes follow dental extraction. The region of the submandibular glands is the site of a large, tender, tense abscess which should be treated in the same way that we have mentioned above.

CHRONIC LYMPHADENITIS

Whereas acute lymphadenitis is characterized by a short, febrile and painful illness, chronic lymphadenitis results in a long-standing, painless enlargement of the cervical lymph glands. Chronic tonsillitis is the most common cause of chronic lymphadenitis, and it is therefore the gland into which the tonsillar lymphatics drain (*the tonsillar gland* which is coloured black in Fig. 33) that is most commonly enlarged.

The general health of children with chronic lymphadenitis is often less robust than other children and a poor appetite, underweight and a general lassitude are often associated findings. Removal of the tonsils, followed by a period of convalescence in the country is usually sufficient to bring about a reduction in the size of these glands and an improvement in the child's general condition.

CHAPTER VI

THE CHEST

THE CHEST WALL

BREAST ABSCESS

NOT infrequently the breasts of newborn infants are slightly enlarged and occasionally they may even secrete a few drops of milk. This is due to the action of some of the maternal hormones upon the infant breast, but the enlargement invariably subsides within the first two weeks of

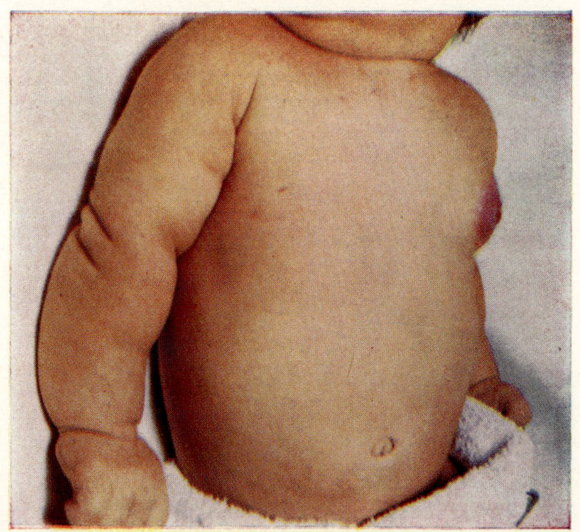

FIG. 34

A left breast abscess in an infant of two weeks of age.

life without any treatment. Sometimes, however, infection of the breast may occur during this period of enlargement, with the formation of a breast abscess. The affected breast enlarges still further, becomes fiery red in colour and acutely tender to the touch (Fig. 34). In boys, a small incision should be made over the most prominent portion of the abscess and the pus

evacuated. In girl infants, however, it is desirable if possible to avoid an incision over the breast and an attempt to aspirate the pus through a wide-bore needle may be made. Once this has been done, 50,000 units of penicillin dissolved in 1 cc. of saline solution should be injected into the abscess through the aspiration needle. This procedure sometimes effects a cure and is always worthy of a trial. If it is unsuccessful, however, a small incision must be made into the breast.

GYNAECOMASTIA

This is an uncommon condition occurring in boys about the age of puberty, in which there is a moderate enlargement of one or both breasts (Fig. 35). The cause of this enlargement is unknown, and as a number subside of their own accord a child with this condition should be observed for a period of six to twelve months in the hope that surgical interference will not be necessary. If, however, the swelling should persist for longer than this it should be excised.

FUNNEL CHEST

This is an uncommon condition occurring more frequently in boys than in girls, in which the sternum and the adjacent rib cartilages are depressed inwards producing the deformity seen in Fig. 36. Mild degrees of this condition seldom cause any organic disability, but severe depression of the sternum may cause displacement of the heart to one side or the other and it may also be responsible for recurring pulmonary infections. In this latter instance a surgical operation should be performed in order to elevate the sternum and the costal cartilages. The operation should be performed under endotracheal anaesthesia, for there is always the danger that, during the operation one or other pleural sac may be opened. Should this eventuality occur positive pressure applied through the endotracheal tube before the pleural sac is closed will cause full expansion of the lung. Post-operatively the child should be nursed either in the horizontal position or sitting upright. Any tendency on the part of the child to slump in bed is liable to interfere with the beneficial effect of the operation.

THE LUNGS

Before considering the individual conditions of the lungs that are amenable to surgical treatment we must first consider the anatomy of the thorax, the mechanism of breathing and the general management of operations within the chest (thoracotomy).

ANATOMY AND PHYSIOLOGY.—The thoracic cavity is divided into two separate air-tight compartments known as the

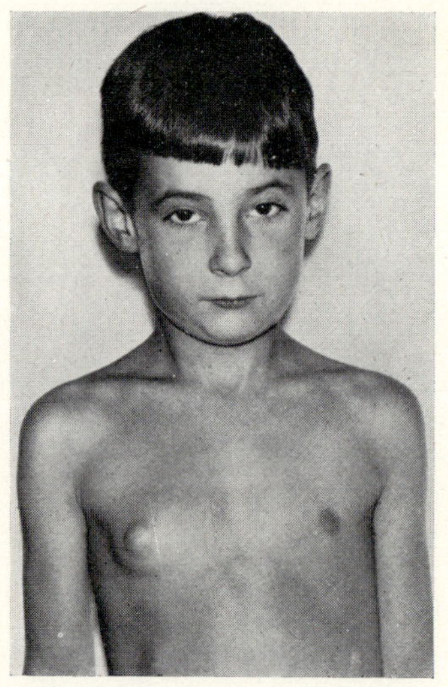

FIG. 35

Gynaecomastia. Note the enlargement of the right breast.

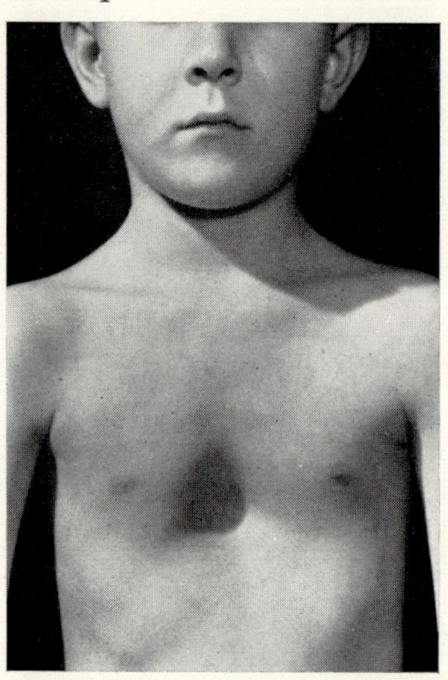

FIG. 36

Funnel chest. Note the deep depression of the lower sternum.

pleural cavities, each of which contains one lung. The central structure which effects this division is known as the mediastinum, and it contains the heart and the great vessels that enter and leave it, and as it is not a rigid structure it may in some conditions be displaced to one side or the other. Each lung is covered by a smooth, shiny membrane (the visceral pleura) which is continuous with a similar membrane which lines the inside of the pleural cavity (the parietal pleura). Between the parietal and visceral pleura (the pleural space) there is a negative pressure (that is to say, a partial vacuum) and thus, when the volume of the chest is increased, by the elevation of the ribs and by the lowering of the diaphragm, the lungs will automatically

7**

follow suit. It is this mechanism which causes air to be sucked into the lungs in the act we know as *inspiration* (Fig. 37), and it is exactly the same mechanism that causes air to enter into a deflated balloon when its sides are forcibly drawn apart. Whereas inspiration is an active effort, expiration is a passive effect and is accomplished by the elastic recoil of the chest wall and diaphragm to their original position. In consequence, the volume of the chest decreases and air is squeezed out of the lungs (Fig. 38). If, as occurs during the course of an operation on the lung, a communication is established between the pleural

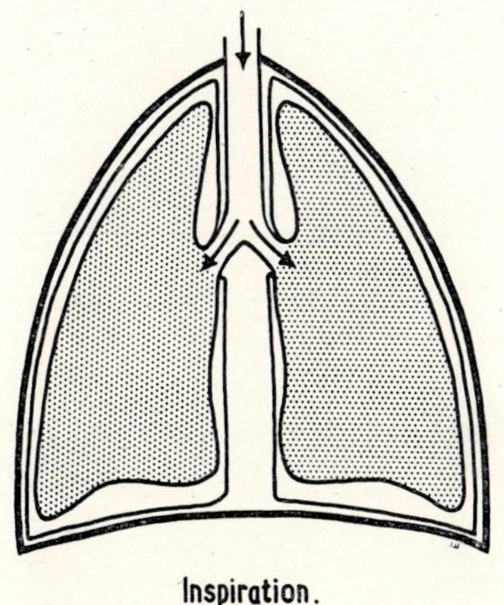

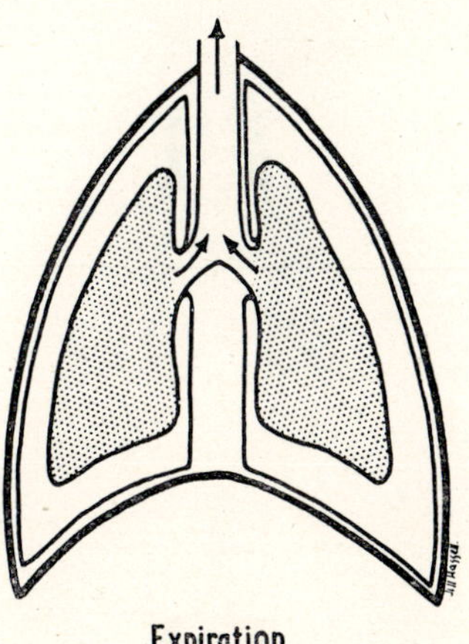

<table>
<tr><td>

Fig. 37

The normal chest in inspiration. The rib cage has been elevated and the diaphragm flattened. The heart is not shown for the sake of clarity.

</td><td>

Fig. 38

The normal chest in expiration. The rib cage and the diaphragm have returned to their original positions.

</td></tr>
</table>

space and the exterior, then air will enter the pleural space and the negative pressure therein will no longer exist (a pneumo-thorax). Thus, when the volume of the chest is increased in the act of inspiration the normal ' sucking out effect ' that this produces on the lung will be absent and the lung will fail to expand (Figs. 39 and 40), and in this event the responsibility of respiratory function will fall entirely upon the other lung.

THE GENERAL MANAGEMENT OF THORACOTOMY

Any operation within the chest (*thoracotomy*) will of necessity produce a pneumothorax and consequent collapse of

the lung. Although this collapse facilitates the operative manoeuvres that are to be performed by giving the surgeon more room in which to work, it is upon the re-expansion of the lung after the chest has been closed that the subsequent progress of the child largely depends. Thus, we may say that the general management of the thoracotomy case is primarily concerned with the measures that are taken to effect this re-expansion.

Pre-operative Measures.—Breathing exercises, designed to ensure full aeration of both lungs, should be practised twice

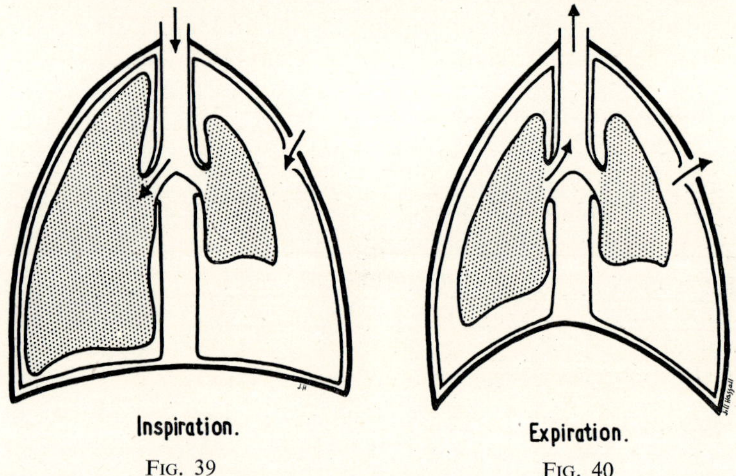

Fig. 39.—The act of inspiration during thoracotomy. Air enters the pleural space through the aperture in the chest wall and the lung, in consequence, fails to expand. Fig. 40.—Expiration during thoracotomy.

daily for a week or so before the operation under the direct supervision of a physiotherapist. In addition, the child should be taught to cough effectively in preparation for the amount of coughing he or she will be required to do in the immediate post-operative period in order to clear the bronchial tree of its secretions.

The Operation.—Once the child has been anaesthetized an endotracheal tube is passed into the trachea. The child is then laid on its side on the operating table with the affected side uppermost. The level of the incision varies according to that part of the thoracic cavity which is to be approached, but at whatever level it is situated it is made parallel to the ribs and

extends almost right round one side of the chest. Some surgeons prefer to make their incision between two ribs, after which they retract the ribs widely in order to obtain adequate entrance into the chest, whereas others prefer to remove the greater part of one rib and then enter the chest through the rib bed. In the case of either pneumonectomy or lobectomy, once the main artery and vein are divided between ligatures the bronchus is carefully closed and over-sewn in order to prevent any leakage of air through its stump once the operation is over. At the close of the operation the layers of the chest wall are closed with catgut and a small rubber tube is left passing through the wound connecting the pleural cavity with the exterior. Once the pleura has been securely closed, the anaes-thetist applies positive pressure through the endotracheal tube and so inflates the lung on the affected side, thus driving the majority of air out of the pleural cavity through the rubber tube. The second this has been done the tube is clamped, in order to prevent air rushing back into the pleural cavity as the deflating lung falls away from the chest wall. The skin is then closed by non-absorbable sutures and the tube is fixed to the skin by a loose ligature to prevent its extrusion from the wound.

Post-operative Measures.—When the child is returned to the ward the tube in the chest is connected to an under-water seal which is placed on the floor beside the bed, that is to say, about two to three feet below the level of the chest. Providing there is a negative pressure in the pleural cavity water will be sucked up the tube for a short distance, and in this way the seal prevents any air from entering the pleural cavity. If, however, there is still some air left in the pleural cavity, it will bubble through the water seal at each inspiratory effort until it is all expelled. In addition any fluid that forms in the chest will easily drain by gravity into the water seal. Whenever the bottle is lifted it is *essential* that the tube be clamped otherwise there is the danger that water will enter the chest. Some authorities prefer to employ two tubes, one being inserted in the lowest portion of the chest (to facilitate drainage of any fluid that may be formed) and the other inserted in the apical region in order to maintain the negative pressure. Both tubes are joined together outside the chest by a Y-shaped glass connection which gives way to a single channel which enters the water seal as in Fig. 41. The

chest should be X-rayed once each day in order to determine the degree of expansion of the lung, and in the normal course of events the lung will expand fully and come to fill the pleural

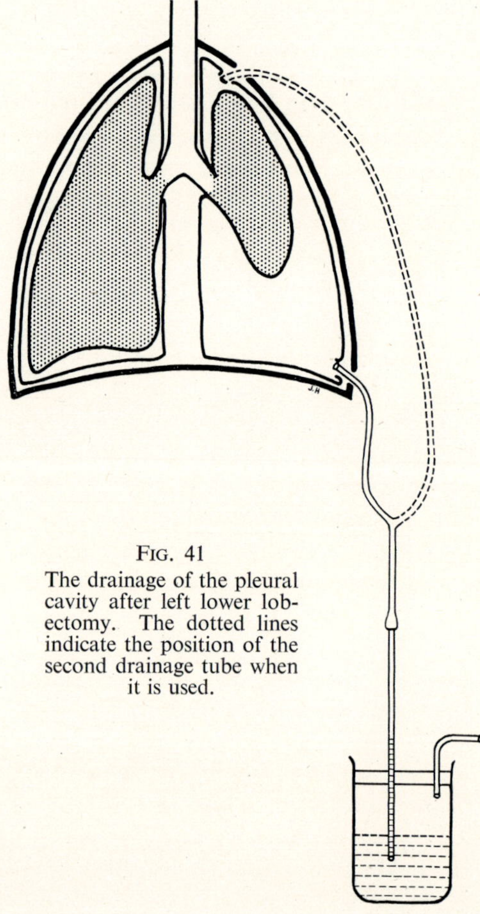

FIG. 41
The drainage of the pleural cavity after left lower lob-ectomy. The dotted lines indicate the position of the second drainage tube when it is used.

space within forty-eight to seventy-two hours. After this has happened the tube (or tubes) may be removed. The breathing exercises that the child has been taught in the pre-operative period should be resumed a few hours after consciousness has been regained in order to encourage expansion of the lung. Painful though it is bound to be, the child should be made to cough as much as possible and should be encouraged to do so

at regular intervals in order to minimize the risk of viscid bronchial secretions blocking a bronchus. In this respect it is often of tremendous help to the child for the nurse to support the upper abdomen with both her hands. Analgesic drugs should be used sparingly and no morphine derivatives should be administered at all as even in small doses they tend to depress the respiratory centre and also to abolish the cough reflex. The nurse will often find herself hard put to insist upon this forceful coughing as it obviously causes the child pain to do so, but it cannot be emphasized too strongly that this is an essential procedure and one that will ensure an uncomplicated recovery.

Complications of Thoracotomy

All the complications of thoracotomy are concerned with the failure of re-expansion of the lung on the side of operation.

(1) **Blockage of the Drainage Tube.**—The level of water which has risen up the drainage tube as a result of the negative pressure in the pleural cavity, rises and falls a few inches with inspiration and expiration respectively. If this fluctuation should cease it indicates a blockage in the tube and this fact must be reported at once. If X-ray examination shows that the lung is almost fully expanded then the tubes may be removed, but if the lung is still collapsed then suction will have to be applied to the tube in order to clear it.

(2) **Blocking of the Bronchus.**—After thoracotomy the bronchial secretions are liable to become excessive in amount and thick in consistency and unless they are coughed up they may block up a bronchus, an event which is followed by absorption of the air in the lung beyond the plug and the subsequent collapse of that portion of the lung. This is revealed by a rise in temperature and pulse rate, difficulty in breathing (*dyspnoea*) and slight cyanosis. The child should be turned on to the unoperated side, the foot of the bed elevated and the back gently slapped in order to promote forceful coughing. This position and procedure should be kept up for ten to fifteen minutes at a time and repeated at frequent intervals, and during each rest period oxygen should be freely administered if there are any signs of respiratory distress. As we have already said, the nurse will naturally feel disinclined to cause the child the amount of pain and discomfort that these

measures will inevitably entail, but if they are unsuccessful in unplugging the bronchus then bronchoscopy will have to be performed in order to aspirate the obstructed bronchus.

(3) **Tension Pneumothorax.**—This complication arises from an air leak through the stump of the sutured bronchus with the result that air will enter the pleural space and bring about a pneumothorax.   If the drainage tube in the pleural space is still *in situ* when this occurs then air will be seen to bubble through the under-water seal. If, however, the drainage tube has already been removed then the air which enters the pleural space from the bronchial stem will have no route of escape and will rapidly build up an increasing positive pressure within the pleural cavity.   In addition to the collapse of the lung that this increasing posi- tive pressure will produce, it will also push the mediastinum over to the other side (Fig. 42) and thus seriously embarrass both the action of the other

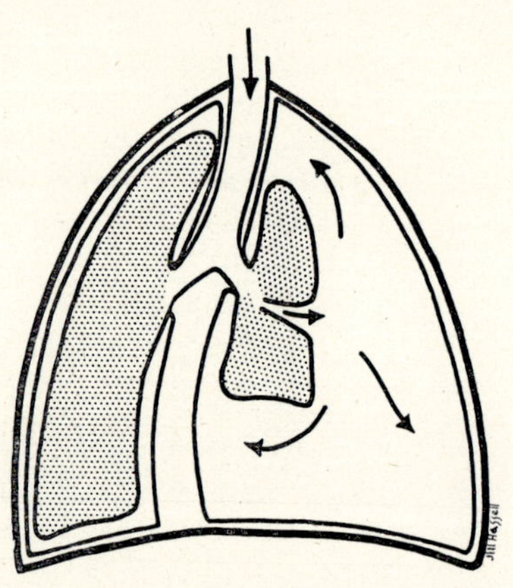

Fig. 42

A tension pneumothorax. In this instance a portion of the lung has been removed and the bronchial stump has sprung a leak.

lung and also the action of the heart.   Such a happening consti- tutes an acute surgical emergency.   The pulse becomes irregular and the child suddenly becomes grossly dyspnoeic and cyanosed. No time should be lost in introducing a wide-bore needle through a convenient inter-costal space on the operated side of the chest in order to release the high pressure of air within. Air then escapes through the needle with an audible hiss and this is followed by an immediate improvement in the child's condition.   A self retaining catheter should then be introduced into the pleural cavity and under-water drainage re-established.

Removal of the whole lung (*pneumectomy*) presents slightly different problems in management as there is no lung tissue left behind which needs to be re-expanded, and the treatment is directed primarily to the obliteration of the pleural space. Authorities differ as to whether under-water drainage, such as we have already described, should be used.   If it is used, a

careful watch must be maintained so that it does not produce too high a negative pressure, for this will only have the effect of sucking the mediastinum across to the operated side and thus interfere with the action of the heart (in other words, the reverse of a tension pneumothorax). If drainage is *not* employed then the empty pleural cavity slowly fills up with fluid and great care must be taken to see that the child is never turned on to the non-operated side, for should there be a small hole in the bronchial stump then the fluid within the pleural cavity will seep into the bronchial system of the remaining lung.

Although thoracotomy is a prodigious undertaking, children seem to stand it remarkably well, and the operative mortality in skilled hands is as small as 4 per cent. From the complications that we have mentioned you will realize that a smooth recovery after thoracotomy is largely dependent upon the continuous observation of the child's comfort, colour, respiration and pulse rate, and thus it becomes obvious that the success of intra-thoracic operations depends primarily upon the nurse who is responsible for this careful and vigilant watch.

EMPYEMA

An empyema is a collection of pus within the pleural cavity. It occurs with equal frequency in both boys and girls and is invariably due to an extension of infection into the pleura from an acute inflammatory process within the lung. Thus it may follow or accompany pneumonia, it may be due to rupture of a small lung abscess, or it may occur secondarily to bronchiectasis. In children, the most common infecting organism is the staphylococcus, although the streptococcus, the haemophilus influenzae and the micrococcus may sometimes be responsible.

The response of the pleura to infection may be divided into three stages:

1. The affected portion of the visceral pleura and the parietal pleura which is opposite to it, lose their shiny, smooth appearance and become red and roughened. This causes the visceral and parietal layers of pleura to rub together. In the early stages of this condition the child may experience acute pain in the chest due to this abnormal friction (a pleural rub).

2. In a short while large amounts of fluid (the inflammatory exudate) accumulate in the pleural cavity (*a pleural effusion*)

and separate the roughened visceral and parietal layers of pleura. Thus the acute pain due to the pleural rub disappears as the fluid is formed. Subsequently the causative organisms gain access to this pleural effusion and convert it into pus.

3. If the out-pouring of fluid is not great in amount then the visceral and parietal pleura around it may adhere to each other and thus localize the collection of fluid. In such an instance the empyema is referred to as a *local* one, but if the fluid production is too rapid for localization to occur then the whole of the pleural cavity is filled up, and a *total* empyema will result. The total variety of empyema is found more commonly in infants and very young children.

The principal effects of an empyema are two-fold:

(*a*) The collection of pus in the pleural cavity interferes with the expansion of the affected lung and indeed, the volume of pus may be so great that the mediastinum may be pushed over to the opposite side and thus seriously embarrass the aeration of the other lung. This may occur in both total and local empyemas and is revealed by a rapid increase in the respiratory rate.

(*b*) The absorption of bacterial toxins from the pus in the pleural cavity produces an intense degree of *toxaemia*, which causes a high, swinging temperature, a rapid pulse, insomnia, anorexia, a rapid loss in weight and an increasingly severe anaemia.

Treatment

The treatment of an empyema is directed to the relief of these two principal effects. That is to say, drainage of the pus from the pleural cavity with consequent re-expansion of the lung, and relief from the intense degree of toxaemia. Before treatment is commenced two X-ray photographs, one in the anterior-posterior and one in the lateral diameter of the chest should be taken, in order to reveal the site and extent of the collection of pus. Once this has been done an *air-tight* aspiration of the pus should be carried out. The best position for the child during this aspiration is sitting up with the arms folded over a bed table, but if the child is too ill to assume this posture then the recumbent position with the affected side uppermost will have to be adopted. The chest wall over the site of the empyema is infiltrated with a solution of 1 per cent

Novocaine and then a wide-bore needle attached to a syringe is introduced into the pleural cavity. It is essential that this needle should have a *two-way tap* at its hilt so that once pus has been withdrawn the tap may be turned and the syringe emptied without the possibility of air gaining access to the pleural cavity. Should air be allowed to enter the chest during the aspiration of a poorly localized empyema then a pyo-pneumothorax will result; what adhesions have already formed will be ruptured and the hitherto local empyema will be converted into a total one, a complication which may well prove to be fatal. The aspiration should be continued until as much pus as possible has been evacuated and a specimen of this pus should be despatched at once to the pathological laboratory so that the causative organism and its sensitivity to the various antibiotics may be determined. Before the needle is withdrawn 25,000 units of penicillin should be injected through it, and some authorities advise the coincident injection of 2 cubic centimetres of lipiodol (a radio-opaque fluid) so that subsequent X-ray examination will reveal the size of the cavity more clearly. Intramuscular penicillin in large doses should be commenced at the same time, and aspiration of the empyema, together with penicillin replacement should be repeated every other day. If the toxaemia is not relieved by these measures; or if the rate of fluid production is greater than can be controlled by aspiration; or should the pus thicken to such a degree that aspiration becomes difficult or impossible, then repeated aspirations should be abandoned and continuous drainage employed in its place. Continuous drainage may be either:

(1) Closed, or

(2) Open.

CLOSED DRAINAGE.—This form of drainage is reserved for those cases in which the pus is still thin in consistency, for this indicates poor and inadequate localization of the empyema. If the child is unduly apprehensive or at all unco-operative a light general anaesthetic should be employed, but in the majority of cases, closed drainage may be performed under a local anaesthetic. The child is placed in the same position as that for simple aspiration, and the chest wall over the lowest part of the empyema is infiltrated with 1 per cent Novocaine solution. The skin is then incised in a vertical direction and

1 or 2 inches of the subjacent rib are removed. A trochar and cannula are then thrust through the parietal pleura into the empyema; the trochar is withdrawn, and a wide-bore rubber catheter is inserted through the cannula. The cannula is then removed and the catheter connected to an under-water drain. The catheter is secured to the wound edge by a silk stitch and the wound is covered by a small dressing held in place by an adhesive dressing. In a small proportion of cases this form of continuous drainage is sufficient to ensure obliteration of the cavity of the empyema but subsequent thickening of the pus may cause a blockage in the catheter and in this event open drainage will have to be substituted.

OPEN DRAINAGE.—Open drainage is employed either as a sequel to closed drainage or in a case where adequate localization has been demonstrated by the thickening of the pus. The empyema is approached in the same manner as we described for closed drainage but instead of employing a trochar and cannula the wall of the empyema is widely opened and a short wide-bore rubber tube is inserted. This is packed around with copious thick dressings into which the pus is allowed to drain. The tube should be removed every second day, cleaned, sterilized and then reinserted. As the size of the empyema diminishes, so the tube is shortened until such time as the cavity is less than $\frac{1}{2}$ to 1 inch deep. After this the tube may be removed and the wound allowed to heal.

The day after either open or closed drainage has been performed the child should be instructed in special breathing exercises designed to increase the expansion of the lung on the affected side and thus help to obliterate the cavity of the empyema. These exercises should be supervised by a skilled physiotherapist. In the event of an open drainage being performed the child should become ambulant as soon as the temperature has returned to normal, as the exertions of walking and playing will help to increase the re-expansion of the affected lung. A high calorie diet with a full complement of vitamins should be given, and the child encouraged to regard the drainage tube more with contempt than with submission.

Empyemas in infancy are usually of the total variety, and as infants do not tolerate the insertion of drainage tubes as well as older children, they should be treated by massive antibiotic therapy and repeated aspirations.

SURGICAL TREATMENT OF BRONCHIECTASIS

Bronchiectasis is a disease of the bronchial tree in which the bronchial walls are permanently dilated and distended, and it may affect either one lobe of a lung, the whole lung itself, or more rarely, it may be present in both lungs. The disease is characterized by a paroxysmal cough and the production of large amounts of mucopurulent sputum. The epithelial lining of the dilated bronchi becomes progressively more insensitive and thus large amounts of mucus and pus are allowed to collect within them without provoking the cough reflex. A change in position, however, causes the sputum to pass from the insensitive bronchi into more normal parts of the bronchial tree with the consequent initiation of a reflex cough. As the clinical course and the investigations and general management of children with bronchiectasis are fully dealt with in medical textbooks, we will confine our interest to the management of those cases which are considered suitable for the surgical removal of either the affected lobe of the lung or the affected lung itself.

As the condition of bronchiectasis is frequently accompanied by chronic sepsis in the upper respiratory tract, the tonsils and adenoids should be removed and the maxillary antra and the ears closely inspected for the presence of chronic inflammation. In addition, any focus of infection in the teeth or gums should also be eradicated. For three months prior to operation the child should undergo postural drainage of the bronchi each morning and evening, and the amount of sputum obtained by these manoeuvres should be measured and a note made of its appearance, particularly as to whether or not it contains any streaks of blood. A high calorie diet rich in vitamins should be given during this time; the child should be weighed regularly, and operation should be postponed until such time as there is a steady gain in weight. If it is found that the causative organisms are sensitive to penicillin some authorities advise the daily inhalation of penicillin delivered from a small spray.

LUNG ABSCESS

Lung abscess is not a common condition of childhood and usually occurs as a complication of either pneumonia, bronchi-

ectasis or occlusion of a bronchus by an inhaled foreign body (such as blood clot following the operation of tonsillectomy). The child suffers a severe degree of toxaemia, and pain in the chest, a high swinging temperature, severe attacks of sweating, anorexia and rapid wasting are common findings. If the abscess ruptures into a bronchus the child suddenly begins to cough up large amounts of foul smelling sputum and as a rule this is accompanied by a dramatic improvement in the clinical condition. In this event the sensitivity of the causative organism should be determined by bacteriological culture and treatment with the appropriate antibiotic instituted, and in addition postural drainage should be carried out at least four times a day. These measures are often sufficient to procure resolution of the condition.

If rupture into a bronchus does not occur, the abscess should be treated conservatively until X-ray examination shows it to be well localized. Then, under a local anaesthetic or a light general anaesthetic, a portion of the rib directly overlying the abscess should be removed and a pack soaked either in iodine or iodoform is laid in the wound in order to stimulate adhesions between the visceral and parietal pleurae, so that when drainage of the abscess is performed at a later date there will be no risk of spreading the infection into the general pleural cavity and incurring the complications of empyema or pyopneumothorax. Four or five days later the wound is re-opened, the pack removed and a needle introduced into the abscess in order to confirm its whereabouts. Once this has been done a bold incision is made into the abscess cavity and a rubber drain is then introduced into its substance. The subsequent treatment does not differ from that of the open form of drainage of an empyema.

Multiple lung abscesses occur as a result of septicaemic or pyaemic conditions and the outlook is usually very grave. Intense antibiotic therapy and drainage of abscesses where and when an opportunity is afforded is the only possible treatment.

CHAPTER VII

THE OESOPHAGUS AND
THE STOMACH

ATRESIA OF THE OESOPHAGUS

THE word atresia literally means 'unbored' or 'uncanalized'. When applied to the oesophagus it describes a number of congenital abnormalities which are characterized by an absent segment in the oesophagus, and which may be further complicated by a fistulous communication between the trachea and the oesophagus (a *tracheo-oesophageal fistula*).

ANATOMY.—The oesophagus is developed from two blind tubes, one growing downwards from the throat and the other growing upwards from the stomach. Normally these two oesophageal components join together to form a single channel but should they fail to unite, the abnormality of oesophageal atresia will result. In addition in early embryological life, the trachea is in wide communication with the upper portion of this primitive oesophagus but later becomes completely separated from it. If this separation is incomplete an abnormal communication, or tracheo-oesophageal fistula, will remain.

There are three main varieties of this abnormality which are illustrated in Fig. 43. In type I the two oesophageal components have failed to unite and in addition the lower component opens into the trachea. This is the commonest variety and is found in about 80 per cent of cases. Type II consists of a simple atresia *without* a fistulous communication between the oesophagus and trachea, and in type III it is the upper oesophageal component which opens into the trachea. Having considered the anatomy of these abnormalities, the symptoms and signs associated with them are the more easily understood.

Clinical Picture

At birth, the child usually appears normal in all respects. The only sign that may lead you to suspect oesophageal atresia

is a persistent efflux of frothy saliva from the mouth, and this is due to the fact that the infant is unable to swallow its saliva into the stomach. At the first feed, however, the diagnosis becomes obvious. The baby sucks for a moment or so and then promptly vomits. This *immediate* vomiting is accompanied by coughing and spluttering and sometimes cyanosis. After a short while the attack passes off only to return when feeding is resumed. Should such an attack occur, feeding should be discontinued at once because of the danger of

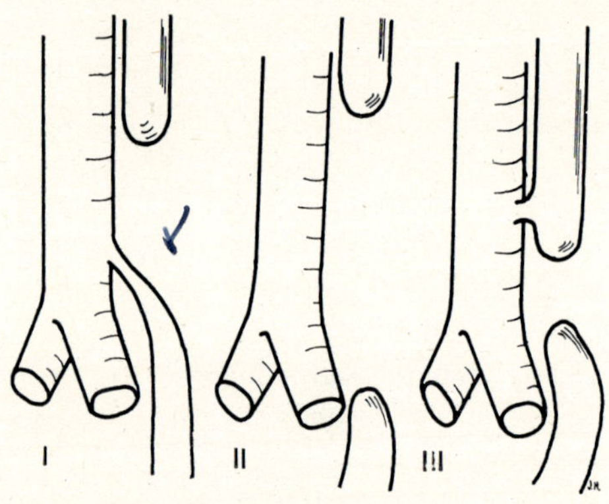

Fig. 43

The three principal types of oesophageal atresia
and tracheobronchial fistula.

introducing milk into the lungs (as, for instance, in type III). In order to confirm the diagnosis, $\frac{1}{2}$ cubic centimetre of lipiodol is introduced through a nasal catheter into the upper oesophageal stump. Subsequent X-ray examination will reveal either a blind ending to the oesophagus (types I and II) or a blind ending together with a fistula (as in type III). A straight X-ray of the abdomen in type I will reveal air in the stomach due to its communication with the trachea, but in types II and III no air will be visible, and in this way the precise anatomy of each particular abnormality may be discovered.

Pre-operative Management.—In all these cases (especially in types I and III) there is always the danger of fluid and infection reaching the lungs via the fistula, and it is for this reason that operation is usually performed within the first forty-eight hours of life. Penicillin therapy is started as soon as the diagnosis is made and an intravenous infusion of 5/N

saline and 4·3 per cent dextrose solution is commenced without delay. In types II and III postural drainage of the bronchi is carried out at regular intervals by tipping the child head downwards and gently patting it on the back. In type I, however, this procedure may cause flooding of the trachea and bronchi with gastric juices and it should not therefore be carried out.

Operation.—As soon as the infant is anaesthetized a bronchoscope is passed and the bronchial passages aspirated of any fluid or mucus. The operation is performed through the right side of the chest and consists of freeing the two blind stumps and then anastomosing the two ends of the oesophagus. Once this has been done the fistula, if it is present, is removed. Should anastomosis prove impossible a gastrostomy must be performed in order to feed the child, and other more complicated methods of anastomosis contemplated when the child is older. At the close of the operation aspiration of the bronchi is once again performed.

Post-operative Management.—The baby is nursed in an oxygen tent and continuous aspiration of the pharynx maintained for forty-eight hours. On the third post-operative day small feeds of expressed breast milk are commenced and provided that they are taken well they should be rapidly increased in amount and the intravenous fluid discontinued on the fourth post-operative day. Penicillin therapy is usually discontinued at the end of the first week.

HIATUS HERNIA

A hernia is best defined as the protrusion of part of an organ through an opening in the walls of the cavity in which it is normally contained. In the normal child the lower end of the oesophagus forms a close fit with the hole in the diaphragm (the oesophageal hiatus) through which it passes in order to reach the stomach. In the condition of hiatus hernia, the oesophageal hiatus is abnormally large and herniation of the upper portion of the stomach through the hiatus and into the chest may thus occur. In addition the normal mechanism which prevents the gastric contents from entering the oesophagus is lost, and as a result the regurgitation of large amounts of the gastric contents is liable to follow each feed.

Clinical Picture

The infant, which appears quite healthy at birth, begins to vomit as a rule within the first week or so of life. The vomiting, which is seldom forceful or projectile in nature but more like a large regurgitation in character, usually occurs at the end of each feed, although in some instances it may be delayed until the child is laid down again. The vomited material consists of gastric juices mixed with milk and occasionally contains a few streaks of fresh or brownish discoloured blood. This persistent

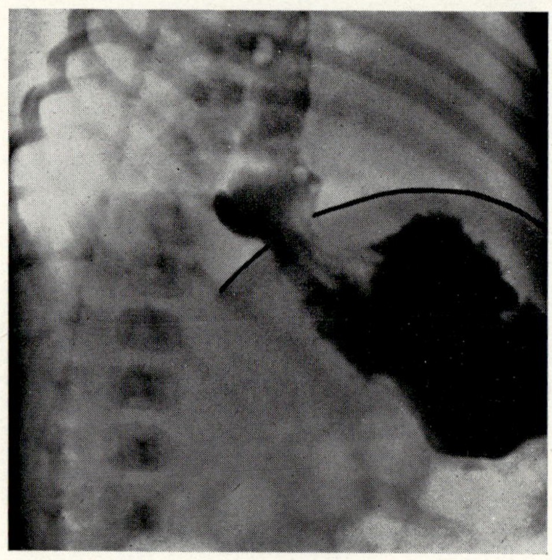

Fig. 44

Hiatus hernia. The line of the diaphragm has been accentuated.

vomiting deprives the infant of a substantial amount of its daily intake of food and thus failure to gain in weight is a common associated finding in this condition.

Diagnosis

The clinical picture described above is extremely suggestive of hiatus hernia but absolute diagnosis is only reached following a barium meal X-ray examination. The barium solution may be introduced into the infant's stomach either through a nasal catheter or by administering the solution in an ordinary feeding bottle. The infant is then placed under a fluoroscopic screen in the X-ray department and the fate of the barium in the stomach observed. If the infant is crying or struggling the

increased intra-abdominal pressure caused by these exertions may be seen to push the upper part of the stomach through the oesophageal hiatus and to cause a regurgitation of barium up into the oesophagus. Similarly, if the infant is tipped head downwards an identical effect is produced. Fig. 44 is an X-ray picture of just such an event. The line of the diaphragm has been inked in to make it more obvious and *above it* can be seen a small portion of the stomach together with some regurgitated barium. It may also be observed that when the infant is sat up in the erect position the herniated portion of the stomach returns from above the diaphragm back through the oesophageal hiatus into the abdominal cavity.

The Complications of Hiatus Hernia

Due to the incessant regurgitation of gastric contents in this condition, the lower reaches of the oesophagus are continually subjected to the action of the acid and the digestive enzymes contained in the gastric juices. As the oesophagus, unlike the stomach, has no protection against the action of these juices, ulceration of its lining eventually takes place and it is this ulceration that is responsible for the occasional streaks of fresh or altered blood that may be found in the vomit. If such an ulcer persists it will increase in size and eventually come to involve the whole thickness of the oesophageal wall. Fibrous tissue is then laid down in the tissues around the oesophagus as a defence against the advancing ulcer. This *fixes* the oesophagus to the surrounding tissues and consequently prevents the herniated portion of the stomach from sliding back into the abdominal cavity. This fixation increases the degree of regurgitation, which in turn increases the severity of the ulceration. This in its turn causes more fibrous tissues to be laid down and in this way a vicious circle of events is produced. The fibrous tissue slowly contracts and in doing so both shortens and narrows the oesophagus. The shortening drags more stomach up into the thorax and the degree of narrowing produces a *stricture* of the oesophagus which may become sufficiently severe to interfere with swallowing (dysphagia).

There are occasional instances in which a short oesophagus or a stricture of the oesophagus are thought to be congenital in origin. It would appear, however, that they are more likely to be the results of a hitherto unrecognized hiatus hernia.

Treatment

The type of treatment used in this condition depends upon whether or not fixation of the oesophagus has taken place. Prior to fixation, whilst the hernia is still able to slide up and down through the oesophageal hiatus, *postural* treatment is employed, but once fixation has occurred *operative* procedures are the only possible forms of treatment. Treatment may therefore be:

(1) Postural.   (2) Operative.

(1) POSTURAL TREATMENT.—The whole aim of this form of treatment is to nurse the infant in a semi-upright

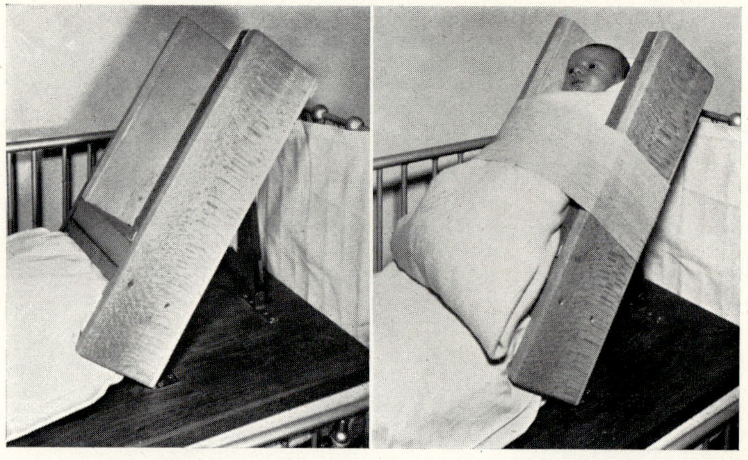

<table>
<tr><td align="center">FIG. 45
A simple form of box for the postural
treatment of hiatus hernia.</td><td align="center">FIG. 46
The child in position.</td></tr>
</table>

position both day and night so that the effect of gravity will maintain the stomach beneath the level of the oesophageal hiatus. In this way the hiatus is no longer constantly stretched by a portion of the stomach sliding in and out of it, and is thus given the chance to narrow down. Many methods have been devised by which the semi-upright position of the infant may be maintained and you will no doubt see a wide variety of appliances used in different hospitals. One of the most simple methods is illustrated in Fig. 45. It can be easily and cheaply made by the hospital carpenter and consists of a solid wooden

platform on which is fixed a wooden box which is kept at the desired angle by an upright bar behind it. The walls are padded with sorbo rubber and the infant merely reclines in the box, its position being secured by a few turns of crepe bandage (Fig. 46). As the child increases in size so increasingly large boxes are made. For the first five to six months of life the child leaves the box only to be changed, bathed and fed, and

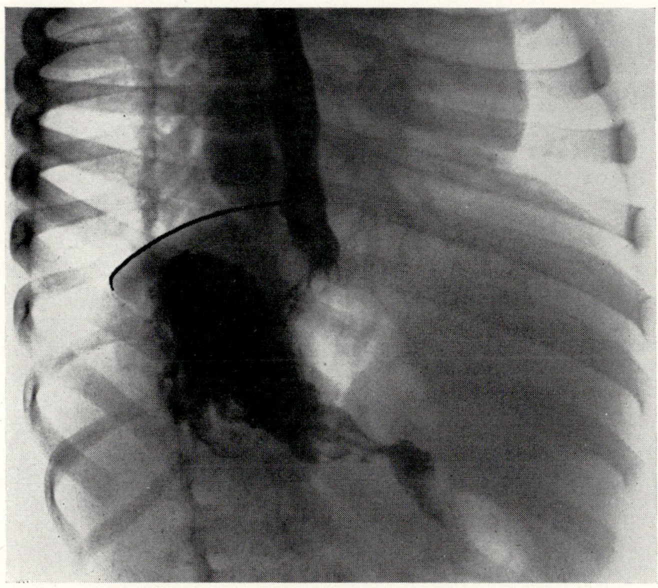

Fig. 47

Hiatus hernia.   The same child as in Fig. 44 after one year of postural treatment.   Note that the stomach is now well below the level of the diaphragm.

during all these procedures the semi-upright position must be maintained at all times. At about six months of age when the child is beginning to sit upright of its own accord it may be transferred from the box to a small cot in which it is supported by pillows arranged in the form of a chair.

Infants treated in this way vomit less frequently and begin to gain weight almost from the first day of treatment. In a successful case such as the one depicted in Fig. 46 a barium meal X-ray at six weeks of age (Fig. 44) shows an obvious hiatus hernia, whereas after nine months of postural treatment an X-ray photograph in the inverted position (Fig. 47) demon-

strates no evidence of hernia whatsoever. This particular child had ceased to vomit altogether within three weeks of commencement of treatment and from then on its weight had always remained normal for its age. In a certain proportion of cases, however, postural treatment is not so successful. The persistence of the vomiting and the failure of the child to gain in weight necessitates barium meal X-ray every few weeks to be certain that fixation of the oesophagus has not taken place. Providing fixation has not occurred, postural treatment should be continued.

(2) OPERATIVE TREATMENT.—Once fixation of the oesophagus has been demonstrated radiologically, operation should be undertaken forthwith. The lower oesophagus and hiatus are approached through the left side of the chest, the oesophagus freed from its surrounding tissues and the herniated portion of the stomach replaced in the abdominal cavity. The hiatus is then stitched together to narrow it as much as possible so that a close fit between it and the oesophagus is established. Post-operatively it is essential that postural treatment should be continued. Operative repair in such cases is by no means a certain method of cure. All too often recurrence of the condition may follow and at the present time it is as yet too soon to assess the ultimate value of operative treatment.

PYLORIC STENOSIS OF INFANCY

Pyloric stenosis is a condition which occurs in infants up to three months of age and which is characterized by vomiting, wasting and progressive dehydration. It is reported to occur in one in every three hundred births and is between five and six times more common in male than in female infants. Although you will occasionally come across cases of pyloric stenosis occurring in both premature infants and babies of four months of age, the usual age of onset is between three and seven weeks. The underlying cause of this condition is a gross increase in size (hypertrophy) of the circular muscle fibres of the pylorus. This hypertrophy has the effect of reducing the pyloric canal to such a narrow channel that the outlet of the stomach is almost completely obstructed. In consequence the infant vomits back all the feeds and in so doing deprives itself of the majority of the daily requirements of food and fluid, with the

result that wasting, dehydration and constipation shortly becomes apparent. Although the vomiting is both copious and forceful it never empties the stomach completely, and as the residue left behind is unable to pass through the pylorus it becomes stagnant and sour and invariably causes a mild inflammation of the gastric mucous membrane (gastritis).

Clinical Picture

The infant with pyloric stenosis is always a *hungry* child. In between feeds he wails with hunger and while feeding sucks eagerly and with enthusiasm. The outstanding feature of this condition is the vomiting, which, on account of the remarkable force with which the vomit is ejected, earns itself the description of *projectile* vomiting. The projectile nature of the vomiting is due to the considerable increase in strength of the gastric musculature which results from its repeated attempts to overcome the pyloric obstruction. The vomited material consists of freshly taken milk mixed together with stagnant curds remaining from previous feeds. As a result of the gastritis induced by the stagnating gastric residue, some mucus and a few streaks of brownish blood may also be present but bile staining of the vomit never occurs, as the degree of pyloric obstruction which is responsible for this condition prevents the regurgitation of bile from the duodenum back into the stomach. Dehydration, which is revealed by depression of the fontanelle, dry inelastic skin and a decrease in the urinary output, is variable in its severity and depends largely upon the duration of the vomiting. Wasting is recognizable by an undue wrinkling of the skin and by the lack of the normal full and well-rounded contours which are so characteristic of a well-nourished child. The infant's weight is always below the expected weight for its age and this is due both to the dehydration and the wasting. Constipation is not always present but is the rule rather than the exception. Sometimes you will hear experienced ward sisters, in referring to a child with pyloric stenosis, say 'it looks like a case of pyloric stenosis'. In saying this they are referring to an expression which is often present on the child's face. It is impossible to describe or depict this expression to you and you will only come to recognize it after seeing a large number of cases. It is often called an 'anxious' expression and is probably due to a combination

of mild dehydration, wasting, a persistent hunger and failure to obtain satisfaction and comfort from a feed.

Diagnosis

Before a feed is given to the infant the stomach should be aspirated through an oesophageal tube and the volume of the residual gastric contents estimated. In the normal infant the gastric residue prior to a meal amounts to little more than a few cubic centimetres of clear gastric juice. In pyloric stenosis, however, the gastric residue may be as high as 5 to 6 ounces and consists mostly of stale curds. Mucus and some streaks of partly-digested brownish blood may also be present due to the coincident gastritis. Although a large gastric residue together with the clinical picture we have already described are in themselves extremely suggestive of pyloric stenosis, the critical point on which diagnosis depends is feeling the hypertrophied pylorus (or pyloric tumour as it is called) through the abdominal wall. When relaxed, the hypertrophied pylorus is not usually palpable but when contracted it readily becomes obvious to the palpating finger as a hard lump about the size of an olive. As contraction of the pylorus only occurs when food is introduced into the stomach, abdominal examination to discover the tumour should always be performed while the child is feeding. In a warm, quiet room the surgeon and nurse both wearing masks, seat themselves as shown in Fig. 48. A feeder is placed around the infant's neck and the abdomen completely uncovered. The baby is cradled by the nurse's left arm and feeding is commenced. The surgeon then gently examines the upper right quadrant of the infant's abdomen until he feels the contracted pyloric tumour. Inspection of the abdomen during the course of this feed may reveal large waves of peristaltic contraction in the stomach passing from left to right across the

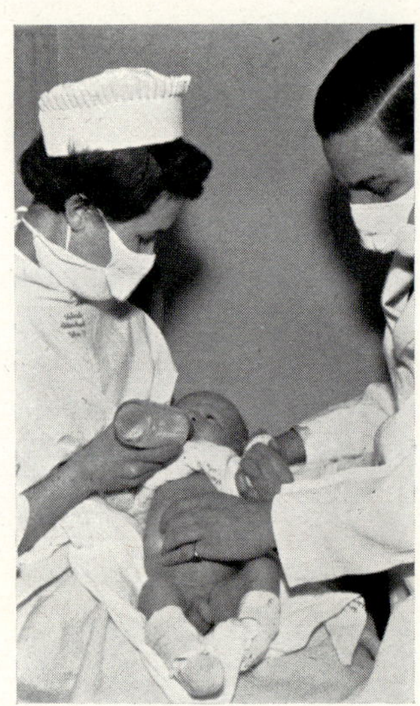

Fig. 48

The examination of a case of pyloric stenosis. (See text.)

baby's upper abdomen. This is known as *visible peristalsis* which, although not confined entirely to this condition, is frequently an associated finding.

Treatment

The methods of treatment used in pyloric stenosis are largely a question of opinion. You will come across cases of pyloric stenosis treated both by surgical operation and also by medicines. What concerns you, however, is that you should understand the principles on which these varying methods of treatment are based.

Surgical Treatment

Treatment of pyloric stenosis by surgery consists of dividing the pyloric tumour in its longitudinal axis so that the constriction of the pyloric canal is alleviated and a normal channel re-established through which the stomach can empty without difficulty.

Pre-operative Management.—Two hours before operation an oesophageal tube is passed and the stomach aspirated. A stomach wash-out with saline solution is then performed and continued until the fluid is *absolutely* clear. This is a most important step, for it removes all the stale curds and mucus from the stomach. If the stomach wash-out is *not* performed or is performed inadequately, once the pyloric obstruction has been relieved by operation the stagnant gastric contents will enter the small intestines and there set up a severe enteritis. Half-an-hour before operation the infant is given 1 minim of Papaveretum by intramuscular injection.

Operation.—The infant is laid between two warm rubber water-bottles on the operating table. The vest is pulled up over each arm and then fixed to the head pillow with safety pins. The surgeon injects between 8 and 10 cubic centimetres of $\frac{1}{2}$ per cent Novocaine solution into the mid-line of the abdomen between the xiphisternum and the umbilicus, distributing it equally between the subcutaneous tissues, the subjacent muscles and the extra-peritoneal tissues. After an interval of five minutes, which is allowed for the local anaesthetic to become effective, he commences the operation by opening the abdomen in the mid-line. As he does so the nurse who is sitting at the head of the table, covers her finger with a rubber finger-stall,

dips it into a little glycerine mixed with a few drops of brandy
and introduces her finger into the baby's mouth.   As she does
so, the infant begins to suck eagerly thus allowing full relaxation

POST-OPERATIVE FEEDING CHART, CONGENITAL PYLORIC STENOSIS   NAME:

Date	Time	Hours after Operation	Feed	Amt.	Treatment, Drugs, etc.	Vomit	P. U.	B.O.	Sig.
		3½	7·5% Glucose in ½ St. Saline	ʒ i					
		4		ʒ i					
		4½		ʒ i					
		5		ʒ i					
		5½		ʒ i					
		6		ʒ i					
		6½		ʒ i					
		7		ʒ i					
		7½	½ St. Milk Food	ʒ i					
		8½		ʒ ii					
		9½		ʒ iii					
		11	Full St. Milk Food	ʒ iv					
		12½		ʒ vi					
		14½		℥ i					
		16½		℥ i					
		18½		℥ i					
		20½		℥ i					
		22½		℥ i½					
		24½		℥ i½					
		27		℥ ii					
		30		℥ ii½					

Fig. 49

The post-operative feeding chart.

of the abdominal muscles.   Once the abdomen is open the
pyloric tumour is delivered into the wound and its wall is slit
from end to end down as far as, but not including, the mucous
membrane of the pyloric canal.   The pyloric tumour is then
returned to the abdomen and the wound closed.   This operation is usually referred to as the Rammstedt operation.

Post-operative Management.—Three and a half hours after
the operation the child is fed with 1 drachm of 5 per cent

dextrose and $\frac{1}{2}$ strength saline solution and thereafter feeding is continued as shown on the chart depicted in Fig. 49. From this chart you will see that full feeding (either breast feeding or a suitable substitute) is re-established within thirty-six and a half hours after operation.

After an interval of a day or so the child rapidly begins to gain in weight. The abdominal sutures are removed on the sixth post-operative day and the child is usually fit to be discharged from hospital a week after operation.

Sometimes you will see Rammstedt's operation performed under a general anaesthetic. In this event any degree of dehydration that is present must always be corrected prior to operation by an intravenous infusion of either 4·3 per cent dextrose and N/5 saline solution or Hartmann's solution. Some surgeons, providing the degree of dehydration is not severe, prefer the *subcutaneous* administration of normal saline solution in doses of 15 cubic centimetres/pound body-weight. In addition to the pre-operative management already mentioned, 1/200th of Atropine is given by intramuscular injection three-quarters of an hour before operation.

Non-Surgical Treatment

This method of treatment is based upon the contention that Atropine, when introduced into the stomach, produces a lessening of the degree of constriction at the pylorus and thus allows freer emptying of the stomach. Twenty minutes prior to each feed 2 minims of an alcoholic solution of Atropine (Eumydrin) is administered by mouth. When vomiting occurs a feed equal to the volume of vomit is given at once. This form of treatment, which requires a much longer and more tedious period of management and supervision than does surgical treatment, usually has to be continued until the child is weaned on to solid foods.

CHAPTER VIII

THE INTESTINES

INTESTINAL OBSTRUCTION

THE term intestinal obstruction describes a state of affairs in which there is an interference with the normal downward progression of the intestinal contents and although a relatively uncommon condition in infancy and childhood it is nonetheless an extremely dangerous one. Intestinal obstruction may be of two principal types:

> (1) Mechanical.
>
> (2) Paralytic.

MECHANICAL INTESTINAL OBSTRUCTION

The mechanical form of this condition may be caused by a congenital blockage such as an atresia, or by obliteration of the lumen of the gut by a plug, a twist (*volvulus*) or by its compression within the neck of a hernial sac. Irrespective of the cause, the effects of intestinal obstruction are:

> (*a*) ABSOLUTE CONSTIPATION.
> (*b*) VOMITING.
> (*c*) PAIN.
> (*d*) ABDOMINAL DISTENSION.

(*a*) ABSOLUTE CONSTIPATION.—The contents of the bowel *beyond* the obstruction are mostly absorbed from the lumen and although there may be a bowel action shortly after the onset of the obstruction, thereafter there will be *absolute constipation*, and a complete absence of *flatus*.

(*b*) VOMITING.—The steady accumulation of bile, gastric and pancreatic secretions and other intestinal contents above the site of the obstruction produces a distension of the gut which can only be relieved by vomiting. If the site of the obstruction is high up in the intestines (i.e. the jejunum or

duodenum) then vomiting will be an early manifestation, but if the blockage is low down (i.e. in the terminal ileum) vomiting will consequently not occur until later. The vomitus is usually clear or bile stained at first but as the condition progresses, blood is liable to ooze from the intestinal wall into the lumen and colour the vomit a dark brown (so-called *faeculent vomiting*).

(*c*) PAIN.—The pain in intestinal obstruction is characteristically colicky in nature and is usually situated around the umbilicus. It is caused by the distension of the bowel above the obstruction and the heroic contractions of the bowel wall in an attempt to overcome it.

(*d*) ABDOMINAL DISTENSION.—As abdominal distension is only a secondary effect due to dilated coils of gut it is most important for you to realize that if the site of the obstruction is high, either in the duodenum or upper jejunum, then there may be no abdominal distension whatsoever. As a general rule we may therefore say that the lower the site of the obstruction the greater the number of dilated coils of intestine, and in consequence the greater the degree of abdominal distension.

The Complications of Intestinal Obstruction

(1) FLUID AND ELECTROLYTE LOSS.—The continued vomiting in this condition has the effect of depleting the body reserves of water and electrolytes, especially chlorides. For this reason rapid dehydration and prostration due to fluid and chloride loss will inevitably occur.

(2) STRANGULATION.—This complication results from local pressure effects cutting off the blood supply of the obstructed portion of gut. Should strangulation remain unrelieved then gangrene, perforation of the gut and general peritonitis is bound to ensue.

The Treatment of Intestinal Obstruction

The treatment of intestinal obstruction is by surgical relief of the obstruction, but there are two important pre-operative measures that we must first consider.

(1) FLUID AND ELECTROLYTE REPLACEMENT.—Any operation for the relief of intestinal obstruction is fraught with additional dangers in the dehydrated and prostrated child. Intravenous replacement of fluid and chloride in the form of

N/5 saline and 4·5 per cent dextrose solution should therefore be instituted as soon as the diagnosis has been made. The volume of all the urine passed should be measured and always tested for the presence of chlorides.

(2) GASTRO-INTESTINAL SUCTION.—In order to decompress the distended intestine a Ryle's tube should be passed into the stomach and either continuous or hourly aspiration performed. In older children some authorities prefer to pass a Miller Abbot tube into the intestine itself. This tube has to be passed under X-ray control to make sure that its end has passed through the pylorus and has come to lie in the lumen of the upper intestine. All aspiration specimens should be saved and neatly labelled with the time of the aspiration and the amount recovered.

PARALYTIC INTESTINAL OBSTRUCTION (PARALYTIC ILEUS)

Paralytic ileus is a condition in which the intestinal muscle is completely paralysed and it most commonly occurs as the result of an infection of the peritoneum (peritonitis). The ability of the bowel to contract is lost and thus the intestinal contents instead of being conducted on their way, merely lie stagnating in the lumen of the bowel. Bile, pancreatic and gastric secretions accumulate within the bowel and it is this accumulation, together with the *gas* produced by the decomposing intestinal contents that causes widespread *distension* of the gut. This is accompanied by effortless vomiting and absolute constipation and there is also a *complete absence of pain*. A straight X-ray photograph of the abdomen taken in the upright position readily reveals the distension of the gut, and it also demonstrates pools of intestinal contents lying in the dilated coils (fluid levels). Due to the paralysis of the bowel musculature there is a complete absence of any bowel sounds and the nurse should always take the opportunity of appreciating this ' deathly ' intra-abdominal silence by using the stethoscope herself.

Treatment

As in all conditions of acute inflammation, *rest* is the first essential in treatment. In order to rest the bowel completely

absolute starvation should be instituted and the child's fluid requirements administered through the intravenous route. Continuous gastric suction, either through a Ryles tube or a Miller Abbot tube is carried out in order to decompress the distended bowel, and intramuscular penicillin and streptomycin should be given in order to combat the infection. This routine is continued until there is a return of function in the intestinal muscle, which is revealed either by the passage of a stool or flatus or by the auscultation of active peristaltic movements within the abdominal cavity.

DUODENAL ATRESIA

At one period during the development of the gut, the duodenum is represented by a solid cord which later becomes canalized into a tube. Duodenal atresia is a rare congenital condition (1 in 20,000 births) in which this canalization has failed to occur and there is therefore a complete block in the duodenum, which is situated either just above or just below the entry of the bile duct. As the obstruction is beyond the stomach, the volume of the first feed or so after birth can usually be accommodated, but after this, vomiting is frequent. The vomit is usually bile stained, but if the site of the blockage is above the entry of the bile duct then bile will of course be absent from the vomit. Visible peristalsis may be present but the abdomen is not distended and little or no meconium is passed. Thus the onset of severe and continual vomiting in a baby only a day or so old is strongly suggestive of duodenal atresia. To confirm the diagnosis a straight X-ray of the abdomen should be taken and this will reveal a complete absence of air in the intestines other than in the stomach and upper duodenum. Such a case is depicted in Fig. 50 where there is a small gas bubble in the stomach and upper part of the duodenum, but none in the intestine. Compare this picture with the amount of air normally seen in the intestines of a two-day old baby (Fig. 51). If confirmation of the diagnosis is required, a few teaspoonfuls of thin barium solution or 2cc. of Lipiodol may be introduced into the stomach through an oesophageal tube. Subsequent X-rays taken up to an hour after the administration of the barium will demonstrate that it has failed to pass beyond the

obstruction and is still lying in the stomach and upper part of the duodenum.

The only possible treatment in this condition is to perform a 'short circuiting' operation between the stomach and the upper part of the small intestine. An intravenous infusion of glucose saline solution should be commenced as soon as the diagnosis is made. In some hospitals you will see the child

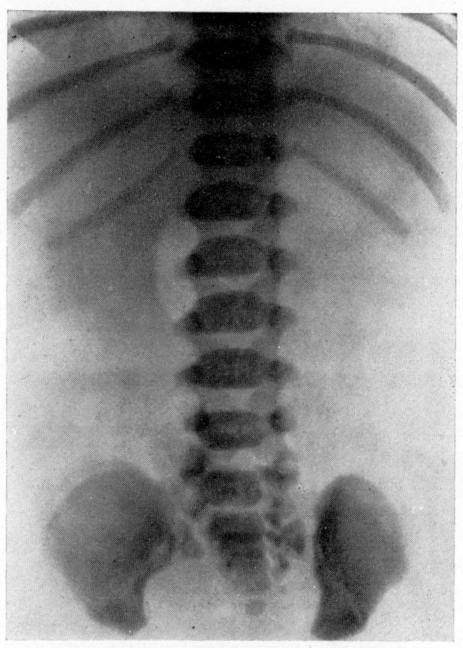

FIG. 50
Duodenal atresia. Note the absence of air in
the intestines. (Compare with Fig. 51.)

lightly bandaged down on to a padded crucifix splint immediately prior to the operation. It is doubtful if this expedient is really necessary for the operation can easily be performed with the infant simply lying flat on the back. The abdomen is opened in the mid-line and a piece of the upper small intestine is anastomosed to the stomach (a *gastro-enterostomy*) or to the upper duodenum. Post-operatively the gastric contents should be aspirated by the passage of a small catheter or polythene tubing every four hours in order to prevent gastric distension and consequent tension at the anastomosis. As the volume of the

gastric aspirations begins to fall so the intervals of aspiration should be lengthened until it is performed only once or twice a day. Once the volume of the aspirate amounts to no more than 2 or 3 cubic centimetres, aspiration should be stopped and feeding with half-strength milk commenced. The intravenous infusion is continued until such time as the child is taking sufficient by mouth to provide the normal fluid requirements.

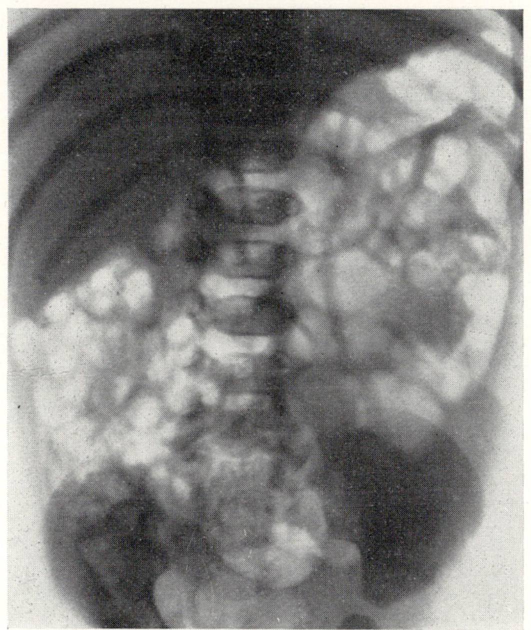

FIG. 51
Air in the intestines of a normal child aged two days.

INTESTINAL ATRESIA

Intestinal atresia may occur in any part of the small intestine, but is most common in the jejunum. The clinical signs of this condition are exactly similar to those of duodenal atresia, but as the obstruction is situated further down the small intestine the interval between birth and the onset of vomiting is usually greater. Similarly a high intestinal atresia may demonstrate little or no abdominal distension whereas it may be pronounced in a low intestinal atresia. A straight

X-ray of the abdomen may show gas bubbles in the intestine, but they are usually limited to the upper abdomen and are infrequent or absent in the lower abdomen. The subsequent introduction of barium into the intestine via the stomach will reveal the presence and the site of the obstruction. The pre- and post-operative treatment is the same as in duodenal atresia, and the operation consists of anastomosing two pieces of the small intestine—one immediately above and one immediately below the atresia.

Occasionally the block may be incomplete (i.e. intestinal stenosis) in which case a few curds may be found in the stools and the signs of complete obstruction are not in evidence. Usually the child is a few weeks or even months old, the only abnormal signs which have been noticed being a failure to thrive and to gain in weight. The presence and the site of the partial obstruction may be demonstrated by barium meal X-ray and the treatment is the same as in the complete variety.

MECONIUM ILEUS

This is an uncommon form of intestinal obstruction, occurring in babies who have been born with fibrocystic disease of the pancreas. In this condition the digestive enzymes normally secreted by the pancreas are very much diminished or indeed absent. In addition, the mucus secreted by the intestinal and pulmonary epithelium is less than normal and is of a thick and sticky consistency. These facts cause children with fibro-cystic disease to suffer under-nutrition (due to the lack of digestive enzymes) and render them particularly prone to the occurrence of pulmonary infections (due to the viscid mucus secreted in the bronchial tree). From this you will see that the treatment of meconium ileus is merely a surgical incident in the course of the prolonged and exacting medical management of the child.

Due to the lack of pancreatic enzymes, the meconium resembles thick tar in consistency, and inspissated masses of this semi-solid and tenacious meconium sometimes cause an obstruction in the lower ileum of the new-born child. Vomiting usually commences during the first three days of life, the vomit at first being clear but becoming increasingly dark and murky. The abdomen becomes distended, and in a large majority of

cases the masses of meconium within the bowel may be felt through the abdominal wall. Under a general anaesthetic the abdomen should be opened and the loop of blocked up ileum delivered into the wound. Some surgeons prefer merely to bring a piece of the terminal ileum to the surface (an ileostomy), whereas others prefer to remove the obstructed and distended loop of ileum and bring both cut ends to the surface (a ' double-barrelled ' ileostomy). This latter procedure has the advantage of actually removing the principal obstruction, and later allows the introduction into the bowel both upwards and downwards of pancreatic enzymes in order to dissolve the inspissated meconium that remains. Post-operatively the child should be placed on oral aureomycin (50 mg. b.d.) as a protection against pulmonary infection, and when normal-looking meconium and curds begin to issue from the bowel opening then the two cut ends of the ileostomy should be re-united and returned into the abdomen.

VOLVULUS NEONATORUM

ANATOMY.—At about the eighth week of foetal development the intestines are growing at such a rate that they can no longer be accommodated in the abdominal cavity. For this reason they extrude outside the body proper through a deficiency in the anterior abdominal wall which is later to become the region of the umbilicus. This *physiological hernia*, as it is called, remains till about the end of the twelfth week of intra-uterine life when the intestines return to the confines of the abdominal cavity. In returning, the bowel normally undergoes a complicated mechanism of rotation whereby the small intestine enters first followed by the large intestine which then takes up its normal position in front of the small intestine. The ascending and descending colon come to be attached to the posterior abdominal wall, and these attachments serve to anchor them in position. (Now before proceeding further, we must consider the meaning of the word *volvulus*. Volvulus merely means a twisting of a loop of bowel. For this to occur it is necessary to have a long loop of bowel with the two ends of the loop situated close together: if they are situated far apart it is impossible for the loop to twist on itself.) The condition of volvulus neonatorum is associated with faulty rotation of the

intestines while they are returning into the abdomen. Instead of the normal anatomy being assumed by the returning gut it just ' piles in ' to the abdomen in a bunch; no anchoring to the posterior abdominal wall takes place, and the whole length of intestines is bunched up together. Thus the pre-requisites for a volvulus are present, and twisting of the mal-rotated gut may occur much in the same way as knots mysteriously appear in a loop of string which has not been correctly coiled but merely put away in a tangled skein.

It is believed that twisting of the gut sufficient to cause intestinal obstruction does not take place before birth but only occurs when peristaltic action begins. It is for this reason that volvulus neonatorum usually occurs within the first few days of life. Absolute constipation, protracted vomiting and abdominal distension make their appearance and should strangulation of the twisted loop occur then sudden collapse of the child due to perforation of the loop will inevitably ensue. The pre- and post-operative treatment do not differ from that we have already described for duodenal atresia. Operation is directed to untying the twists and attempting to return the bowel to the abdomen in such a way that retwisting does not subsequently recur. If strangulation has occurred, then the strangulated segment should be excised and the two ends of healthy bowel anastomosed together.

INTUSSUSCEPTION

The normal method of propulsion of the intestinal contents is called *peristalsis*. The muscle of the intestinal wall grips the intestinal contents and by squeezing them in a distal direction causes them to pass downwards on their journey to the exterior. In addition there are a variety of other intestinal movements which are largely responsible for mixing the intestinal contents with the digestive juices, but, in considering intussusception, it is principally the movement of peristalsis with which we are concerned. If a small tumour attached to the inside of the intestine is treated by the muscle wall as intestinal contents, then the intestine will endeavour to push it onwards and in so doing, that portion of the bowel to which the tumour is attached will become telescoped into the lumen of the gut and itself be dragged onwards as the tumour is pushed further

and further down the alimentary canal. This is just one way in which an intussusception may occur, and although it is an extremely uncommon form in childhood it serves as the most simple explanation of how an intussusception is produced. (Fig. 53).

Intussusception in childhood occurs up to the age of two years and is most commonly encountered between the ages of five and nine months. This age incidence corresponds with the time in an infant's life when it is being weaned on to solid foods, and thus when the intestine is having to deal with a much larger bulk of intestinal contents than it has previously been used to accommodate. The intussusception commonly occurs in the region of the ileocaecal junction and in this area the lumen of the bowel is markedly decreased due to large aggregations of lymphoid tissue in the gut wall. In its effort to push the increased contents through a decreased lumen the bowel wall itself may then become infolded, with the production of an intussusception.

Clinical Appearances

Sudden acute abdominal pain in a child who has previously been in normal health is the commonest mode of onset of this condition. The pain lasts for only a few moments and then passes off completely, so that the child may once again appear to be perfectly normal. Within half an hour, however, an identical attack occurs and again passes off. These attacks continue to recur every twenty minutes to half an hour, and after a few hours the child becomes increasingly pale in the interval between each attack. Vomiting does not commonly occur until the condition has been present for twelve hours or more. Shortly after the attacks begin a normal stool may be passed, but thereafter there is absolute constipation. As the piece of intussuscepted bowel is forced further and further on it becomes more and more congested with blood—so much so, in fact, the blood may ooze out of its tip into the lumen of the bowel in which it finds itself, and this is revealed by the passage of a mixture of blood and mucus from the rectum, which, because of its similar appearance is sometimes referred to as a ' red currant jelly stool '. It is important for you to realize, however, that a red currant jelly stool does not contain *any faeces whatsoever*, for by the time the intussusception has

become sufficiently congested to produce red currant jelly the bowel distal to it has been emptied by the passage of a normal stool.   Thus a child with recurrent abdominal pain who passes

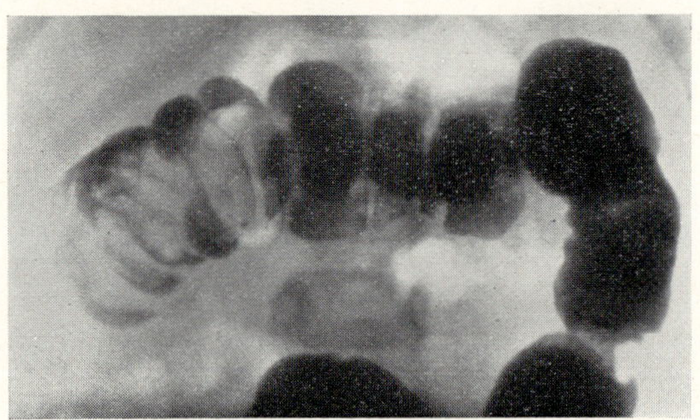

Fig. 52
A barium enema X-ray of an intussusception.

a *blood-stained* stool (i.e. blood mixed with faeces) is clearly *not* suffering from an intussusception.   As the intussusception consists of an ingoing layer of bowel, a returning layer of bowel and the ensheathing layer of bowel into which they have both

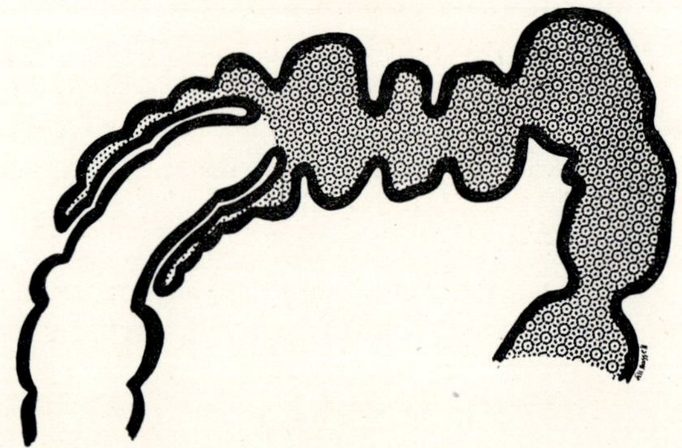

Fig. 53
To demonstrate the anatomy of the intussusception
shown in Fig. 52.

passed, it forms an easily palpable lump in the abdomen, and the history that we have described, taken together with the palpation of such a lump, is conclusive evidence of an intussusception.   Sometimes, however, the lump may have passed up underneath the ribs, in which case it will become impalpable.

A thin solution of barium should then be run into the rectum and visualized under a fluoroscopic X-ray screen as it passes upwards in the colon. When it reaches the tip (apex) of the intussusception it will be prevented from flowing any further: the barium flows just around the tip and the succeeding piece of bowel, but thereafter stops completely. This is well illustrated in Fig. 52. The accompanying diagram (Fig. 53) has been drawn to demonstrate the local anatomy which is responsible for the X-ray appearance.

Treatment

An intussusception is most commonly and most satisfactorily reduced by surgical operation, but occasionally you may see it treated by hydrostatic pressure.

Surgical Operation.—As soon as the diagnosis has been made operation should be carried out as soon as possible for fear that the intussusception may become *irreducible*. Under a general anaesthetic the abdomen is opened in the mid-line beneath the umbilicus and the tip of the intussusception is gently squeezed until the intussuscepted bowel has returned to its normal position. After this the abdomen is closed. Post-operatively the child should receive fluid requirements by the oral administration of glucose saline solution for the first twenty-four hours, half-strength milk for the second twenty-four hours, and normal feeding should be resumed on the third day. Alternate stitches are removed on the sixth and eighth post-operative days and the child may be discharged from hospital on the tenth day. About 5 per cent of all intussusceptions are liable to recur, in which instance the clinical appearance and the treatment do not differ from that already described.

Occasionally it may be found at operation that the tumour has become irreducible and this is especially likely when the condition has been present for more than twenty-four hours. In such an instance the only course open to the surgeon is to remove the intussusception and then anastomose the cut end of the ileum to the cut end of the colon (*an ileocolostomy*). This procedure naturally lengthens the time of the operation and the chances of infection of the peritoneum are also increased due to the transection of the bowel. Intramuscular penicillin and streptomycin should be commenced as soon as the child

has been returned to the ward in order to provide a defence against any such infection that may have occurred, and for the first three post-operative days all fluids should be administered by the intravenous route in the form of 4·5 per cent dextrose and N/5 saline solution.   On the fourth day feeding should be resumed in the manner we have already described.

HYDROSTATIC PRESSURE.—The advocates of this form of treatment wish to avoid a surgical operation and seek to reduce the intussusception by pressure on its tip exerted from within the lumen of the bowel.   In the same way as we mentioned in the diagnosis of this condition, a catheter is introduced into the rectum and a thin solution of barium is run in from a can suspended *not more than* 18 inches above the level of the child's abdomen.   Under the fluoroscopic screen the barium is visualized as it flows upwards to the apex of the intussusception, and providing the intussusception is easily reducible, the hydrostatic pressure of the 18 inches of barium solution may be seen to push the apex down the ascending colon and ultimately reduce the intussusception.   Once this has been accomplished barium is seen to flow through the ileocaecal valve and into the ileum.   The advantage

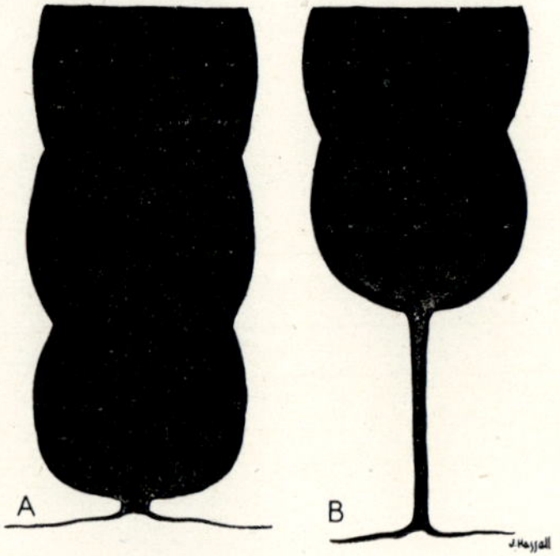

FIG. 54

To illustrate the X-ray appearances of idiopathic megacolon (A), and Hirschsprung's disease (B).

of this method is that surgical intervention is avoided, but the disadvantages are firstly, that if the intussusception is too tight to be reduced in this manner valuable time has been wasted and the child unnecessarily exhausted prior to operation, and secondly, that it is not always easy to tell if full reduction has in fact been obtained.

MEGACOLON

The term megacolon merely means a large colon, and it is the immense increase both in size and content of the colon that is the predominent feature of both types of the condition that we are about to consider.

IDIOPATHIC MEGACOLON

Idiopathic megacolon may occur at any age but is more commonly encountered in children of three to five years and upwards. The presenting symptom is severe constipation, and there may be intervals of up to two weeks between the passage of each stool. When it is eventually passed the stool is large

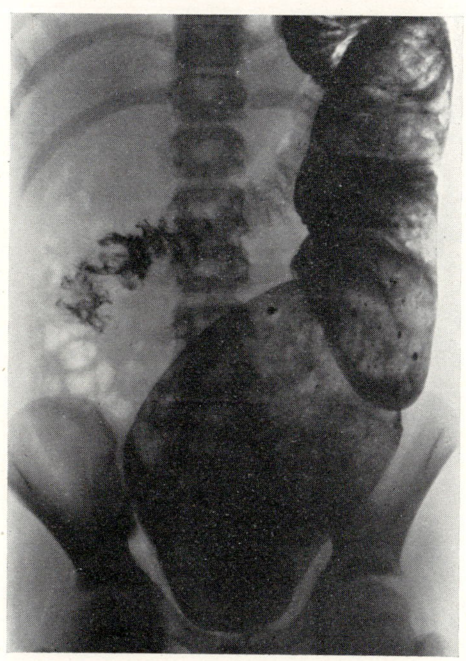

FIG. 55

A barium enema X-ray of idiopathic megacolon.

and hard, but is small in comparison with the large amount of faeces that remain behind in the colon. Abdominal pain does not occur and rectal sensation and the desire to defaecate are usually absent. Rectal examination discloses a distended rectum packed tight with faeces, and if a barium enema is performed it demonstrates a gross distension of the rectum and colon which extends right down to the *anal canal* (Figs. 54 A and 55). The precise cause of this condition is unknown, but it is now generally conceded that psychological factors may be responsible for the child's lack of enthusiasm to open its bowels,

and that the gross dilatation of the colon may in fact be a secondary effect rather than of primary significance.

Treatment is purely a question of adequate management, both of the child and of the colon. In order to allow the stretched colonic muscle to recover its tone the colon should be emptied by a series of high colonic washouts, and the child thereafter sent to the lavatory at least twice a day, with instructions to concentrate entirely on the act of defaecation and nothing else. The administration of enemas in this condition is quite valueless, for the success of enema administration is entirely dependent upon the ability of the colonic and rectal muscles to contract. In idiopathic megacolon the bowel is already grossly distended and its ability to contract is almost lost. Therefore, if an enema is administered it will never be returned and its fluid content will slowly be absorbed through the bowel wall. The whole point of giving colonic washouts in this condition is to convert some of the faecal material to silt and having done so to syphon the silt back to the exterior. This is a long and protracted business, and in order to empty the colon of a child with idiopathic megacolon it may take the nurse two hours each day, for sometimes as much as two or three weeks, before the colon is finally emptied.

Hirschsprung's Disease

This condition more commonly affects boys than girls and is usually revealed within the first year or so of life. The presenting symptom is again protracted constipation, and the colon becomes so grossly distended that it may produce quite a considerable enlargement of the abdomen. Waves of peristalsis may be seen coursing over the colon and abdominal pain and even episodes of intestinal obstruction may also occur. The child does not continue to thrive and there may be marked wasting of the body which is thrown into greater relief in comparison with the grossly distended abdomen. When the stools are passed they are often flattened like a piece of tape, and rectal examination discloses a narrow channel quite empty of faecal material.

It is only within the last few years that the true nature of this condition has been discovered. In the muscle of a normal piece of intestine—be it large intestine or small intestine—there

are small nerve ganglia which initiate and maintain peristaltic action. In Hirschsprung's disease it has now been found that there is a small segment of bowel, usually in the upper portion of the rectum or lower sigmoid colon, which is completely devoid of these ganglia. This is called the *narrow* or *aganglionic segment*, and it is quite incapable of any form of peristaltic activity. Any faeces that do reach the exterior get there after being pushed through the aganglionic segment by the normal bowel above it, and barium enema X-ray examination reveals this narrow strip-like aganglionic segment lying beneath a grossly distended and overburdened colon (Fig. 54 B).

No amount of dilatation or stretching of this narrow segment will result in any benefit, and surgical removal of the segment is the only treatment of value. This is usually performed in two stages. Before the first stage is undertaken the bowel is sterilized by the administration of succinyl-sulphathiazole, given over a period of five days in four-hourly doses of $\frac{1}{2}$-1 gram according to the age of the child. Under a general anaesthetic the abdomen is opened and the narrow segment is visualized. Two black silk stitches are placed in the wall of the gut at the upper limit of this segment in order to serve as markers when the second operation comes to be performed. The transverse colon is then transected and both cut ends brought to the surface (a double transverse colostomy). This allows the ready discharge of faecal contents and the consequent return of the colon to normal dimensions. Following this operation the child's nutrition readily improves and a gain in weight, together with a happier disposition are obvious in a short time. After an interval of between three to six months the intestinal tract is again sterilized in the same manner as we have previously mentioned and for three days prior to operation the isolated piece of colon between the colostomy and the rectum should be irrigated with a solution of succinyl-sulphathiazole. Under a general anaesthetic the abdomen is re-opened and the marking sutures placed in the bowel at the first operation are located, for due to the decompression of the colon the narrow segment is no longer so obvious as it was at the first operation. The whole of the narrow segment together with a cuff of colon above it is now removed and the normal colon brought down to be united to the anal canal (the operation of *rectosigmoidectomy*). At the end of this operation the transverse

colostomy is left undisturbed, and two weeks later, when the suture line between the colon and the anal canal is healed, the transverse colostomy is closed and the normal route of the intestinal contents restored. In the post-operative period, particular attention should be paid to maintaining a regular bowel action, for although the cause of the condition has been removed the child's previous experience of constipation may remain as a bad habit.

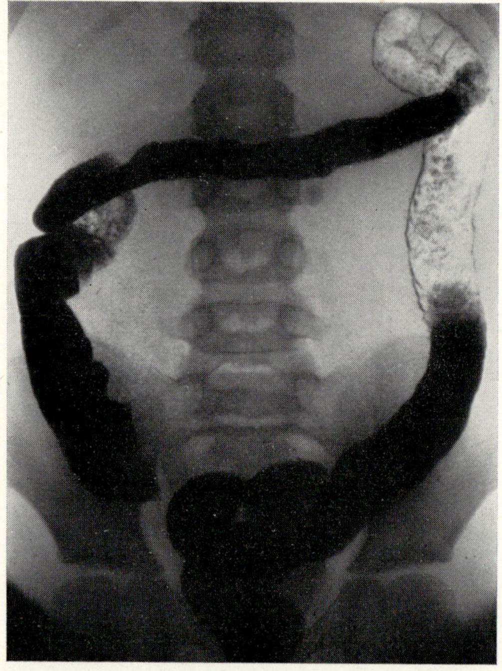

FIG. 56

A barium enema X-ray in ulcerative colitis. Note the smoothness of the walls of the colon.

ULCERATIVE COLITIS

This condition is most uncommon in children and is characterized by a progressively severe diarrhoea. The passage of blood and pus in the stools accompanies the diarrhoea and as many as fifteen to twenty motions may be passed during twenty-four hours. A multitude of causative agents have been incriminated, but the true cause of the condition is still unknown.

There is invariably a pyrexia and as a result of the colonic bleeding there is a progressively severe anaemia. Barium enema X-ray examination reveals that the normal contour of the colon is lost and that it now appears almost as smooth as a lead pipe (Fig. 56), and sigmoidoscopy reveals an acutely inflamed bowel wall with a number of small shallow ulcers on its surface.

The treatment of this condition in childhood consists primarily of careful medical management, and surgery is restricted to dealing with perforation of the colon should it occur. Rarely, in spite of the most expert medical care, the child's condition may continue to deteriorate and in this event the acutely inflamed colon is put at rest by performing an ileostomy. As the contents of the ileum are fluid and excessively irritant to the abdominal wall, the skin around the ileostomy should be painted with aluminium paint in order to provide a barrier between the intestinal contents and the skin, and an ileostomy belt, designed to collect as much of the faecal discharge as possible, should then be glued to the skin around the ileostomy. Re-establishment of the continuity of the bowel at a later date is frequently followed by recurrence of the condition, and for this reason removal of the whole colon (total colectomy) may eventually have to be performed.

RECTAL POLYP

Rectal polyps may be either single or multiple and consist of small buds of excessively friable rectal mucosa which often bleed during the act of defaecation. The blood usually appears during the passage of the stool or immediately afterwards and removal of the polyps is the only effective treatment. The pre-operative treatment is designed to empty the colon, and consists of an aperient given forty-eight hours before operation, an enema twenty-four hours later, and a high colonic washout twelve hours before the operation is performed. Under a general anaesthetic a sigmoidoscope is passed up the rectum and a search made for the polyp; once found it is twisted off the rectal wall with a long pair of forceps.

RECTAL PROLAPSE

The rectal mucosa in some children is only loosely attached to the underlying muscle and small fringes of it may be extruded

through the anus during defaecation. When this occurs these fringes are easily reduced manually, and by softening the faeces with liquid paraffin (4 drachms t.i.d. by mouth) the prolapse may occasionally fail to reappear. If, however, it should persist, then one of two procedures may be carried out. Some authorities advise threading a piece of chromic catgut just underneath the skin right around the anal orifice. It is then tied so that the external orifice of the anus is slightly narrowed. Others again advise injection of a 5 per cent solution of Phenol in almond oil into each lateral rectal wall about 1 inch up from the anal verge. This produces a fibrous reaction between the mucous membrane and the muscle wall and may succeed in preventing a recurrence of the prolapse. Both these procedures should be preceded by the same preparation of the bowel as we mentioned in the case of rectal polyps, and after the operation has been performed the buttocks should be strapped together for four days. Liquid paraffin should be administered during this period, and after the four days have passed the child is allowed to open the bowels spontaneously.

ANAL FISSURE

This is a small tear of the mucosa of the anal canal and is usually situated in the mid-line posteriorly. It is invariably the result of the passage of hard, constipated faeces. The tear in the anal mucosa causes an intense degree of spasm in the anal sphincter, with the result that any attempt at defaecation is accompanied by severe pain. The faeces should be softened by the liberal administration of liquid paraffin, and if this is insufficient to allow the fissure to heal then an anaesthetic ointment such as 1 per cent Deccicane should be smeared on to the anus every four hours. This application takes away the pain which accompanies defaecation and allows the fissure to heal of its own accord.

IMPERFORATE ANUS

ANATOMY.—At one time during the development of the foetus the rectum and the bladder are in wide communication. These two cavities are finally separated into individual compartments by a septum which grows down between them. When this has been completed the rectum still does not

10

communicate with the exterior, but ends as a blind stump just short of the skin. A small dimple then appears in the skin opposite this rectal stump and continues to deepen in extent until it finally enters into communication with the rectum. This invaginated piece of skin becomes the anal canal, and its site of union with the rectum becomes the ano-rectal junction.

Failure of this normal process of development may result in one of two principal deformities:

(1) Imperforate anus.

(2) Ectopic anus.

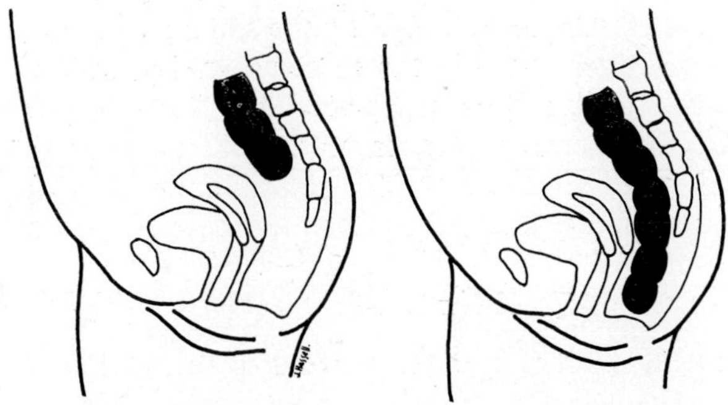

<table>
<tr><td align="center">Fig. 57
Imperforate anus with wide separation between the rectal stump and the skin.</td><td align="center">Fig. 58
Imperforate anus. The rectal stump is only separated from the skin by a thin diaphragm.</td></tr>
</table>

(1) IMPERFORATE ANUS.—In this condition the communication between the anal canal and the rectum has failed to take place. The rectal stump and the anal canal may be widely separated or may only be separated by a thin diaphragm (Figs. 57 and 58). The distance of the rectal stump from the anus can quite easily be determined by X-ray examination. Air is not present in the intestines of a child until it has been born but after birth air is swallowed, and as it reaches the rectum in about six hours the child should be turned upside down and an X-ray photograph taken of the lower abdomen. Air will then ascend into the rectal stump and demonstrate the site of its termination. This is clearly illustrated in Fig. 59, in which a small metal bead has been placed in the anus to

demonstrate its position. If the rectal stump is more than 3 centimetres from the anus it is usually impossible to perform an anastomosis between the two, and in such an instance a left inguinal colostomy has to be performed. If, however, it is less than 3 centimetres distance away, an operation under a general anaesthetic may be performed in the region of the anus. The rectal stump is first located, freed of its local attachments and

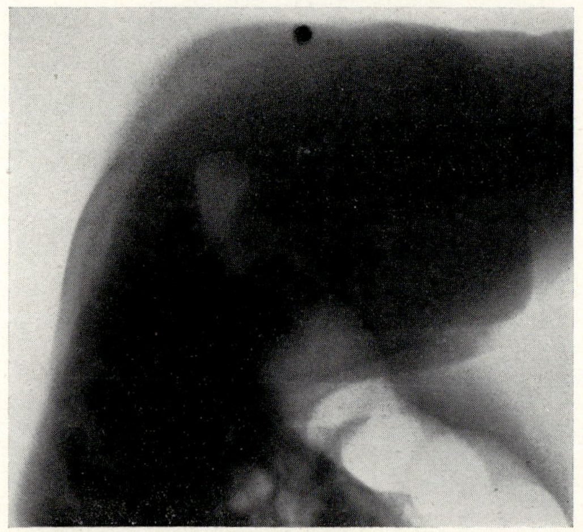

FIG. 59

Imperforate anus. An X-ray of the infant in the inverted position showing air in the rectal stump.

then brought down and sutured to the anal margin. In the event of only a thin diaphragm being present, this can quite easily be excised without the necessity of a general anaesthetic. In both instances dilatation of the anus should be performed three times each day by inserting a finger, covered by a well lubricated finger cot, into the anal canal. This dilatation should be continued for several weeks.

(2) ECTOPIC ANUS.—In this condition, not only is the anus imperforate but the rectal stump communicates with the exterior by a fistulous track, which may end either in the vagina or on the skin of the perineum just in front of the imperforate anus. Treatment is directed to dealing with the imperforate anus in the manner we have described. If faeces should subsequently be discharged through the fistulous track it will have to be excised.

FOREIGN BODIES IN THE INTESTINAL TRACT

A large number of children frequently enjoy sucking various non-digestible objects in their mouths and not uncommonly

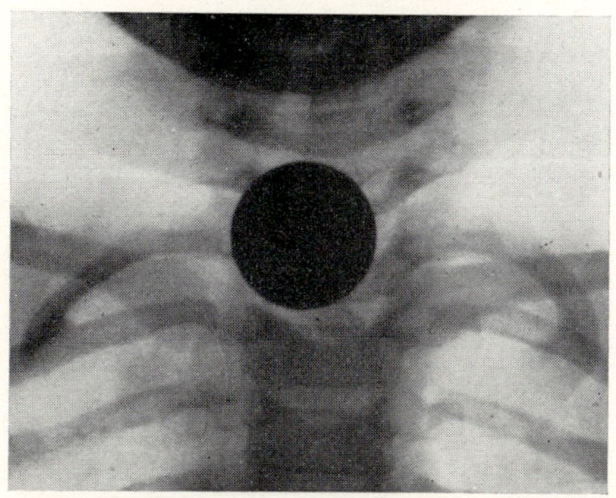

FIG. 60
A coin stuck in the upper oesophagus.

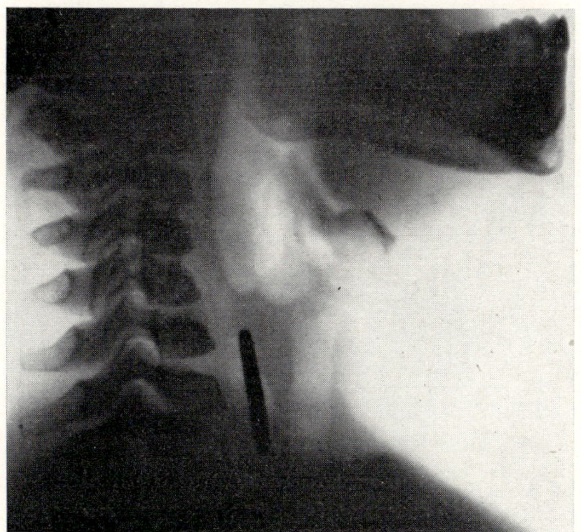

FIG. 61
A lateral view of the same case shown in Fig. 60.

such objects are swallowed. The subsequent management of such cases depends largely on the composition, shape and size of the ingested foreign body. Foreign bodies which fail to

reach the stomach but get stuck in the oesophagus should be retrieved without delay as they may cause local ulceration and even perforation of the oesophagus. Under a general anaesthetic an oesophagoscope should be passed, the foreign body visualized and then grasped with a pair of long forceps and gently manoeuvred into the oral cavity. Figs. 60 and 61 show

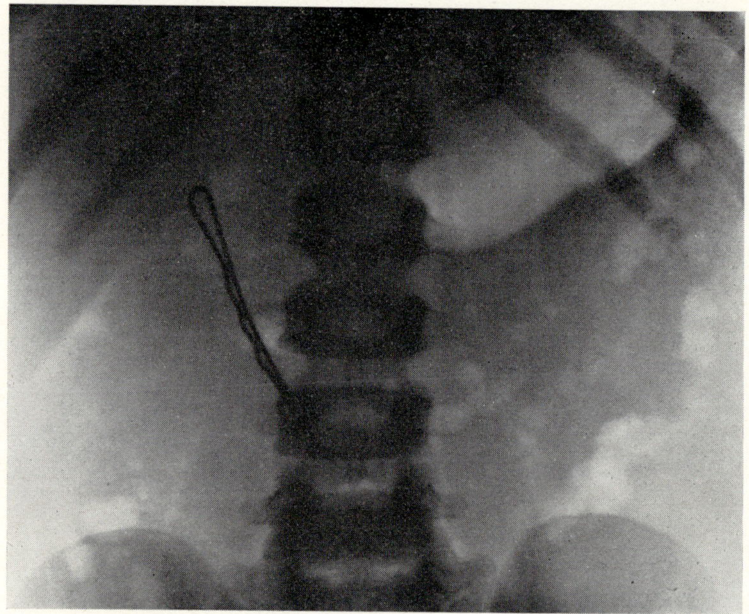

FIG. 62
A hair grip lying in the duodenum.

a coin stuck in the upper oesophagus which was easily removed through an oesophagoscope within a few hours of being swallowed.

Once a foreign body has reached the stomach it should be visualized every other day by means of an X-ray examination, and in this way its progress can be observed. All the stools should be kept for thorough examination until the foreign body has been discovered. The diet should be a normal one and the age-old recipe of cotton wool sandwiches have little or nothing to commend them. No purgatives should be given for fear of increasing the peristaltic activity of the gut and causing impaction of the foreign body and possibly perforation of the

intestinal wall.   It is quite remarkable how objects, both sharp and blunt, can pass through the intestine without causing any upset.   Figs. 62 and 63 show a hair grip in the duodenum and a drawing pin in the caecum, respectively.   Fig. 64 reveals a hair grip lying in the rectum immediately prior to its passage in the stool.

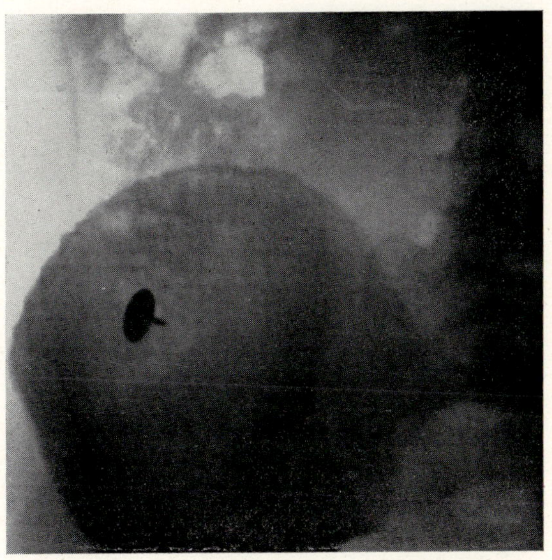

FIG. 63

A drawing pin in the caecum.   It caused no symptoms
and was passed the following day.

If the foreign body is known to be composed of lead and has not been passed within three days, it should be removed by surgical operation in order to prevent the absorption of lead into the system.

Generally speaking, the majority of foreign bodies pass through the intestinal canal without incident and up to three weeks should be allowed for them to do so.   If, however, after this period a foreign body has not been passed then surgical removal should be undertaken. The sudden onset of abdominal pain indicates that either perforation of the intestinal wall or blockage of the intestinal lumen has occurred, and in this event the abdomen should be opened forthwith in order to deal with these complications.

CONGENITAL ATRESIA OF THE BILE DUCT

This is a rare congenital condition in which there is a complete blockage or absent segment in the common bile duct. As a result the bile, instead of entering the duodenum, is dammed up in the liver thus causing an increasingly severe degree of *obstructive jaundice*.   The liver, which is usually two to three times its usual size, causes some degree of abdominal enlargement and the absence of bile in the intestines results in

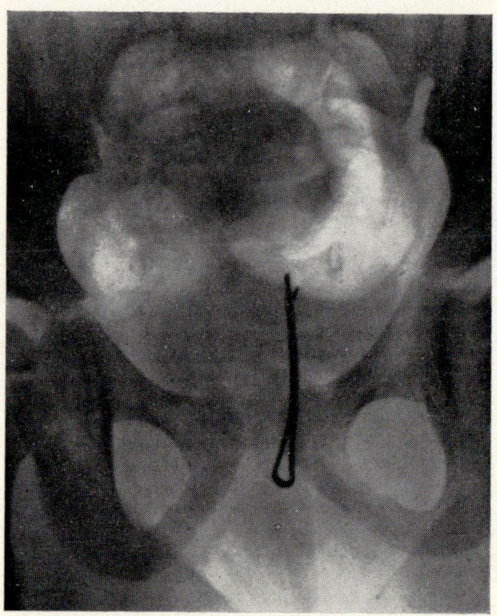

FIG. 64
A hair grip in the rectum.

the stools being white or clay coloured from birth. The jaundice in atresia of the bile duct must always be differentiated from the other causes of jaundice in the new-born child. Whereas the so-called physiological jaundice (icterus neonatorum) is seldom particularly deep and gradually disappears during the first week or so of life the jaundice in atresia of the bile duct may or may not be present at birth but thereafter becomes severe and progressive in character. The discovery of a difference in the Rhesus factor between the mother and child is sufficient to differentiate the jaundice of haemolytic disease of the new born (erythroblastosis foetalis) from that of

atresia of the bile duct. If left untreated the jaundice will continue to deepen until the child eventually dies of liver failure.   The aim of treatment is to bring the stump of the bile duct to the duodenum and then to anastomose these two structures together so that the bile may find its way into the alimentary tract.   Very occasionally the site of the atresia is too high for any operative repair to be undertaken but this state of affairs can only be discovered at operation.   Any degree of anaemia should be corrected by blood transfusion before the operation and an intramuscular injection of Vitamin K in doses of 5 milligrams should be administered in order to restore the clotting time of the blood to normal.   The operation itself is an exceptionally difficult one and is invariably associated with a high mortality but it is none the less the only procedure which can afford any hope for the survival of the child.

CHAPTER IX

THE APPENDIX

ACUTE inflammation of the appendix is one of the most common and certainly one of the most dangerous diseases of childhood that you will ever encounter. It is for this reason that we shall devote the whole of this chapter to a detailed study of acute appendicitis, together with a consideration of the other causes of abdominal pain that may be mistaken for it. Every child from time to time complains of 'tummyache' and although the cause of these transient attacks of abdominal pain is not always determined you will see in this chapter how important it is that each case *must* be regarded as a potential attack of acute appendicitis until the contrary has been proved.

Anatomy and Physiology

Before we consider the manner in which the various symptoms and signs of acute appendicitis are produced we must first revise a few facts concerning the anatomy of the appendix and peritoneum, and the physiology of abdominal pain.

The caecum and the appendix are normally situated in the *right iliac fossa* of the abdomen and the appendix is either tucked up behind the caecum (the *rectro-caecal position*), lying just beneath it, or hanging down into the pelvis (the *pelvic position*). As a result of faulty rotation of the gut, however, the caecum and the appendix may be located high up underneath the liver or out in the region of the right loin, and very rarely indeed they may be situated on the left, instead of the right side of the abdomen.

The peritoneum is a continuous membrane which lines the whole of the inside of the abdominal cavity and which also provides a covering for the intestines. Its surface is beautifully smooth and glistening and is kept lubricated by a very thin film of fluid. In the normal state all the intestines are in constant motion and it is the smooth lubricated surface of the peritoneum which allows this movement to proceed without friction. The

peritoneum is divided into that portion which provides a covering for the intestines (the *visceral peritoneum*), and that portion which lines the inside of the abdominal walls (the *parietal peritoneum*), and whereas the visceral peritoneum contains no nerve fibres which transmit the sensation of pain, the parietal peritoneum has an abundant supply of pain fibres and is acutely sensitive to both trauma and inflammation.

Abdominal pain due to distension of the gut (and thus distension of the visceral peritoneum) is characteristically *generalized* in distribution, *colicky* in nature, and is always associated with a sensation of *nausea* which may or may not cause actual vomiting. In contrast to this form of pain, inflammation of the parietal peritoneum produces an actue pain which is *localized* to the site of the infection and is *constant* in nature.

With these facts at our disposal we may now consider the course and the ultimate fate of inflammation of the appendix, together with the clinical symptoms and signs that may be produced.

Pathology

The walls of the appendix are composed almost entirely of lymphatic tissue and it is within this tissue that infection of the appendix always commences. Frequently the onset of infection is associated with obstruction of the lumen of the appendix by a hard piece of faeces (a faecolith), and even if obstruction is not present to start with, it may subsequently result due to occlusion of the lumen of the appendix by the inflammatory oedema in its walls. Once obstructed the lumen of the appendix distal to the obstruction becomes distended and thus causes a generalized, colicky form of abdominal pain, which is accompanied by a sensation of nausea. As the infection increases in extent it comes to involve the whole thickness of the appendix wall and as a result of this, inflammatory exudate appears on the visceral peritoneum covering the appendix and converts this smooth and slippery membrane into a rough and sticky surface. (As omentum and coils of intestine rub against this sticky surface they tend to adhere to it, and if the course of the infection is not particularly rapid, then the appendix may come to be completely enclosed by adhering omentum and coils of intestine.) The inflammation of the visceral peritoneum in turn inflames the parietal peritoneum

with the result that the previous generalized and colicky abdominal pain becomes overshadowed by an acute and constant pain which is localized to the abdominal wall over the right iliac fossa.

If at this point the wall of the appendix should give way (*perforation*), the subsequent events depend largely upon how well the appendix has been isolated from the rest of the abdominal cavity by the adherence of omentum and neighbouring coils of gut. Should the appendix be completely surrounded in this way then perforation will result only in local peritonitis and local abscess formation. If, on the other hand, localization is either inadequate or absent, then perforation will result in the dissemination of infection throughout the whole peritoneal cavity and the infinitely more grave condition of *general* peritonitis will supervene.

Clinical Picture

Acute appendicitis is most common after five to six years of age and rare before the age of two, but it is very much more common between the ages of two and five than is generally recognized. At the onset of the disease the child usually appears listless and irritable and loses the usual enthusiasm for meals. Shortly after this (due to distension of the appendix) intermittent generalized abdominal pain is experienced, during the course of which the child feels sick and may vomit one or more times. The temperature is raised to between 99° and 100° F., the tongue is usually furred and the breath may become increasingly foul. If at this time the child is asked to point to the site of the pain the hand is passed over the whole of the abdomen (but principally around the umbilicus) in a vague and inconclusive manner. After about twelve hours or so, the pain becomes constant in character and localized to the right iliac fossa (due to secondary involvement of the parietal peritoneum) and in addition, the abdominal wall in this area becomes tender and resistant to palpation (Fig. 65).

VARIATIONS OF THE CLINICAL PICTURE.—This ' classical ' history and appearance of acute appendicitis may be varied in a number of ways. If the appendix is situated high up underneath the liver or out in the loin, the usual localized abdominal pain may be absent or situated much higher up in the abdomen. Similarly, a retro-caecal appendix may fail to

inflame the parietal peritoneum and thus localized pain may again be absent. A pelvic appendix may cause secondary inflammation of the wall of the bladder or the rectum and in such an eventuality, abdominal pain may be largely absent, the only presenting signs being either pain on micturition (due to

THE ONSET OF ACUTE APPENDICITIS

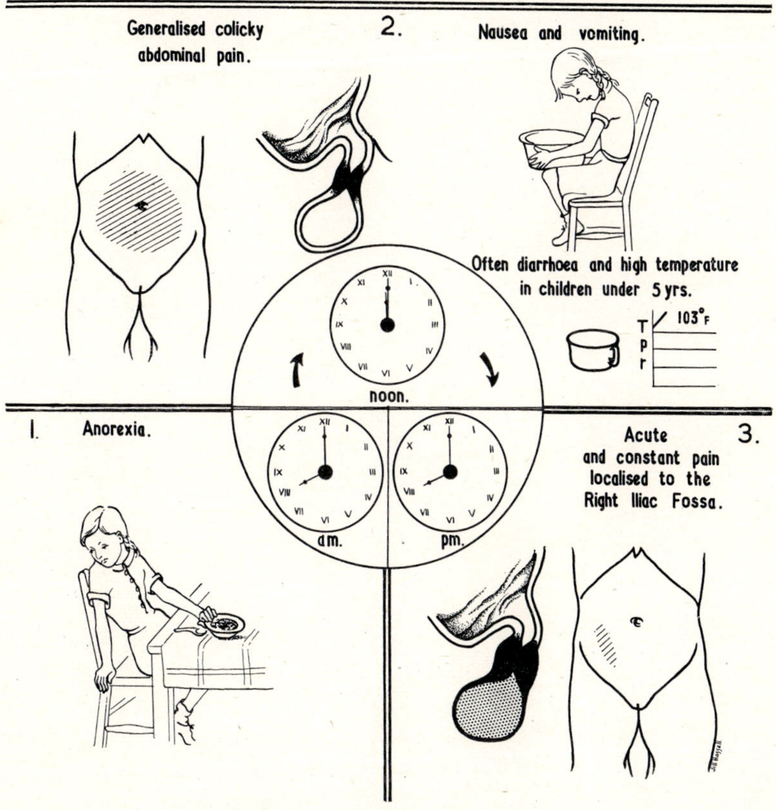

Fig 65

The onset of acute appendicitis.

secondary inflammation of the bladder) or diarrhoea (due to secondary inflammation of the rectum).

In children under five years of age the onset of acute appendicitis may be most misleading, and it is largely due to this fact that complications are much more common in this age group than in any other. In the first place, young children

with abdominal pain are not only poor witnesses but they are frequently most unco-operative whilst being examined. Rather than lie on the back and submit to examination they prefer to curl up on one side (a most difficult position in which to examine the abdomen) and if disturbed from this position they may struggle and scream until they are allowed to resume it. Secondly, the pelvis of a child under five years of age is comparatively smaller than that of the older child and thus *diarrhoea* due to secondary inflammation of the rectum may be the presenting symptom, and suggest to the examiner a diagnosis of food poisoning or enteritis rather than that of acute appendicitis. Finally, the slightest inflammatory disturbance in a young child is capable of causing a considerable elevation of the temperature, and whereas acute appendicitis in older children is seldom associated with a temperature of more than 101° F., in young children it may reach 103° to 104° F. and thus confound the diagnosis still further. These facts, which are often responsible for a delay in reaching the correct diagnosis in a young child, should impress upon the nurse the dangers that may attend abdominal pain at this age.

Treatment

The treatment of acute appendicitis is appendicectomy. Once the diagnosis has been made, no time should be lost in preparing the child for immediate operation for there is no telling in any given case whether perforation will take place in a few minutes, a few hours or a few days. Acute appendicitis must therefore be regarded as a true emergency and operation should be carried out as soon as possible. One of the most common forms of surgical approach to the appendix is through a small, oblique incision in the right iliac fossa, known as a *muscle splitting incision*. Its chief advantage lies in the fact that as the muscles are split in the direction of their fibres and not actually cut across, the strength of the abdominal wall is not imperilled as a result of the operation. Post-operatively, sips of glucose water may be taken shortly after the child recovers from the anaesthetic and a fluid diet should be commenced twelve hours after operation. If the temperature has been raised prior to operation, it may take two or three days to subside completely and providing a gradual fall in temperature is shown on the chart there is no cause for anxiety. If a muscle

splitting incision has been used in order to remove the appendix, then the child may be allowed up during bed-making on the evening of the second or third post-operative day and should become fully ambulant by the sixth day when the skin stitches are removed. In the case of a long mid-line incision, which is commonly employed in order to deal with a pelvic appendix, the child should be confined to bed until the seventh post-operative day, in order to prevent any undue tension on the wound.

THE COMPLICATIONS OF ACUTE APPENDICITIS

All the complications of acute appendicitis are characterized by the presence of pus in the peritoneal cavity, the nature and severity of each of them depending to a large extent on how successfully the appendix has been localized by the adherence to it of the omentum and loops of small intestine before perforation has occurred. As the peritoneum is an excellent absorbing surface the absorption of bacterial toxins from the pus into the general circulation always causes a state of *toxaemia*. The degree of toxaemia depends upon the amount of pus in the peritoneal cavity and will therefore be minimal in a small well localized abscess and will be maximal and indeed sometimes overwhelming if the whole of the peritoneal cavity is involved.

The complications of acute appendicitis are:

(1) Wound abscess.
(2) Appendix abscess.
(3) Pelvic abscess.
(4) Sub-phrenic abscess.
(5) General peritonitis.

(1) Wound abscess

Wound abscess is perhaps the commonest suppurative complication of appendicectomy. It results from inoculation of the sides of the incision by the infected wall of the appendix during the course of its removal. It usually reveals itself about the third or fourth post-operative day by a swinging temperature and an increase in pulse, together with a swelling beneath the abdominal incision, increasing redness of the surrounding skin and acute local tenderness. If the elevation of temperature is not severe, then hot fomentations should be applied to the

wound and the abscess allowed to burst in its own time. If, however, the constitutional symptoms and signs are more severe then the abscess should be opened by simple incision through the original wound and the pus allowed to drain to the exterior.

(2) Appendix Abscess

If the acutely inflamed appendix has been completely localized by the adherence to it of the omentum and coils of small gut, then subsequent perforation will result in an *appendix abscess*. As a rule the child has been ill for up to a week and the symptoms and signs of acute appendicitis have failed to be recognized. The temperature is elevated to 100° to 102° F. and later becomes 'swinging' in character, and the pulse is also raised. The child complains of a constant pain in the right iliac fossa where, with care and gentleness, the mass of the abscess may be felt through the abdominal wall.

An appendix abscess is treated in one of two principal ways:

(*a*) Operative.

(*b*) Non-operative.

(*a*) OPERATIVE.—If, in the opinion of the surgeon, the abscess is in danger of rupturing into the rest of the peritoneal cavity then operation should be carried out at once. Under a general anaesthetic the abdomen is carefully palpated in order to discover that part of the abscess which is closest to the anterior abdominal wall and an incision is made at this point. The abscess cavity is then opened, the pus sucked out and, if possible, the appendix is removed at the same time. Whether or not the appendix is removed a small, soft, rubber drain is left in the abscess so that the pus may drain to the exterior and allow the abscess cavity to collapse. The child is fed on a high calorie fluid diet and after forty-eight hours the drainage tube is shortened a little each day until it finally drops out altogether. Pus may continue to discharge from the wound for several days after this, but usually ceases by the end of a week, and following this the abdominal wound heals of its own accord. Once the abscess has been opened, antibiotics such as aureomycin by mouth or streptomycin and penicillin by intramuscular injection should be given, but it is unwise to administer these powerful anti-bacterial agents before operation as they are liable to cause

an apparent improvement in the condition and thus obscure the true clinical picture.

(*b*) NON-OPERATIVE.—This form of treatment is reserved for cases in which the abscess is well localized, constitutional disturbance slight and the chances of extension of the abscess seemingly remote. It is designed to allow resolution of the abscess without running the risk of disseminating the infection by surgical intervention. The intestines are put at rest by instituting *absolute starvation* by mouth and by administering the fluid requirements by the intravenous route. Streptomycin and penicillin are given by intramuscular injection and the size of the abscess is estimated each day and its limits drawn on the abdominal wall with a skin pencil. The temperature is taken every four hours and the nurse in charge should try to estimate whether there is an increase or decrease in the pain that the child is feeling. In a large majority of such cases the size of the abscess gradually diminishes, the pain decreases and the temperature falls to normal in the course of a few days. Oral feeding may be resumed on the third or fourth day, the child is allowed up one week after the abscess has become impalpable, and three months later the child should be readmitted to hospital for appendicectomy. If, however, during the course of this treatment the pain should get worse, the size of the abscess increase, or the temperature fail to decline within forty-eight hours, then it becomes obvious that the abscess is extending and in this event the non-operative form of treatment should be discontinued and operation as described above carried out forthwith.

The decision required to advise one form of treatment or the other is a difficult one, and one which requires considerable skill and experience. Although you will never have to make

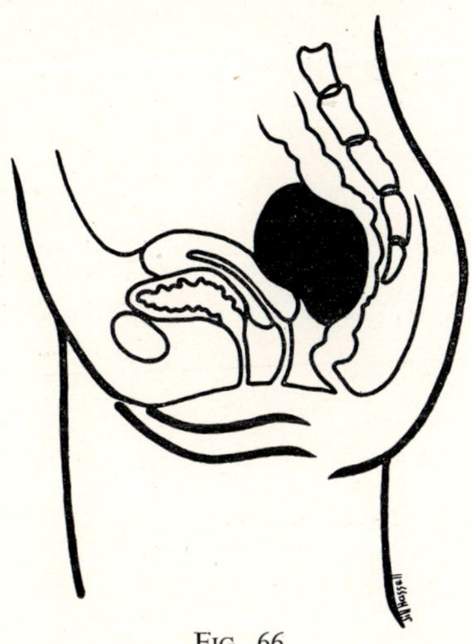

FIG. 66

A pelvic abscess. Note how it bulges into the anterior wall of the rectum.

the decision yourself it is nonetheless essential that you should understand the principles upon which both forms of treatment are based.

(3) Pelvic Abscess

This is a collection of pus in the pelvis, and usually draws attention to itself by a swinging temperature, an increase in the pulse rate, increasing girth of the abdomen, and the onset of diarrhoea which may contain both blood and mucus. If the pelvic abscess is bulging into the wall of the rectum, it may be safely opened through the rectal wall, thus allowing the drainage of pus into the rectum itself (Fig. 66).

(4) Sub-phrenic Abscess

This is a collection of pus occurring in the vicinity of the liver, usually between the dome of the liver and the diaphragm, and may follow the removal of a recently perforated appendix or be a legacy of general peritonitis. It is one of the most difficult abscesses to diagnose, and its presence is usually revealed first of all on the ward chart. The temperature, having subsided following the operation, begins, about a week later, to climb and assume a swinging character. The pulse also increases in rate and, due to the interference with the diaphragm as a result of the collection of pus beneath it, the respiratory rate may also be raised. Exploration of the sub-phrenic area with a wide-bore needle attached to a syringe is carried out under a general anaesthetic, and once pus is discovered, a drainage tube is inserted into the abscess cavity.

(5) General Peritonitis

General peritonitis is the most serious complication of acute appendicitis and is always associated with severe *toxaemia*. It results from perforation of the appendix when little or no attempt at localization of the inflamed organ has taken place prior to this event. The subsequent sequence of events may be divided into three principal phases:

(1) The child's condition immediately following perforation often appears to be improved. The pain is usually less and the child appears more comfortable than previously. The intestines, however, are still in motion and as the result of this they

11

disseminate the pus from the perforated appendix throughout the peritoneal cavity.

(2) After a few hours there is a rapid increase in both pulse and temperature and, due to the infection of the parietal peritoneum, the abdominal muscles become rigid and tender. The child lies in the cot motionless and apprehensive and often with the knees drawn up.

(3) Due to the inflammation of the visceral peritoneum the intestines become paralysed and distended (*paralytic ileus*). Effortless vomiting and absolute constipation make their appearance and the rigidity of the abdominal muscles gradually gives way to an increasing abdominal distension.

In all cases of general peritonitis, providing the child is considered strong enough to withstand operation, the abdomen should be opened and the appendix removed, for in this way only can the causative focus of the disease be eradicated. If there is much pus in the peritoneal cavity a drainage tube is left *in situ*. As paralytic ileus is invariably an accompaniment or an immediate sequel to the condition, fluids should be administered by the intravenous route, gastric suction instituted, absolute starvation by mouth observed and streptomycin and penicillin given by intramuscular injection. This regime should be maintained until there is evidence that the bowel musculature has recovered from its state of paralysis. If the degree of tox-aemia is so intense that it renders the child a grave operative risk the abdomen may be opened under a local anaesthetic and a drainage tube inserted in order to allow the pus to drain to the exterior. Recovery from general peritonitis is frequently interrupted by the incidence of residual abscesses (such as a sub-phrenic or pelvic abscess) and the child should be nursed in the Fowler position in order to encourage the pus to collect in the pelvis and thus form a pelvic, rather than any other form of abscess.

ABDOMINAL PAIN IN CHILDHOOD

Abdominal pain is perhaps the most common symptom of which children ever complain and it is most important for you to have a general knowledge of the possible causes together with the ways in which they either simulate or differ from those of acute appendicitis.

(1) Constipation

Chronic constipation is exceptionally common in childhood. The passage of a normal sized stool each day is not sufficient evidence on which to suppose that chronic constipation is not present. Even after passing a quantity of faeces each morning, a considerable quantity may remain behind in the lower colon. The constant presence of hard faeces in the lower colon causes a mild back pressure with the result that the thinner walled caecum becomes distended and pain and tenderness may be felt in the right iliac fossa. Furring of the tongue and foul breath are commonly present and the pain itself may be sufficiently severe to cause confusion with a diagnosis of acute appendicitis. If, however, in such a case an enema is administered, the lower colon will be cleared, the distended caecum will collapse and the child will be relieved of discomfort. Should the diagnosis in fact be acute appendicitis the symptoms will not be relieved but no harm will have been caused by the enema. It is important to draw a wide line of distinction in this respect between an enema and a purgative. The administration of an enema merely distends the lower colon and excites a reflex contraction of the gut. Following this the enema fluid and the constipated faeces are returned to the exterior and the gut returns to its previous peaceful existence. On the other hand, a purgative puts the whole intestinal canal into a state of turmoil and greatly increased peristaltic activity, and although this may eventually empty the lower bowel the risks of perforation of the appendix and the subsequent dissemination of pus throughout the peritoneal cavity is a far more likely result. It is for this reason that the administration of purgatives to children with abdominal pain cannot be too strongly condemned, and it is a regrettable fact that a large majority of children who succumb to general peritonitis have been given an irritant purge at the onset of the abdominal pain.

(2) Non-specific Mesenteric Adenitis

In this condition the lymph glands within the abdomen become mildly inflamed and greatly enlarged and may cause recurrent attacks of acute generalized abdominal pain associated with a mild pyrexia and sometimes with vomiting (see Chapter V). Although they may be intense in character the attacks of

pain are usually short lived. The condition frequently occurs either during or just after a mild attack of tonsillitis and it would appear that there is ' sympathetic ' enlargement of the abdominal lymph glands resulting from infection of the faucial tonsils. Removal of the tonsils reduces the severity and the frequency of the attacks in a proportion of cases but has little effect in others.

(3) Tuberculous Mesenteric Adenitis

In this condition the abdominal lymph glands are the site of tuberculous inflammation. Abdominal pain is generalized and colicky in character and comes and goes over a period of weeks or months. Straight X-ray examination of the abdomen may reveal calcification in these glands but this is seldom observed during the period in which the child is suffering abdominal pain. Calcification is usually the end result of tuberculous inflammation and may be taken in the majority of cases as an indication that active inflammation has ceased (see Chapter XIV). Treatment is directed to increasing the general resistance of the child against the infection, and a period of convalescence, preferably at the seaside, for a period of two or three months is usually sufficient to ensure the cessation of abdominal pain.

(4) Renal Tract Disease

A right hydronephrosis may cause attacks of right-sided abdominal pain, though the site of the pain is usually higher than that in acute appendicitis (see Chapter XI). Characteristically a hydronephrosis always causes one-sided pain and is never preceded by an attack of generalized abdominal pain. A urinary infection on the right side is usually associated with a much higher temperature (103° to 104° F.) than in acute appendicitis, and pus cells and albumen are always present in the urine.

(5) Meckel's Diverticulum

Inflammation of a Meckel's diverticulum may cause generalized abdominal pain of gradually increasing intensity and be associated with a mild pyrexia and attacks of vomiting (see Chapter X). As such it may be indistinguishable from acute appendicitis. If a normal appendix is removed at the subsequent operation the last few feet of small intestine should

be searched and if an inflamed Meckel's diverticulum is discovered it should be removed.

(6) Primary Peritonitis

Primary peritonitis occurs with equal frequency in both boys and girls and usually results from a septicaemic condition arising from either an otitis media or an infected umbilical stump. The onset of the condition is usually rapid and is characterized by vomiting and diarrhoea in the early stages, a high swinging temperature and increasing abdominal distension. The causative organisms are usually either the haemolytic streptococcus or the pneumococcus. A small opening should be made in the abdominal wall under a local anaesthetic in order to recover some of the pus so that the causative organism and its sensitivity may be discovered. Apart from this no further operative treatment should be undertaken except in order to drain any residual abscess that may be formed, and treatment is confined to the administration of the appropriate antibiotic. When occurring in girls this condition is sometimes thought to have ascended through the uterus and Fallopian tubes and thus gained access to the peritoneum cavity. Although an attractive theory, there is little evidence to support this contention.

(7) Pneumonia

Pneumonia associated with inflammation of the pleura over the diaphragm (diaphragmatic pleurisy) may cause reflex pain and tenderness in the region of the appendix. The chest signs of pneumonia, together with a high temperature (104° F.), dilatation of the nostrils on inspiration and a raised respiratory rate are usually sufficient to distinguish abdominal pain in pneumonia from acute appendicitis, but you must remember that pneumonia is a septicaemic condition in its early stages, and thus acute inflammation of the appendix may be present in addition to the pulmonary manifestations of the disease.

(8) Iliac Adenitis

In this condition the iliac lymph glands are secondarily inflamed due to a primary septic focus either in the lower limb or in the region of the buttocks or genitalia. If it is the right iliac glands that are affected then the child commonly complains

of pain and tenderness situated just above the right groin. With care and gentleness, however, the inflamed glands can usually be palpated thus distinguishing the condition from acute appendicitis.

From what we have said you will see that there are a wide variety of conditions which may present themselves as abdominal pain, and the close similarity in the appearance of these various diseases should impress upon you the difficulties in accurate diagnosis and should teach you to regard the symptom of abdominal pain with the high respect that it deserves.

CHAPTER X

THE ABDOMINAL WALL

ABDOMINAL INJURIES

INJURIES to the abdominal wall and the abdominal contents are uncommon in childhood and usually result from falls and road accidents. We may conveniently divide them into:

(1) Injuries of the abdominal wall.

(2) Injuries of solid organs.

(3) Injuries of hollow organs.

(1) Injuries of the Abdominal Wall

Such injuries seldom amount to more than simple bruising. With rest and the application of cold compresses to the affected area, the pain and tenderness associated with these injuries usually pass off in the course of a few days. Innocent though such injuries may appear on the surface, it is essential that close observation of the pulse rate, the child's colour and general condition should constantly be observed for there is always the possibility that associated intra-abdominal injuries may also be present but as yet unrevealed.

(2) Injuries to Solid Organs

The two solid intra-abdominal organs that are most commonly damaged by abdominal injuries are the liver and the spleen. Rupture of these organs may produce such violent intra-abdominal haemorrhage that the child dies before treatment can be instituted. Less violent haemorrhage is revealed by a slowly increasing pulse rate, increasing pallor of the skin, restlessness and even air hunger, but little or no abdominal pain. The pulse should be recorded every ten minutes by the same nurse so that any alteration in the *volume* of the pulse is more easily appreciated. Blood should be withdrawn from one of the arm veins so that the child's blood group may be determined and a supply of blood made available should transfusion

become necessary. If intra-abdominal haemorrhage is suspected the abdomen should be opened under a general anaesthetic in order to discover the site of the bleeding. If the liver is found to be ruptured the wound in its surface is brought together with catgut sutures and this is usually sufficient to arrest the bleeding. If the spleen is ruptured, then removal of the whole organ (splenectomy) rather than an attempt at its repair, is carried out. Whichever organ is damaged, blood transfusion should be commenced whenever possible before the operation, and it is essential that an amount of blood roughly equal to that which has been lost should be replaced.

Occasionally the onset of bleeding from a damaged liver or spleen may be delayed for a day or so, and during this time close observation should be maintained so that the signs of concealed haemorrhage may be discovered as soon as they occur.

(3) **Injuries of Hollow Organs**

Rupture of the intestine causes the peritoneal cavity to be flooded with intestinal contents. This produces a marked increase in the pulse rate and acute, widespread abdominal pain and tenderness, with rigidity of the abdominal muscles. Unless operation is carried out within a few hours a fulminating and frequently fatal peritonitis will ensue. Operation is performed in order to repair the rent in the intestinal wall and to remove all the intestinal contents from the peritoneal cavity. Intramuscular penicillin and streptomycin should be commenced at once, and, after the operation is over, absolute starvation by mouth together with intra-venous fluid administration should be instituted until the danger of paralytic ileus is passed.

THE UMBILICUS

The umbilicus is one of the most important, and frequently one of the most neglected structures in the baby's body. It may be the seat of several congenital abnormalities and it may also be the starting point of some of the most severe infections of infancy. The stump of the umbilical cord (which contains one umbilical vein and two umbilical arteries) usually separates from the umbilicus by the end of the first week of life and, although the lumens of the umbilical vessels usually close within the first two days of life they may occasionally remain

patent for one or two weeks. Once the umbilical cord has separated the umbilical scar should be gently cleaned with sterile saline solution and swabbed dry with sterile wool. Boracic powder should then be dusted on to the umbilicus and the area covered with a sterile dressing. This routine should be carried out after bath time each day until the umbilical scar is completely covered by normal skin.

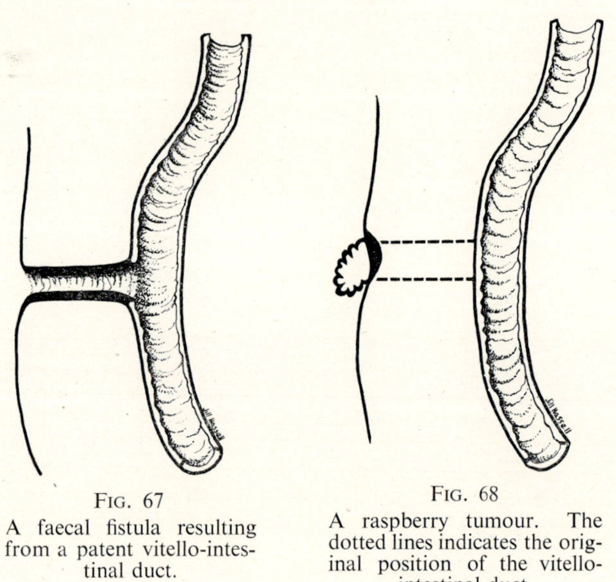

FIG. 67

A faecal fistula resulting from a patent vitello-intestinal duct.

FIG. 68

A raspberry tumour. The dotted lines indicates the original position of the vitello-intestinal duct.

CONGENITAL ABNORMALITIES

Exomphalos

In this condition the child is born with a wide deficiency of the abdominal wall where the umbilicus should normally be. The intestines, covered only by a thin layer of peritoneum, protrude through this gap, and unless treatment is carried out promptly rupture of the peritoneal covering may occur and peritonitis supervene. Treatment should therefore be carried out as soon as possible. It is seldom possible at this time to unite the muscles of the abdominal wall, but it is of the first importance that the skin should be brought together to cover the exomphalos. In this way the protruding intestines are given the added protection of a covering of skin, and the danger

of rupture of the peritoneum is avoided. Some months later, when the abdomen is capable of accommodating all the intestines, a second operation may be performed in order to restore the integrity of the muscle wall of the abdomen.

Faecal Fistula and Raspberry Tumour

At one time in the development of the foetus there is communication between the terminal portion of the ileum and the exterior through the umbilicus (the vitello-intestinal duct). Normally this communication is obliterated and disappears but if it should remain patent then intestinal contents will be discharged at the umbilicus. This is what is known as a *faecal fistula* (Fig. 67), and treatment is directed to its removal. If, however, only the umbilical end of the duct remains intact, then a small pocket of intestinal mucosa will be present at the umbilicus. This mucosa hypertrophies and produces a red lobulated lump known as a *raspberry tumour* (Fig. 68). It is treated by applying a silver nitrate stick to it twice or three times a week until it has completely disappeared.

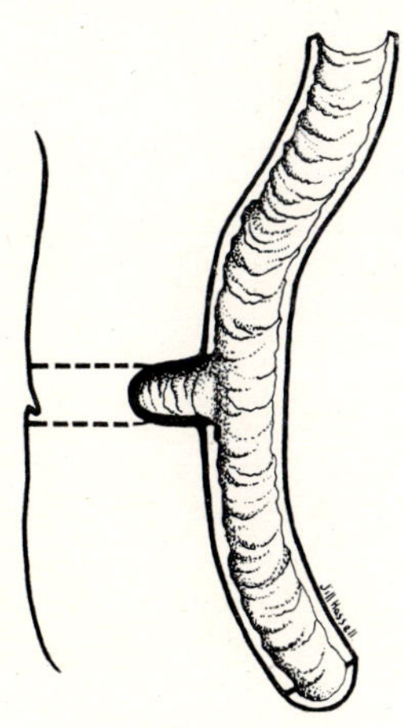

FIG. 69
A Meckel's diverticulum.

Meckel's Diverticulum

A Meckel's diverticulum is the persistence of the intestinal end of the vitello-intestinal duct and it consists of a small blind bulge about the size of a finger tip which is situated on the wall of the small intestine a foot or so above the ileo-caecal junction (Fig. 69). It is lined with intestinal mucosa and its walls have fully developed muscle coats which are capable of expelling intestinal contents should they enter the lumen. A Meckel's diverticulum may therefore exist throughout life as a local abnormality without causing any symptoms or signs whatsoever. Sometimes, however, it may contain islets of gastric mucous membrane and as these islets are capable of secreting both hydrochloric acid and gastric digestive enzymes (pepsin), local ulceration of the adjacent intestinal wall may occur.

The Complications of a Meckel's Diverticulum

INFLAMMATION.—Very occasionally a Meckel's diverticulum may become inflamed and cause attacks of acute abdominal pain and vomiting which may be indistinguishable from acute appendicitis. It is for this reason that when a normal appendix is discovered in an operation for a suspected acute appendicitis, the last few feet of the small intestine should always be searched for the presence of an inflamed Meckel's diverticulum.

ULCERATION.—Ulceration of the intestinal wall resulting from the secretion of hydrochloric acid and pepsin from islets of gastric membrane in a Meckel's diverticulum may occur at any age, but is most common at about two years of life and results in either:

(1) Intestinal haemorrhage.

(2) Perforation.

(1) INTESTINAL HAEMORRHAGE.—Of the two complications of a Meckel's diverticulum due to ulceration this is the most common, and results from erosion of a large blood-vessel in the floor of the ulcer. The subsequent haemorrhage is usually *sudden, profuse and painless* and is revealed by the passage of large quantities of either fresh or dark blood from the rectum. Constitutional signs of haemorrhage, such as pallor, listlessness and an increased pulse rate are also present and may be sufficiently severe to necessitate blood transfusion.

(2) PERFORATION.—Perforation of the intestinal wall through the base of the ulcer allows the intestinal contents to flood into the peritoneal cavity, with the production of a general peritonitis (see Chapter IX, Peritonitis).

The treatment of a Meckel's diverticulum, irrespective of the manner in which it has presented itself, is by complete removal.

Urinary Fistula

In addition to the intestinal communication with the exterior during foetal development, the bladder also has a similar connection. Very rarely indeed this communication (the *urachus*) remains patent and, if it does so, then urine is

discharged at the umbilicus. Treatment consists of ligating this patent channel just above the fundus of the bladder and just below the umbilicus, the intervening portion either being removed or left *in situ*. Rarely only the mid portion of the urachus remains patent, and this may cause a cystic swelling in the mid-line, just beneath the umbilicus; it is quite simply and easily removed.

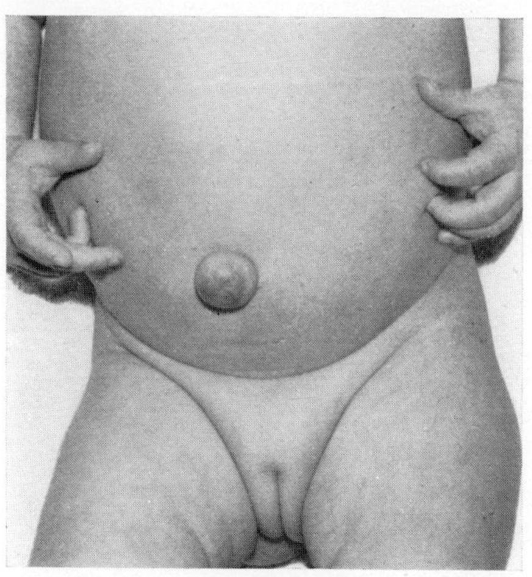

FIG. 70
An umbilical hernia.

Umbilical Hernia

At birth the central portion of the umbilicus is patent in order to allow the entry and exit of the umbilical vessels. Shortly after birth, however, this heals by scar formation which normally obliterates the hole that was there. Should this scarring be incomplete, then a small protrusion may appear at the umbilicus, and this is what is known as an umbilical hernia (Fig. 70).

A large number of these umbilical herniae are cured by non-operative measures designed to allow contraction of the umbilical scar tissue. A length of *non-extensible* adhesive strapping is stuck to the infant's lumbar region opposite the umbilicus; both ends of this strapping are then brought round to the front. Before they are overlapped, the forefinger should be placed in the umbilicus, in order to reduce the hernia, then

two folds of skin are picked up on either side of the umbilicus by the thumb and the second finger and are approximated together as soon as the forefinger is withdrawn. The two ends of strapping are then wrapped over the umbilicus with the two folds of skin still in apposition, in this way maintaining reduction of the hernia. The strapping should be renewed every three weeks, and in a large majority of cases the hernia will not recur after about three months of this treatment. Some authorities advise placing a small button over the umbilicus before applying the strapping. Although this keeps the hernia reduced it also keeps the hernial orifice open and thus prevents the contraction of the scar tissue.

Should an umbilical hernia persist in spite of the strapping treatment, it should be dealt with by surgical operation once the child has begun to walk. It is a very simple operation: a small incision is made just beneath the umbilicus, the protrusion of the peritoneum through the umbilical orifice is removed, and the orifice itself obliterated by catgut sutures. The skin stitches are removed on the sixth day, and recurrence of the hernia is infrequent.

INFECTIONS OF THE UMBILICUS

When the umbilical cord separates from the umbilicus, there may be a little moist granulation tissue left behind. This usually disappears of its own accord in the course of a few days, but it is of the highest importance that it should be kept scrupulously clean until complete healing has taken place. Should the umbilicus become infected during this period of healing, serious and widespread dissemination of the infection may occur. The two organisms most commonly responsible for such infections are the Staphylococcus aureus and the haemolytic Streptococcus.

Cellulitis

Umbilical cellulitis presents as a fiery red discoloration of the skin surrounding the umbilicus and pressure on the skin may cause a few drops of pus to be exuded at the umbilicus itself. The infant's temperature is elevated, sometimes to as much as 104° F., and vomiting and diarrhoea from the effects of the toxaemia may also be present. Treatment is of the

greatest urgency. A bacteriological swab of the pus should be sent to the laboratory for culture and also for determination of the sensitivity of the organism to antibiotics. Large doses of intramuscular penicillin are then commenced, and if there is not an obvious response to this treatment in twenty-four hours, incision into the infected area in order to provide more adequate drainage of the pus may become essential.

Epigastric Abscess

Infection travelling from the umbilicus may spread up the umbilical vein, causing an abscess just beneath the liver. In addition to a high, swinging temperature, there may also be a fullness in the epigastrium, and varying degrees of jaundice may also be present. Treatment is the same as in the case of cellulitis.

Septicaemia

This is the most dreaded complication of umbilical sepsis. The organisms causing the infection gain access to the blood-stream along the umbilical vein and are disseminated throughout the body. In addition to the effects of the septicaemia, widespread metastatic foci of infection may also occur, and each of these may necessitate separate incision and drainage.

INGUINAL HERNIA

A hernia is defined as the protrusion of a viscus, or part of a viscus, through an abnormal opening in the walls of the cavity in which it is normally contained.

ANATOMY.—Shortly before birth, the cavity of the scrotum communicates with the peritoneal cavity by a small finger-like process of peritoneum (the processus vaginalis) (Fig. 71). Normally this processus vaginalis completely disappears, except just around the testicle, where it forms a covering tunic for this organ (the tunica vaginalis) (Fig. 72). Should the processus vaginalis remain patent or persist only in its upper reaches (Figs. 71 and 73), then it will provide a passageway through which abdominal contents can pass out from the normal confines of the abdominal cavity. This passageway is referred to as the hernial sac, and its presence is the anatomical ab-

normality which is responsible for the clinical condition of inguinal hernia.

CLINICAL APPEARANCES.—An inguinal hernia may be unilateral or bilateral; it may occur at any age and though very much more common in boys it may also occur in girls. It appears as a small lump to one or other side of the upper margin of the pubic bones and is very much more in evidence when the child is straining or coughing (due to the increased intra-abdominal pressure during these exertions). If the processus vaginalis has remained patent in its whole extent,

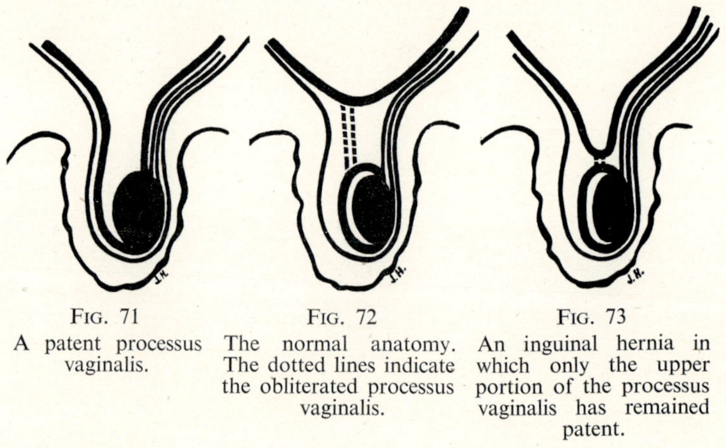

FIG. 71	FIG. 72	FIG. 73
A patent processus vaginalis.	The normal anatomy. The dotted lines indicate the obliterated processus vaginalis.	An inguinal hernia in which only the upper portion of the processus vaginalis has remained patent.

then the swelling will enter the scrotum. The hernia is usually noticed by the mother when she is washing the child, and she will frequently tell you that the lump becomes larger when the child is standing and that it usually disappears when the child lies down.

Irrespective of the age of the child, all cases of inguinal hernia should be treated by surgical removal of the hernial sac. Although not a dangerous condition in itself, the complications of inguinal hernia may be attended by serious and even fatal results, and it is for this reason that operative cure of inguinal hernia should be carried out as soon as it is convenient. A small incision is made in the skin crease over the hernia, and deepened until the spermatic cord is reached. The hernial sac lies in an intimate relationship with the spermatic cord and sometimes a prolonged and delicate dissection is necessary before these two structures can be separated. Once the hernial

sac has been isolated the neck is transfixed by a stitch and that portion of the sac distal to the stitch is excised.

Occasionally you will see inguinal hernia treated by a rubber horseshoe-shaped truss, which is designed to keep a pad on the point of exit of the hernia and so keep it permanently reduced. This adds to the difficulty in management of the child, and as the operation for removal of the hernial sac is a simple and safe procedure, even in young infants, the use of a truss does not appear to afford any advantage in the treatment of this condition.

Complications

(1) IRREDUCIBILITY.—The opening into the hernial sac from the abdominal cavity (the neck of the sac) is frequently small compared with the rest of the sac and for this reason intestines that have entered the hernial sac may be prevented from returning into the abdomen. This constitutes an *irreducible inguinal hernia*. The child, if it is old enough, invariably complains of pain over the hernia, especially on walking, and the lump itself becomes increasingly tender to the touch. This condition should first of all be treated by *taxis*. The child is put to bed and the foot of the bed raised about 6 inches from the floor. An intramuscular injection of Papaveretum should be given and the child allowed to remain perfectly quiet for three-quarters of an hour. In this way the child's abdominal muscles are relaxed and the effect of gravity on the intestines may be sufficient to withdraw the imprisoned loop out from the hernial sac. If satisfactory reduction follows this treatment, then formal operation for the removal of the sac should be carried out in the course of the next day or so. If, however, at the end of three-quarters of an hour reduction has not taken place, then immediate operation should be performed.

(2) STRANGULATION.—The word strangulation means that the gut in the neck of the sac has become so tightly constricted that the blood-supply to the imprisoned loop has been cut off and that the loop is in imminent danger of dying. Thus you will see that strangulation constitutes a grave surgical emergency. (See Chapter VIII, Intestinal Obstruction.) The strangulated hernia becomes exceedingly tender and the skin over the swelling may become red and inflamed. The usual increase in the size of the swelling when the child coughs or strains

(the cough impulse) is no longer present and operation should be carried out as soon as possible. At operation the hernial sac is opened and the tight neck of the sac is cut through. The colour of the herniated portion of the bowel is usually a deep blue due to the intense congestion, and you will see the surgeon wrap this piece of bowel in warm, moist towels in an attempt to restore the circulation. If the loop of bowel is still alive it will shortly become pink again, in which case it is returned into the abdominal cavity and the neck of the sac is closed with catgut sutures. If, however, the strangulated loop of bowel is a deep green or greeny-black, it means that the loop has become gangrenous, and in this event the dead loop must be excised and a normal piece of bowel above it and below it anastomosed together in order to restore the continuity of the intestinal canal. Following this procedure, large doses of penicillin and streptomycin should be given by intramuscular injection in order to combat any infection of the peritoneal cavity that may have occurred due to the leakage of intestinal contents through the gangrenous bowel wall. The child should be fed on fluids only for the first three days, but if there are any signs of dehydration then fluid should be administered by the intravenous route.

HYDROCELE

As we mentioned when dealing with the anatomy of inguinal hernia, the tip of the processus vaginalis remains as a small tunic or sac surrounding the testicle (the tunica vaginalis). (See Fig. 72.) Sometimes, in children of any age, this sac becomes distended with fluid, producing a pear-shaped swelling in the scrotum (Figs. 74 and 75). The cause of this accumulation of fluid is unknown, and quite frequently, after being present for a few months, it will subside completely. For this reason a hydrocele, unless it is sufficiently large to cause the child discomfort, is not operated on until it has been given an adequate chance to disappear of its own accord. The child should therefore be kept under observation for about six months and if at the end of this time the hydrocele has not disappeared, operation should be performed.

There are a variety of operations for this condition. Some surgeons prefer to remove the greater part of the tunica

12

vaginalis, whereas others are content merely to make a small hole in it, deliver the testis through the hole, and so turn the whole tunica vaginalis inside out. Whichever method is used, the results are always satisfactory and the condition does not recur.

Simple aspiration of a hydrocele should not be performed in children, for as soon as the sac has been emptied it merely fills up again.

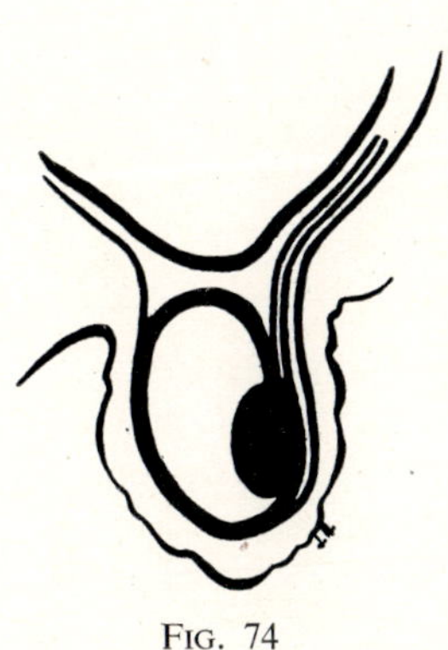

FIG. 74
The anatomy of a hydro-
cele.

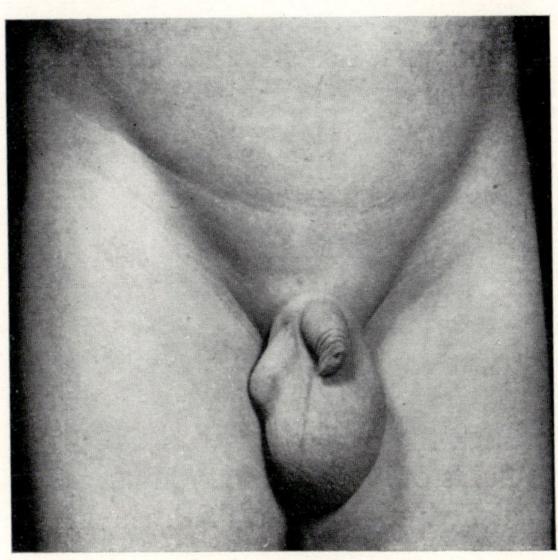

FIG. 75
A left hydrocele.

MAL-DESCENT OF THE TESTICLE

THE DESCENT OF THE TESTICLES.—Early on in foetal life the testicles are found lying high up on the posterior abdominal wall, just below the kidney. During the latter half of pregnancy they move in a downward direction and, having passed through the layers of the abdominal wall in a small canal in the inguinal region (the *inguinal canal*), come to lie beneath the skin just above the commencement of the scrotum. Finally, during the ninth month of pregnancy, the testicles descend to the bottom of the scrotum where they are normally found at birth.

Errors in descent of the testicle may be divided into two principal types:

(1) Ectopic testicle.

(2) Undescended testicle.

(1) ECTOPIC TESTICLE.—When the testicle has reached the level of the pubic bones, it may miss the opening into the scrotum altogether and either pass:

(*a*) upwards beneath the skin (an *inguinal* testicle);
(*b*) into the upper part of the thigh (a *femoral* testicle);
(*c*) into the perineum (a *perineal* testicle). (Fig. 76.)

A testicle found in any of these positions is clearly *off course* and, as such, is referred to as an *ectopic testicle*, and as it is unable to retrace its steps and enter the scrotum of its own accord, surgical operation is always indicated in this condition and should be carried out soon after the diagnosis has been made, irrespective of the age of the child.

(2) UNDESCENDED TESTICLE.—In this condition, although the testicle is still *on course*, it has failed to complete its journey. It may therefore lie anywhere along the normal route of descent.

In order of frequency, it may be:

(*a*) just above the neck of the scrotum;
(*b*) inside the inguinal canal;
(*c*) still inside the abdomen. (Fig. 76.)

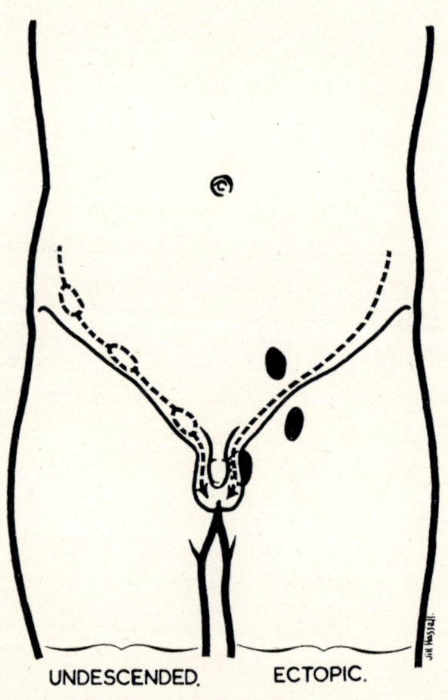

FIG. 76.

To illustrate the various positions of ectopic and undescended testicle. The dotted line on each side indicates the normal route of descent.

The treatment of this condition is governed by the fact that the production of spermatozoa (*spermatogenesis*) can only occur in the fully descended testicle. The reason for this is obscure, but it would appear that the slightly lower temperature in the scrotum is of significance in this respect. If the child should attain the age of puberty and the testicle remain undescended,

further development will not occur. As spermatogenesis normally commences at, or just before the time of puberty, it will be obvious to you that surgical correction of this condition should be performed in advance of this time. Occasionally a testicle that is undescended at birth may succeed in completing its journey during the first few years of life but if full descent has not occurred by the age of ten years, then operative correction should be performed forthwith.

The Complications of Undescended Testicle

(1) HERNIA.—About 80 per cent of undescended testicles are associated with a small hernial sac. Frequently this sac is so small the clinical evidence of a hernia does not occur. If, however, herniation does occur, then an operation to cure the hernia and bring the testicle down into the scrotum at the same time should be carried out, irrespective of the age of the child.

(2) TRAUMA.—Not infrequently boys with undescended testicles who have started to play football and similar games at school, complain of aching pains in the region of the undescended testicle due to the incessant minor trauma to which it is being subjected. Should these pains be sufficiently severe to cause the child real discomfort, then the testis should be brought down to the scrotum by surgical operation without waiting for the child to attain ten years of age.

(3) TORSION.—Occasionally the undescended testicle and the spermatic cord may become twisted. In this event the testicle becomes swollen and acutely tender. Operation designed to untwist this torsion should be performed, and at the same time the testicle should be brought down into the scrotum.

(4) MALIGNANT CHANGE.—This only very rarely occurs in childhood, but in adults it is estimated that the incidence of malignant disease of the testicle is ten times greater in the undescended testicle than it is in the descended one. For this reason, people who have reached adult life with a testicle that is still undescended are always advised to have that testicle removed.

Treatment

Although there are several types of operation designed to correct both ectopic and undescended testicles there are only two that are in common use. These are the *Keetley-Thorëk*

and the *Bevan* operation, and they differ from each other only in the method that they employ to fix the testicle in the scrotum in order to prevent it returning to its original position. In both operations an oblique incision is made through the skin, parallel to and about $\frac{1}{2}$ an inch above the inguinal ligament. The testicle is then located and any coincident hernia is dealt with in the manner we described when considering inguinal hernia. The spermatic cord is then dissected free from the adjacent tissues until the testicle can be placed in the scrotum without tension and it is when this has been achieved that the two types of operation differ in their procedure. In the Keetley-Thorëk operation a hole is made in the bottom of the scrotum, the testicle is passed through it and then buried in a small incision in the adjacent thigh. The wounds in the scrotum and thigh are then united together and the testicle is left in this situation for a period of three to six months. At the end of this time the union between the scrotum and the thigh is reopened, the testicle returned to the scrotum and the scrotal and thigh wounds are closed individually. In the Bevan operation, once the testicle has been placed in the scrotum a nylon stitch is passed through both the scrotum and the testicle and tied to a piece of strapping on the thigh. This anchoring stitch effectively prevents the testicle from returning to its original position and is maintained for a period of fourteen days. At the end of this time it is removed and the child is allowed out of bed.

Both these operations have their advantages and their disadvantages. Whereas the Keetley-Thorëk operation is a two-stage procedure requiring two separate operations, it provides the most secure form of fixation of the testicle. The Bevan operation necessitates only a single admission to hospital but employs a method of fixation that sometimes allows the testicle to retract upwards.

HORMONE THERAPY.—This form of treatment is restricted to the *undescended testicle* only. Although its use is a controversial issue you should know the principles upon which it is founded. It has been discovered that a temporary increase in the size of an undescended testicle will sometimes result in its full descent into the scrotum. This temporary increase in size can be brought about by the intramuscular injection of Pregnyl (a sex hormone recovered from the urine of pregnant

women), in doses of 300 units twice a week for six weeks.   The disadvantages of this form of treatment are twofold.   Firstly, it may fail to effect descent of the testicle, and secondly, when it is discontinued the consequent decrease in the size of the testicle may allow it to return to its original undescended position.   Although some authorities condemn this form of treatment outright on the ground that it may produce an unnecessary psychological upset in the child, other authorities employ the use of Pregnyl as a routine measure.

Retractile Testicles

Retractile testicles are not unusual, nor are they in any way abnormal.   Both in cold weather and also in the unfamiliar surroundings of a hospital consulting room, the testicles of a child with this condition may retract right up into the confines of the inguinal canal, and thus become invisible and impalpable. This condition has in the past frequently been confused with undescended testicles, and the diagnosis of undescended testicle should never be made until the child has been examined on more than one occasion by the same person, in a warm room and with a warm hand.   Retractile testicles need no treatment whatsoever, and their ' disappearing act ' ceases once puberty has been attained.

CHAPTER XI

THE GENITO-URINARY SYSTEM

THE URINARY SYSTEM

BEFORE considering the individual abnormalities and diseases that affect the urinary system we must first describe the tests that the nurse will be required to perform on the urine; and we must also consider the basis upon which the more complicated investigations are based.

THE INVESTIGATION OF THE URINARY SYSTEM

The Ward Tests

The detailed investigation of the urinary system commences first of all with the simple ward tests for abnormalities of the urine. Remember that complete reliance is placed upon you to carry out these tests accurately. Inconclusive results are just as important as obviously positive or negative ones and they must be reported as such.

The first thing to do is to look at the urine and to decide whether it is clear or cloudy and whether there is a deposit lying at the bottom of the flask. Such deposit may be made up of mucus, phosphates or urates. Phosphates only occur in alkaline urine, and once the urine is acidified they will disappear. Urates are usually of a pinky-red colour (*brickdust deposit*) and are often found in febrile conditions. After observing the urine, tests for the following abnormal constituents should then be carried out:

ALBUMEN AND PHOSPHATES.—Fill a test-tube about three-quarters full with urine and place the upper portion of the test tube over a spirit lamp until the urine begins to boil. If albumen or phosphates are present, the upper portion of the urine will become cloudy. Now add a few drops of 5 per cent acetic acid. If the cloudiness disappears it indicates that phosphates are present, but if it persists then the test is positive for albumen. Albumen may be an incidental finding in febrile

conditions but it may also be indicative of organic diseases such as nephritis, tuberculous disease, malignant growths, stones or a urinary infection. Occasionally it may be a constant constituent of the urine in rapidly growing, poorly developed children.

SUGAR.—Add 8 drops of urine to 5 cubic centimetres of Benedict's solution in a test-tube and boil the mixture for two minutes. If there is a very slight amount of sugar present (*glycosuria*) the solution will turn to a cloudy green. Higher concentrations of sugar in the urine will result in a yellow coloration, and if the sugar content amounts to as much as 1 or 2 per cent a deep orange or red precipitate is formed. When you enter the result of this test on the ward chart it is most important that you should state to what colour the reagent has changed, for this is a rough indication of the amount of sugar that is present and it also serves as a standard against which further tests may be compared.

ACETONE BODIES.—Acetone bodies appear in the urine in both diabetes mellitus and following prolonged vomiting and starvation. About an inch of ammonium sulphate crystals should be placed in a test-tube and the tube then half filled with urine. This should be thoroughly shaken and a few drops of Rothera's reagent and about 10 drops of strong ammonia should then be added. If there are acetone bodies in the urine a deep purple ring will appear on the surface of the fluid.

BLOOD.—Blood in the urine (*haematuria*) may result from a variety of conditions, such as malignant disease of the kidney, tuberculous disease and calculi in the urinary tract. There are a number of tests for blood in the urine, all of which are unreliable. If haematuria is suspected, then the urine should be sent to the laboratory where it is examined under a microscope in order to confirm the presence of red blood-cells.

BILE SALTS AND BILE PIGMENTS.—One of the commonest tests for bile *salts* is Hay's test. A pinch of powdered sulphur is sprinkled on to the surface of the urine and whereas it normally remains on the surface, if bile salts are present it will sink to the bottom of the test-tube. The presence of bile *pigments* is revealed by pouring a 10 per cent solution of tincture of iodine down the side of a test-tube containing urine. If bile is present a green layer is formed at the junction of the two fluids.

Pus.—The most reliable test for pus—a specialized laboratory test—consists of the visualization of pus cells with a microscope.

Clean and Catheter Specimens of Urine

If a urinary infection is suspected the urine should also be inoculated on to a culture medium to determine the nature of any infective organism. For this purpose sterile specimens of urine will have to be obtained from the child. In boys this specimen is usually referred to as a 'clean' specimen. The foreskin should be well retracted and the glans penis cleaned thoroughly with a 1 per cent solution of cetavlon. The child should then be encouraged to pass water and once the urethra has been flushed through by a moderate amount of urine the remainder is passed into a sterile bottle. In infants and young boys who cannot micturate to order, the end of the penis should be cleaned as before and a sterile test-tube strapped on to the organ until an adequate specimen is obtained. In girls a catheter specimen is essential. Meticulous attention to aseptic technique in these procedures is of paramount importance. Should only one organism from the skin of the patient or the nurse gain access to the specimen of urine it will render the investigation valueless and the diagnosis worthless.

Intravenous Pyelography

This investigation consists of introducing into a vein a radio opaque dye which is subsequently excreted by the kidney. During the course of its secretion, being radio opaque it will delineate the architecture of the renal tract in X-ray photographs. One of the safest and most widely used drugs for this purpose is 35 per cent diodone solution. For eight hours immediately prior to an intravenous pyelogram the child should be deprived of all fluids so that the excretion of the radio opaque dye will be as concentrated as possible in the renal tract. Rather than starve the child of fluids for this purpose during the daytime, it is much more satisfactory if the intravenous pyelogram is performed first thing in the morning so that fluids need only be restricted from the time of waking. Notorious in young children is the fact that pronounced gas and faecal shadows in the intestines may mask the revelation of the urinary tract in intravenous pyelography. For this reason a

thorough preparation of the bowel, comprising an enema each day for two days prior to X-ray examination, should be performed and a straight X-ray of the abdomen should be taken before the dye is injected in order to make sure that the preparation has been adequate. Should repeated purgation and the administration of an enema fail to clear these obstructive shadows, a useful dodge is to encourage the child to drink a bottle of

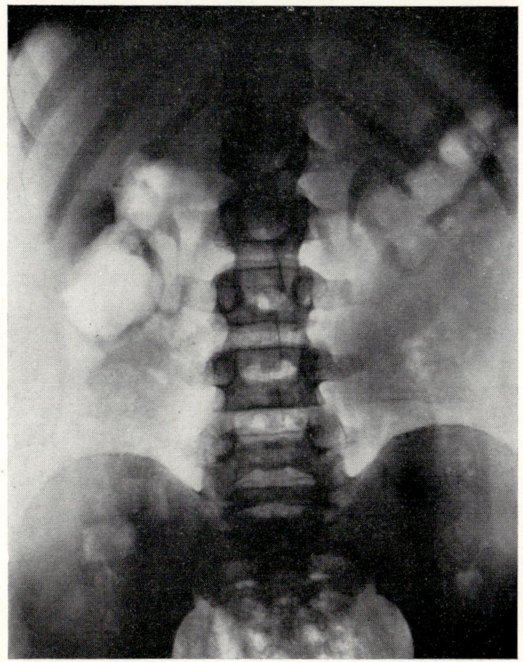

FIG. 77

Intravenous pyelogram obscured by the shadows of faeces and gas.

ginger beer through a straw; this has the effect of distending the stomach which, as it distends, displaces the large and small intestines in a downwards direction. This frequently produces an excellent picture of the renal pelvices and upper portions of the ureters, but quite naturally does not improve the pictures of the lower portion of the ureters. Fig. 77 is an X-ray picture taken during the excretion of a radio-opaque dye and you will notice that the gas and faecal shadows obscure the renal pelvices. Fig. 78 was taken one minute after the child had consumed a

bottle of fizzy ginger beer and the kidneys are clearly visualized now that the intestines have been pushed downwards by the distended stomach. Intravenous pyelography is useful, not only to outline the renal tract on both sides but it also gives a good indication of the renal function on one side as compared

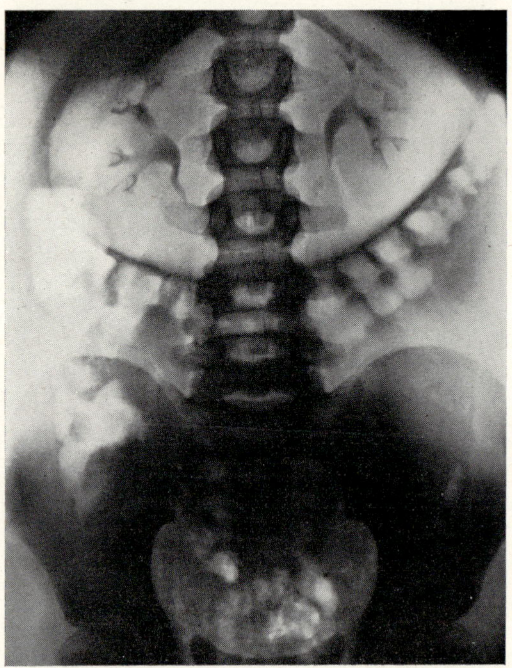

FIG. 78

The same case as in Fig. 77 after the ingestion of a
bottle of fizzy ginger beer. The dye excretion shadows
are now plainly visible.

with the other. If the shadow on one side is very much fainter or takes longer to appear than on the other, then it may be assumed that the renal function on that side is correspondingly diminished.

Cystoscopy and Retrograde Pyelography

Cystoscopy consists of passing a cystoscope through the urethra into the bladder in order to visualize its interior. Copious amounts of fluid should be given to the child, prior to the examination, so that the efflux of urine through the ureteric

orifices may be observed. If the preceding intravenous pyelogram has been inconclusive then ureteric catheters may be passed through the cystoscope and up into each ureter so that a solution of dye may be injected directly into each renal tract in order to procure a clearer definition on X-ray examination. This latter procedure is known as retrograde pyelography.

Cystography

This method of investigation is employed to reveal the size and shape of the bladder in X-ray photographs. A small rubber catheter is passed into the bladder, and a 15 per cent solution of diodone injected until the child receives the sensation of wishing to pass his water. This indicates that the bladder is now full. The catheter should be slightly withdrawn and then clipped and the necessary X-ray photographs taken at once. Once this has been done the catheter should be undone and the bladder completely emptied of the radio opaque fluid. In the rare instances where an obstruction is suspected to be present in the upper reaches of the urethra in boys, a *micturating* cystogram may be performed. The bladder is filled as before and the catheter then withdrawn. The child then passes his water into a receptacle during which time an X-ray photograph is taken. This reveals the anatomy of the urethra as outlined by the radio opaque fluid.

Tests of Urinary Function

The only one of these tests that you will be required to perform yourself is the determination of the variations in the specific gravity of the urine. With normal urinary function the specific gravity should be at least 1 : 1020 in the first specimen of the day before any fluids have been taken and this value should fall to at least 1 : 1010 following the oral administration of half a pint of fluid. Any decrease in this variation of the specific gravity is indicative of impaired renal function and further corroborative investigations should then be carried out.

The other tests of urinary function are specialized laboratory investigations and you need only know them by name. The blood urea value is a good indication of the state of the renal function and does not exceed 45 milligrams per cent in the normal. The urea clearance and the urea concentration tests

are performed to determine the ability of the kidney to deal with known amounts of urea which have been given by mouth. As we mentioned before, the speed with which dye appears in intravenous pyelography and the rapidity with which it is eliminated is also a useful indication of the function of the individual kidney.

CONGENITAL ABNORMALITIES OF THE URINARY SYSTEM

RENAL AGENESIS

Bilateral agenesis (bilateral absence) of the kidneys is of academic interest only. The infant may be still-born or may die shortly after birth, and post-mortem examination reveals no kidney substance whatsoever.

Unilateral agenesis is compatible with normal existence but should any disease subsequently affect the child's one and only kidney the outlook is correspondingly worsened.

HYDRONEPHROSIS

The term hydronephrosis literally means water (hydro) on the kidney (nephros); it describes a condition characterized by distension of the pelvis and the calyces of the kidney which is due to back-pressure resulting from complete or incomplete obstruction in the lower urinary tract. Thus, if the site of the obstruction is beyond the bladder the back-pressure that it produces will affect both kidneys, and the hydronephrosis will consequently be bilateral. If, on the other hand, the obstruction is in the ureter before it enters the bladder, then unilateral hydronephrosis will be present in the corresponding kidney.

Bilateral Hydronephrosis

Compared with unilateral hydronephrosis, the bilateral variety is a rare condition and results either from a congenital narrowing of the neck of the bladder or from the presence of a valve in the male urethra. It is more commonly encountered in infants and young children and the clinical appearances depend largely upon the degree of advancement of the obstruction. In cases of severe obstruction the infant passes only very small amounts of urine and unless the condition is recognized and

dealt with early, then death either from uraemia or from infection of the dammed-up urine may occur in the course of a few weeks or months. If, however, the child manages to survive a year or so, then dwarfism, chronic nephritis, or delayed rickets may become apparent. An intravenous pyelogram in children with this condition demonstrates gross distension of the bladder and of both ureters and kidneys. Treatment is directed to surgical relief of the obstruction.

If the obstruction is less complete then the condition may escape recognition until the child is several years of age. The clinical appearances in such an instance, and the appropriate treatment are dealt with under the subject of prostatic valves.

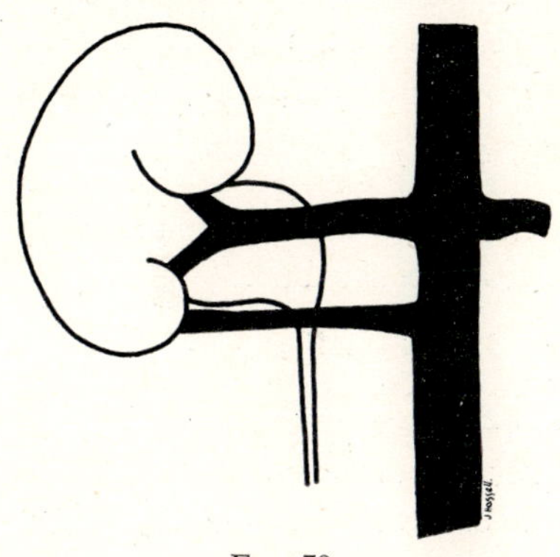

Fig. 79

Hydronephrosis due to an aberrant renal artery.

Unilateral Hydronephrosis

Unilateral hydronephrosis is more commonly found in children over five years of age and it may result from one of three primary obstructive lesions:

(1) Congenital stenosis of the ureter. In this condition there is a narrowing at the junction of the pelvis of the kidney and the ureter (the pelvi-ureteric junction) which offers a degree of obstruction to the emptying of urine from the renal pelvis.

(2) Congenital valves. These also occur at, or just below the pelvi-ureteric junction.

(3) An aberrant renal vessel. Normally arterial blood reaches the kidney through one large artery (the renal artery) which arises from the aorta. Occasionally an additional vessel (an aberrant renal vessel) may enter the *lower* part of the kidney and on its way either compress or hitch up the ureter and thus produce an incomplete obstruction of it. (Figs. 79 and 80.)

Unilateral hydronephrosis may become clinically apparent in one of two ways. Most commonly, the child suffers attacks

of pain which are sudden in onset and confined to one or other side of the abdomen. The attacks usually last from between a few hours to a day in duration, and when due to hydrone-phrosis of the right kidney may sometimes be mistaken for the onset of acute appendicitis. As a rule, the attacks are not particularly severe, but occasionally they may be suffi-ciently intense in character to cause the child to cry out and

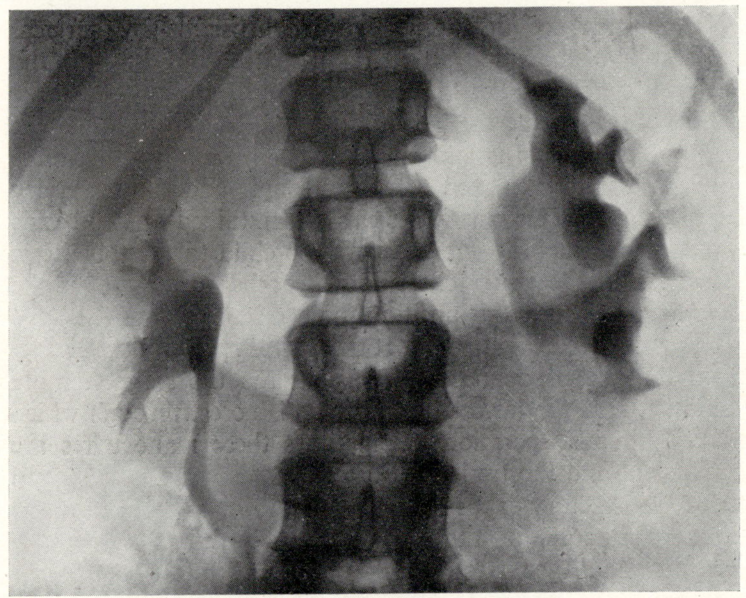

FIG. 80

Intravenous pyelogram of a left hydronephrosis due to an
aberrant renal artery.

writhe with the pain. In attacks of such severity, vomiting and profuse sweating are often present. Hydronephrosis may also be revealed by recurrent attacks of urinary infection. It is a cardinal principle in the human body that whenever a natural route of conduction is blocked, then the cavity that has been blocked off together with its contents invariably becomes infected. The renal tract is perhaps the best example of this. The stagnant urine in a hydronephrotic sac becomes infected and as it overflows into the ureter and the bladder it causes a secondary infection of these structures (a descending urinary infection). Such attacks of urinary infection, which are

revealed by a high temperature, an increased frequency of micturition, and sometimes a dull aching abdominal pain, rapidly respond to chemotherapy. Once cured of the attack the child invariably suffers further almost identical episodes and it is for this reason that all cases of urinary infection should, following recovery, be investigated by intravenous pyelography in order to exclude the presence of a hydronephrosis.

TREATMENT OF UNILATERAL HYDRONEPHROSIS.— The treatment of unilateral hydronephrosis is by surgical exploration of the kidney in order to discover and deal with the obstructing agent. The kidney is approached through the loin, and in order to give the best possible exposure in the field of operation, the child is laid on one side on the operating table with the under leg flexed to a right angle and the upper leg kept straight. This position is easily maintained by two bands of adhesive strapping which secure the child to the table, one passing over the upper chest and the other passing over the buttocks. Once in this position the head and feet of the table are then lowered slightly so that the child's spine is flexed away from the site of operation. This affords the surgeon more room between the lowest rib and the iliac crest through which to perform his operation. Sometimes these manoeuvres are insufficient and the twelfth rib itself may have to be removed before satisfactory exposure of the kidney can be obtained. In cases of stenosis of the pelvi-ureteric junction the narrow portion should be removed and the cut end of the ureter resutured into the renal pelvis. Ureteric valves are most easily dealt with by opening the renal pelvis and then passing a small gum elastic bougie down the ureter. This is usually sufficient to break down the structure of the valve, and after the bougie has been withdrawn the opening in the renal pelvis is closed with catgut sutures. Aberrant vessels are dealt with by removal between stout ligatures. The kidney does not, as a rule, suffer deprivation of its blood-supply as a result of this procedure, but occasionally the aberrant vessel is discovered to be larger than the renal artery itself. As ligature of the aberrant vessel might cut off the blood-supply to the lower portion of the kidney, removal of the kidney (nephrectomy) may be the only alternative. If it is discovered at operation that the hydro-nephrosis has advanced to such an extent that the kidney substance has been compressed into a functionless ' rind '

surrounding the hydronephrotic sac, then nephrectomy should always be performed.

If, during the course of operations on the kidney, either the pelvis of the kidney or the ureter has been opened, there is always a slight leak of urine between the cat-gut sutures that have been used to repair them. For this reason a rubber drainage tube is always stitched into the wound in order to conduct any leak of urine to the exterior. This tube should remain in place until there has been no drainage of urine from it for twenty-four to forty-eight hours, after which it should be removed.

Megalo-ureter (hydro-ureter)

This term merely means a wide ureter, and it is the usual accompaniment of obstruction at the lower end of the ureter or obstruction at or beyond the bladder neck. Treatment is directed to the removal of the obstructing lesion. Not infrequently, megalo-ureter is also produced by infections of the urinary tract, but in the absence of an obstruction the dilated ureter usually returns to its normal dimensions once the infective process has been overcome.

Pylon Duplex (Double Kidney)

Pylon duplex is an uncommon congenital anomaly which may be either unilateral or (more rarely) bilateral, and there are two principal varieties:

(1) There may be a complete reduplication of the urinary system with two separate renal pelvices and two complete ureters which open individually into the bladder. When this configuration is present the ureter from the upper renal pelvis always enters the bladder at a lower level than the one from the lower renal pelvis (Fig. 81). Providing both ureters drain satisfactorily, this state of affairs usually causes no symptoms or signs and is often only discovered on routine intravenous pyelography performed for some other condition. Urinary infections are, however, more likely to develop in a pylon duplex (even in the absence of obstruction) than in the normal. The reason for this is not known. Occasionally in the female, the lower ureteric orifice may be

13

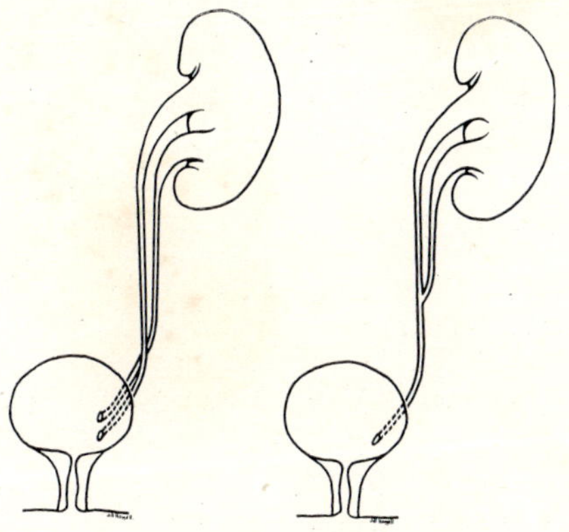

FIG. 81   FIG. 82

FIG. 81.—A complete pylon duplex.   FIG. 82.—A pylon duplex in which the two ureters have united into a single channel before entering the bladder.

situated *outside* the confines of the bladder. In this event the 'ectopic ureter', as it is called, may empty into the vault of the vagina, or even into the vulva and thus there will be no control over the efflux of urine from it. This from of abnormality is characterized by persistent dribbling of urine from the external genitalia throughout both the day and the night, and unless it is recognized for what it is, a hasty diagnosis of enuresis is liable to be made.   Once discovered the ectopic ureter should either be excised or re-implanted into the bladder.

(2) There may be two renal pelvices and two complete ureters which unite together before entering the bladder through a single ureteric orifice (Fig. 82).

In both the varieties we have described the kidney substance secreting urine into one of the renal pelvices may be of poor functional quality and therefore not provide sufficient urine to 'flush' the pelvis and the ureter properly. In such a case infection of the pelvis and ureter invariably supervenes. As recurring episodes of infection are bound to result, treatment is directed to removal of the offending components once the infection has been overcome.

URETEROCELE

A ureterocele is a prolapse of the mucous membrane lining the termination of the ureter through the ureteric orifice into the bladder. It is liable to cause an obstruction to the drainage of urine with the usual sequel of stagnation and infection of the urine above it. Thus, like all the obstructive lesions we have described, it is usually revealed by a urinary

infection.   There are two methods of attack on a ureterocele. If it is small enough, then it may be destroyed by a diathermy electrode applied to it through a cystoscope.   If it is too extensive for this procedure then the junction between the ureter and the bladder will have to be cut across and the cut end of the ureter re-implanted into the dome of the bladder.

ECTOPIA VESICAE

This is fortunately a rare congenital abnormality occurring predominantly in male infants (one in fifty thousand births) in which both the anterior wall of the bladder together with that portion of the anterior abdominal wall which usually covers it, are absent.   In severe cases the neck of the bladder is wide open, the penis is cleft and deformed (see Epispadias), and X-ray examination demonstrates wide separation of the pelvic bones.   The condition is obvious at birth and as a result of the deficiency in the lower abdomen, the buttocks, groins and thighs are constantly bathed in urine discharging from the open bladder.   Severe irritation of the skin caused by the ammonia liberated from the decomposing urine causes ammoniacal dermatitis, and ascending infection of the kidneys through the open bladder frequently occurs in spite of the most careful hygiene.   The skin around the deformity should be gently smeared with boric ointment in order to counteract the effects of the ammonia and sterile gauze pads, kept in place by a T bandage, should be applied over the deficiency in order to absorb the urine.   These pads should be changed at four-hourly intervals.   This routine should be continued until the child is about two years of age when surgical intervention may be considered.

Surgical treatment is largely dependent upon the severity of the condition.   When the deficiency is small and the bladder neck is intact, then an attempt can be made to repair the bladder in the hope of restoring normal urinary function.   More often, however, this is not possible and the only course is to transplant both ureters into the lower bowel so that the urine enters the rectum and thereafter continence is achieved by the anal sphincter.   This procedure is usually performed when the child is two years old, though some surgeons prefer to operate as soon as possible after birth.   For five days before operation the large

13*

bowel is sterilized by the oral administration of succinyl-sulphathiazole in doses of 1 gram given every six hours. As a rule, each ureter is transplanted at a separate operation with about two weeks interval in between, but in some instances the two stages may be performed together. The redundant bladder remnant is removed as soon as the child has recovered from the transplantations and the abdominal wall is repaired at the same time. Once continence has been achieved the child usually desires to void urine from the rectum about every three to four hours.

Following transplantation of the ureters there are three main post-operative complications to be considered. Firstly the kidneys may fail to continue to function (*anuria*) and as a result the child will rapidly die from uraemia ; secondly, infection may ascend to the kidneys from the colon and finally, as the rectal wall is an excellent absorbing surface, the urea in the urine may be re-absorbed into the blood-stream. To overcome these complications a tube is left in the rectum for the first post-operative week and allowed to drain into a bottle beneath the cot. In this way the urinary output is conveniently measured ; the possibility of an ascending urinary infection is reduced, and the re-absorption of urea is decreased to a minimum until the child's excretory apparatus has recovered from the alteration to its anatomy.

PROSTATIC VALVE

In this condition there exists in that portion of the urethra that passes through the prostate gland, a valve of mucous membrane so placed that, although it will allow fluid or instruments to be passed upwards in the direction of the bladder, it offers either complete or partial obstruction to urine on the way down. If the obstruction is complete, or almost complete, the infant is born with gross distension of the bladder and the ureters and the pelvices of both kidneys, and unless the obstruction is relieved in a short time the infant will die of uraemia or urinary infection or both. When the obstruction is only partial the condition may escape recognition until the child is several years of age. In this instance the act of micturition is accompanied by such grunting and straining, and the stream of urine that the child passes is thinner and less forceful

than normal. Diagnosis is made by performing a micturating cystogram which reveals distension of the urethra above the valve and a wide funnel-shaped neck to the bladder. Owing to the small size of the urethra in a young male child it is only very occasionally that the valve can be destroyed under direct vision through a special instrument introduced into the urethra (a urethroscope). The more usual method of treatment is to open the bladder through the abdominal wall (a supra-pubic cystotomy) and to introduce a metal bougie *down* the urethra in order to destroy the valve. Following this procedure, the incision into the bladder is closed but a small rubber drain is always left in the pelvic tissues just in front of the bladder in order to conduct any subsequent leakage of urine to the surface. In addition to this a urethral catheter should be left in the bladder for a few days in order to keep the bladder empty and so reduce still further the possibility of a leak.

INFECTIONS OF THE URINARY SYSTEM

As we have already mentioned, in the presence of obstruction to the drainage of urine, infection is the rule rather than the exception, so much so in fact, that a urinary infection may be the first sign that some obstructive lesion is present. Urinary infections, however, frequently arise in the absence of an obstruction and in such cases it is often difficult and sometimes impossible to determine the route by which the infective organisms have reached the urinary system. In very young infants, both male and female, a urinary infection may result from the spread by the blood-stream of a primary infection of the umbilicus. In infants between five and nine months of age, however, females are affected far more frequently than males. This is believed to be due to the comparative ease with which organisms from a soiled napkin can ascend the short female urethra and gain access to the bladder, from which they may ascend still further to the kidneys. Although without proof, this would appear to be the most satisfactory theory to account for the increased susceptibility of female children to urinary infections occurring after the first few weeks of life. Malnutrition and chronic ill-health are often associated findings.

Though the Staphylococcus albus and aureus are responsible for a few cases of urinary infection, the majority (about

13**

90 per cent) are due to the Bacillus coli and whereas the urine in staphylococcal infections is alkaline in reaction, in Bacillus coli infections the acidity of the urine is increased beyond its normal value.   In addition to the change in its reaction, the urine always contains an abundance of pus cells and the causative organisms are usually present in profusion.

PYELITIS AND PYELONEPHRITIS.—Some authorities still prefer to regard these two conditions as separate clinical entities.   Pyelitis literally means infection of the renal pelvis and pyelonephritis means infection of the kidney substance, but as it is unlikely the one can exist without the other, we will consider them merely as different aspects of one and the same condition.   In infancy the clinical diagnosis is usually obscure until such time as pus cells and organisms have been demonstrated in the urine.   Screaming attacks, toxaemic vomiting, rigors, high temperatures and even convulsions are the usual modes of onset, and symptoms directly referable to the urinary tract are *absent* in the majority of cases.   It is for this reason that the clinical investigation of an infant with the symptoms and signs that we have mentioned can never be considered complete until the urine has been examined.   In older children the diagnosis at first may be equally obscure, but an aching pain in the region of the affected kidney usually appears within the first few days of the illness.   Although the temperature may be elevated to 103°-104° F. the child's general condition seldom seems as severe as one would expect with such a fever. Frequency of micturition due to secondary irritation of the bladder is invariably present, and in Bacillus coli infections the increased acidity of the urine may cause scalding pain in the urethra during the act of micturition.   When this is severe the child, rather than suffer the pain associated with micturition, often refuses to pass water for long periods of time and when micturition finally becomes inevitable, she will pass only sufficient urine to relieve the discomfort associated with her distended bladder and thus fail to effect complete emptying of the bladder.

CYSTITIS.—Inflammation of the bladder is invariably present to a greater or lesser degree when the kidneys are the seat of an infection.   Cystitis may, however, be the predominant feature in infections ascending from the perineum.   There is usually a mild pyrexia and the principal clinical features are

an almost continual and urgent desire to pass water and a scalding pain during the act of micturition.

The Treatment of Urinary Infections

(1) Chemotherapy and Antibiotics. The sulphonamides are still the most effective therapeutic drugs in the majority of urinary infections. The more soluble the sulphonamide, the less likelihood there is of it crystallizing in the kidneys during the course of excretion. Sulphamezathine and sulphafurazole (Gantrisin), being the most soluble type of the drug, are thus the safest in use and should be given in doses of 0·5-1 gram every four or six hours depending upon the age of the child and the severity of the infection. Penicillin is reserved almost entirely for cases due to the staphylococcus which have been proven by bacteriological means to be penicillin sensitive. The use of streptomycin, though normally highly effective against the Bacillus coli, is not recommended as a routine because of the likelihood of producing resistant strains of the organism. Aureomycin and Chloramphenicol should not be used in routine cases but reserved for infections that do not respond to the use of other drugs. Irrespective of the drug used, the course of treatment should be continued for one or two weeks after which further examination of the urine should be carried out in order to prove that it is bacteriologically sterile.

(2) Fluid intake. Abundant oral fluid administration in the form of bland fluids is the rule in all cases of urinary infection. When ill, the majority of children naturally feel disinclined to drink sufficient fluid and the nurse will often find her resources of tact, perseverance and coercion severely taxed in order to persuade the child to drink the prescribed amount. In infants the task is even more difficult, and if there are any signs of dehydration that cannot be corrected by the oral administration of fluid, then intravenous N/5 saline and 4·3 per cent dextrose solution should be given until such time as the infant can maintain a normal fluid balance by oral feeding.

(3) Alteration of the reaction of the urine.   This procedure is designed, by changing an acid urine to alkaline and vice versa, to discourage the multiplication of the infecting organisms.   When the urine is strongly acid, as in Bacillus coli infections, the child should be given from 20 to 30 grains of potassium citrate every four hours until the urine becomes alkaline to litmus paper.   Once an alkaline urine has been produced in this fashion the amount of potassium citrate should be decreased until just sufficient is given to maintain the alkalinity of the urine.   To make the urine acid, as in staphylococcal infections, either 10 to 20 grains of ammonium sodium phosphate or 20 to 30 grains of ammonium chloride should be given every four hours and gradually decreased in amount until the minimum dose required to keep the urine acid to litmus is discovered.   These procedures are less easy in practice than they may sound in theory, for all the compounds we have mentioned share in common a distinctly unpleasant taste and the nurse may have to employ both camouflage and subterfuge in order to succeed with their administration.

Chronic Urinary Infections

Chronic infections of the urinary tract may be the legacy of an untreated or insufficiently treated acute infection, or they may be chronic from the start.   Symptoms referable to the urinary system are seldom in evidence and such cases are usually first brought to their doctors because of failure to gain in weight and stature, chronic ill health, poor appetite and sometimes ' enuresis '.   A full urinary investigation should be carried out in order to exclude the presence of a congenital abnormality which may be responsible for the condition.   A course of treatment along the lines we have already mentioned should be prescribed for two to three weeks but all too often a relapse occurs a short time after the treatment is concluded. Some authorities prefer to use a combination of Mandelic acid and hexamine (Mandelamine) as a urinary antiseptic, for this drug has the advantage that it may be administered for long periods up to two to three months without producing any ill effects.   Attention should also be paid to the general condition of the child and a period of convalescence in the country or at the seaside is always beneficial though not always curative.

Perinephric Abscess

This is an uncommon condition of childhood, in which there is a collection of pus in the tissues immediately surrounding the kidney. It may arise for no apparent cause or it may be secondary to some other focus of suppuration elsewhere in the body. As it is a deep-seated abscess, diagnosis is in consequence often difficult to make. The child suffers high, swinging temperatures, rigors, vomiting and frequently an aching pain in the affected loin. The urine is normal but the white blood count is raised to 20,000 to 30,000 per cubic millimetre. Treatment consists of exploring the peri-renal tissues through an incision in the loin, and passing a wide-bore rubber drainage tube down to the abscess once it has been opened.

Tuberculosis of the Urinary System (see Chapter XIV)

URINARY CALCULI

As urinary stones are most uncommon in childhood in this country and almost unheard of in infants, you do not require a detailed knowledge of their chemical composition nor of the theories advanced for their formation. There are, however, two significant facts of which you should be aware. Firstly, there is no doubt that chronic urinary infection plays an important part in the formation of urinary calculi and secondly, there is a great deal of evidence that avitaminosis, especially of vitamin A, may also be responsible. This is particularly so in India and southern China where urinary calculi are still a common childhood complaint. Stones composed of calcium phosphate and ammonium-magnesium phosphate (triple phosphate) more commonly occur in children who have of necessity had to spend long periods in the recumbent position (e.g. during the treatment of tuberculosis of the spine) and it is thought that the stagnation of the urine in the renal pelvis and possibly a co-incident mild chronic infection are probably causative factors. Calcium oxalate stones are reputed to occur more commonly in the summer months due to the high concentration of oxalate in summer foodstuffs such as rhubarb and strawberries. Stones composed almost entirely of cystine only occur in children who have inherited a rare error of metabolism in which cystine (a breakdown product of protein) is excreted

as such, instead of being broken down into urea and inorganic sulphates. Whether or not urinary calculi are visible on a straight X-ray photograph of the urinary tract is dependent upon the amount of calcium that they contain and thus, whereas calcium phosphate and calcium oxalate stones are readily visible (radio-opaque), ammonium urate and cystine stones are not.

Although they may remain symptomless for long periods of time, urinary calculi sooner or later become stuck (impacted) either in the renal pelvis or in the ureter. When this occurs, the child suffers a sudden agonizing pain which, in renal stones is situated over the affected kidney (renal colic) and which in ureteric stones is usually felt chiefly in the lower abdomen and groin and may radiate into the testicle (ureteric colic). These attacks of colic may be from a few hours up to a day in duration and may be sufficiently intense to cause the child to writhe about the bed in agony. Vomiting and sweating are also commonly present. Haematuria is a constant feature and although blood in the urine is not always visible to the naked eye, microscopic examination will always reveal the presence of red blood corpuscles. In the acute attack copious fluids should be administered by mouth and Papaveretum should be given by intramuscular injection. In addition either 6 minims of tincture of belladonna should be given by mouth or 1/100 grain of atropine by intramuscular injection, in an attempt to relieve the spasm of the renal pelvis or ureter around the stone.

Renal stones are approached through the classical kidney incision and either removed through the kidney substance (nephrolithotomy) or through the pelvis of the kidney (pyelolithotomy). In both these operations a rubber drain is left in the wound in the manner we have already described. Once in the ureter a stone stands a good chance of passing into the bladder and the child should be kept under observation and X-rayed every other day in the hope that this will occur. If, however, no progress occurs for a week or so the stone should be removed (ureterolithotomy), and as in kidney operations a drain should be left in the wound. When any of the three operations that we have mentioned are about to be performed the child should be X-rayed *on the way* to the theatre in case the stone should have moved since the previous picture was taken. Stones in the lower end of the ureter can sometimes be persuaded to enter the bladder

by manipulation with a ureteric catheter introduced through a cystoscope. Once in the bladder, stones seldom cause colic, but frequent micturition is common due to irritation of the base of the bladder by the stone. Large stones can only be removed by opening the bladder through the abdominal wall (supra-pubic cystotomy) but as very small stones may be passed through the urethra, an adequate opportunity should be allowed for them to do so.

WILM'S TUMOUR

(Embryoma. Adenomyosarcoma)

Wilm's tumour is a rare but exceedingly malignant growth of the kidney which occurs in the first two years of life, and occasionally appears in children up to five years of age. Although rare, it nonetheless accounts for half the malignant tumours of infancy and nearly a quarter of the malignant tumours of childhood. In the early stages of its growth the tumour is invariably symptomless, and pain, which is seldom severe, only occurs in about one-third of all cases. Haematuria is also uncommon and when it does occur, it does so late in the progress of the condition when the tumour has eroded and entered the renal pelvis. The predominant sign in Wilm's tumour is the presence of an abdominal swelling. This is frequently so great that it causes gross distension of the abdomen. Pallor, weakness and loss of weight are common accompanying signs and in about half the cases there is also a mild pyrexia. Intravenous pyelography usually demonstrates distortion and ' stretching ' of the calyces of the kidney.

The treatment of Wilm's tumour is still most unsatisfactory and however energetically it is applied, it is uncommon for a child to survive more than five years after the discovery of the tumour. A pre-operative course of deep X-rays is given until the tumour has decreased to such a size that it can barely be felt. Following this the tumour is approached through the abdomen, rather than through the loin, so that any extensions of the growth, either into the surrounding tissues or along the renal vein, may be more easily removed. Post-operatively a further course of X-ray irradiation is given during which time close observation of the white blood count and the haemoglobin

level must be maintained as leucopenia and severe anaemia are prone to develop.

THE GENITAL SYSTEM

THE PENIS

Epispadias

This is a congenital deformity in which the penile urethra instead of being in the normal position on the ventral surface of the penis is represented by a shallow gutter on the dorsal surface of the organ. There is also a pronounced dorsal curvature of the penis itself. Epispadias may occur as a single clinical entity or it may be present in association with ectopic bladder in which case, as continence is seldom if ever possible, the only course of treatment is transplantation of both ureters (see Ectopia Vesicae). When occurring without ectopic bladder there is no telling in a given case whether continence will develop or not and it is for this reason that treatment is delayed until such time as the child should have become continent, that is to say, until three to four years of age. If continence is finally obtained, the dorsal curvature of the penis is first corrected by a plastic procedure and at a second operation some weeks later the penis is split in two, the urethra displaced downwards to the ventral aspect of the organ and the two halves of the penis re-united. If, however, the child does not become continent, then transplantation of the ureters is the only possible course of surgical treatment.

Hypospadias

Hypospadias is a congenital deformity which may be regarded as being almost the complete opposite of epispadias. There is pronounced *ventral* curvature of the penis, and the urethra instead of reaching as far as the external urethral meatus opens somewhere along the ventral surface of the penis. The abnormal urethral opening is most commonly situated either on the glans penis just short of the normal opening (glandular hypospadias), along the underside of the shaft of the penis (penile hypospadias), less commonly at the junction of the penis and the scrotum (peno-scrotal hypospadias) or most rarely of all in the perineum (perineal hypospadias). The sphincteric mechanism at the neck of the bladder is intact and

continence always develops normally. The surgical correction
of the condition is divided into two principal stages. Firstly,
at about eighteen months of age, the penis is straightened by a
plastic operation, and secondly, at about four years of age an
operation is performed to restore the normal length of the

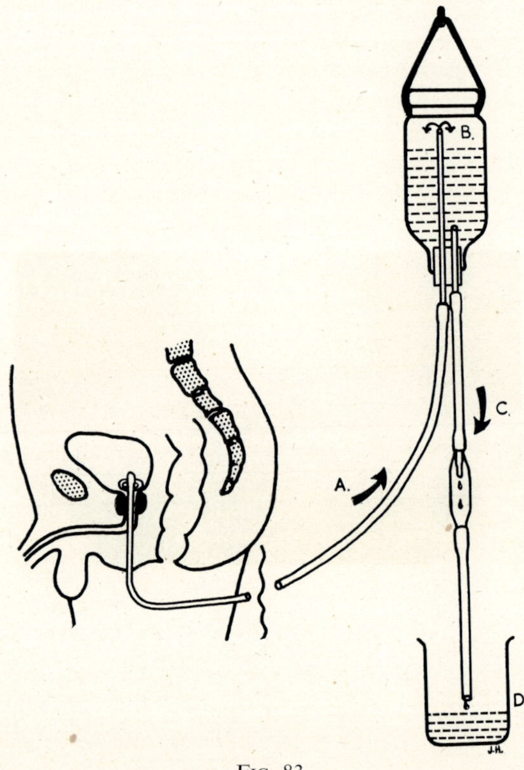

FIG. 83

To illustrate a perineal urethrostomy and a convenient
method of continuous drainage.

urethra. For this latter procedure there are a number of
operations and although the details of these need not concern
you, the success of all of them is dependent upon a temporary
alteration in the direction of the urine flow until healing of the
penile urethra has taken place. This diversion is carried out
by means of a perineal urethrostomy. A self-retaining catheter
is passed through the perineum and up the posterior urethra
into the bladder and is secured to the skin of the perineum by a
stitch. The catheter is then connected up to a continuous

drainage apparatus, one of the most simple forms of which is depicted in Fig. 83.   The fluid in the bottle drips away through the tube C, thus creating a partial vacuum at B, which in turn sucks urine up the tube A.   In this way the fluid in the bottle is slowly but continuously replaced by urine.   Once the apparatus is working the amount of fluid in the receptacle D is equal to the urinary output.   It is not necessary to place a clip anywhere along the course of tube C, providing the bottle is placed only a foot or so above the level of the bladder. After about two weeks, when the operation site has healed, the perineal stitch is removed and the catheter gently withdrawn, after which the child commences to pass urine through the

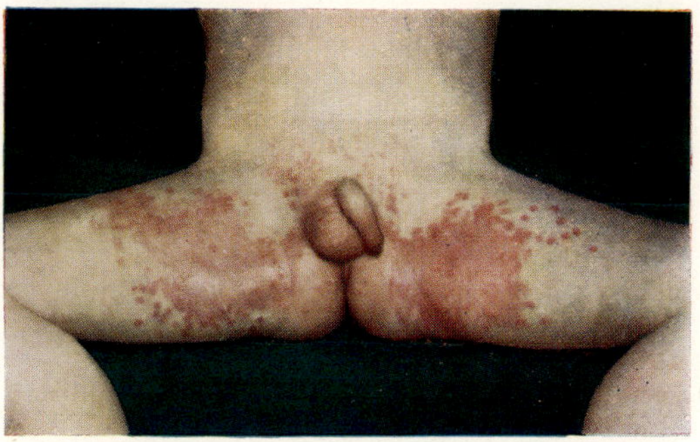

FIG. 84

A napkin rash.   Note particularly the involvement of
the foreskin (posthitis).

newly fashioned urethra.   The wound in the perineum usually leaks urine for a few days but it heals of its own accord in the course of a week without any further attention.

Ammoniacal Dermatitis (Napkin Rash)

One of the principal constituents of urine is a chemical substance known as urea.   When urine and faeces become mixed together in a soiled napkin, certain bacteria which are normal inhabitants of the lower bowel break down the urea and liberate ammonia.   If the napkins are not changed sufficiently frequently or are inadequately washed, then the accumulation of this ammonia causes an inflammation of the skin within the napkin area known as ammoniacal dermatitis (Fig. 84).   You will often hear mothers of infants suffering from this condition remarking ' his water smells so strong, nurse '.

What in fact they are referring to is not the urine, but the smell of ammonia. The foreskin becomes swollen, bright pink in colour (posthitis) and acutely sensitive, and when urine is passed through it the child cries out with a sudden excruciating pain. This is one of the commonest causes of ' night crying ' in babies and is easily and effectively cured by the following measures. Once the napkins have been thoroughly boiled, washed and wrung out they are soaked in a solution of boric acid (about two tablespoonfuls of boric acid crystals to the pint of boiling water) after which they are wrung out and dried *without* any further rinsing. When ammonia (which is a weak alkali) is liberated into a napkin treated in this fashion it is neutralized by the boric acid and ammoniacal inflammation of the skin is thus prevented. The condition always subsides in the course of a week or so, providing strict adherence to the above regime is observed and if the inflammation fails to subside, it is always due to careless observance of the rules we have laid down. Some authorities in addition to treating the napkins in this fashion advise smearing boric acid ointment over the inflamed patches of skin.

Phimosis

In the vast majority of male infants the inside of the foreskin (the prepuce) is firmly adherent to the glans penis at birth. During the first few years of life, however, this dense adherence slowly breaks down and by the time the child is between two and three years old, complete separation between the two structures has usually occurred and the foreskin in consequence becomes retractable to its full extent. Very occasionally the meatus of the foreskin is so small (pin-hole meatus) that the foreskin ' balloons out ' during the act of micturition, and in such cases circumcision is of course the only rational procedure. The term *phimosis* is without doubt the most loosely applied and inaccurate diagnosis that is made in children's surgery. The correct diagnosis of phimosis is only applicable in cases where the foreskin cannot be retracted after the age of three years. All too often, a non-retractile foreskin or one with ammoniacal dermatitis is labelled phimosis and promptly removed. The inadvisability of this peremptory attitude to a non-retractile foreskin is as short-sighted as it is unreasonable. The foreskin is primarily a structure designed to protect the sensitive glans

penis and if it is removed, then the glans penis and the external urinary meatus are liable to suffer the consequences (see below —meatal ulcer). Attempts at forcible retraction before full separation has occurred, apart from causing the child unnecessary pain, are also liable to cause splitting and subsequent scarring of the foreskin and thus render it less retractile than it would otherwise have been. Once full retraction of the foreskin has occurred and the child is old enough to understand, he should be taught to retract his own foreskin at bath times and wash behind it, in order to prevent the accumulation of irritant secretions with the same regularity and thoroughness as he is taught to wash behind his ears.

Paraphimosis

This condition results from the inability to replace the foreskin in the normal position after full retraction has been obtained, and it not infrequently follows the attempts of incorrectly instructed mothers to retract it each day. Due to the constricting effect of the rolled back foreskin, venous congestion and swelling of the glans penis occurs and the longer this condition is allowed to continue the more difficult reduction is liable to become. The first step in treatment is to push the glans penis down beneath the constricting band and at the same time to attempt to roll the retracted foreskin forwards into its normal position. No anaesthetic is necessary for this method of reduction, which usually meets with instant success. Occasionally, however, it is unsuccessful and in such cases the constricting band of foreskin must be divided with a pair of scissors before the foreskin can be returned to its normal position. Once the oedema of the foreskin has subsided formal circumcision should be carried out in order to prevent a similar recurrence.

Circumcision

The operation of circumcision is frequently performed for a variety of reasons few of which are dictated by surgical indications; the only conditions for which it is the correct treatment are ballooning of the foreskin during the act of micturition, paraphimosis and true phimosis (that is to say, failure of the foreskin to retract after three years of age). Under a general anaesthetic the foreskin is forcibly retracted

and all adhesions to the glans penis are broken down. The foreskin is then removed, the bleeding vessels are ligated and the inner lining of the foreskin is sutured to the remaining fringe of skin with cat-gut. (In infants who are only a few days old a simplified form of this operation is easily performed without an anaesthetic.) The site of operation is covered with a few turns of ribbon gauze soaked in Friars' balsam. This dressing is soaked off in the bath on the fourth post-operative day after which no further dressings are required. The cat-gut sutures do not need to be removed as they fall out of their own accord within a week to ten days. The only serious complication of circumcision is reactionary haemorrhage and a close watch must be kept on the pulse rate and the penis itself for twenty-four hours. If bleeding should occur the ribbon gauze should be reapplied and if this is not sufficient to arrest the haemorrhage a further anaesthetic must be given and a search made for the bleeding vessel, following which a ligature is applied to it. It is a most regrettable fact, that throughout the country each year a score or so of male children die as a result of reactionary haemorrhage following circumcision.

Meatal Ulcer

This condition results from ammoniacal inflammation of the external urinary meatus and never occurs in the uncircumcised infant. The lips of the meatus become reddened and ulcerated and a small scab sometimes forms over it. Each time the infant passes water it causes a scalding pain, and children of six months to a year in age frequently delay passing their water as long as possible in order to avoid the pain they have learned by experience to expect. Treatment is difficult and often prolonged, as any form of medicament applied to the meatus will be washed away the next time the child voids his urine. The napkins should be treated with boric acid in the manner we mentioned when dealing with ammoniacal dermatitis and boric acid ointment should be applied to the tip of the glans penis.

The Surgical Aspects of Enuresis

The term enuresis is unfortunately used rather loosely at times. It is best defined as an involuntary voiding of large amounts of urine, often during the period of sleep, for which

14

there is no anatomical abnormality to account for it. The surgical aspect of enuresis is confined to excluding abnormalities such as hydronephrosis, urinary calculi, chronic urinary infection, urethral valves and ectopic ureters in the manner we have already described in this chapter, and it is not until this has been done that the true diagnosis of enuresis can be entertained. For a full discussion on the subject and management of enuresis, the reader is referred to a textbook of Paediatrics.

The Vagina

ATRESIA OF THE LABIA MINORA.—This is an uncommon congenital condition in which the labia minora are fused together in the mid-line. The line of fusion is devoid of any blood-vessels and is easily divisible with a scalpel or a pair of scissors.

FOREIGN BODIES.—Foreign bodies provide the most common cause of a vaginal discharge in female children over about five years of age, and no case of vaginal discharge should be treated until the presence of a foreign body has been excluded. The easiest way of examining the interior of the vagina is by means of a laryngoscope and as the examination is liable to be both uncomfortable and disconcerting to the child, a light general anaesthetic is usually advisable. Most foreign bodies are easily removable and once this is accomplished a warm vaginal douche of a mild antiseptic solution such as 1 : 100 Dettol solution, should then be administered through a fine catheter. Following this no further treatment is necessary and the discharge ceases of its own accord.

BOTRYOIDES SARCOMA.—This is a rare but highly malignant tumour occurring in female children up to the age of about five years. It appears as a mass of pale pink cysts which protrude from the vaginal orifice. Treatment usually consists of local applications of radium within the vaginal cavity though some authorities prefer to excise the whole of the genital tract. Whichever method is employed the mortality from the disease is very high indeed and there are only a very few cases of long-term survival.

CHAPTER XII

THE BRAIN AND SPINAL CORD

CONGENITAL ABNORMALITIES

HYDROCEPHALUS

BEFORE we proceed to a consideration of this condition we must first describe the ventricular system of the brain and the circulation of the cerebro-spinal fluid. Within the substance of each cerebral hemisphere there is a space

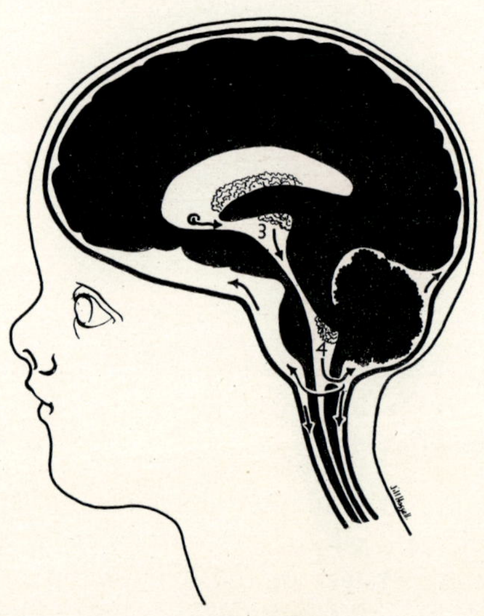

FIG. 85
The circulation of the cerebrospinal fluid.

known as the *lateral ventricle*. At their anterior ends both lateral ventricles communicate with each other and also enter into a third space (the *third ventricle*) which lies in the mid-line immediately beneath them. From the third ventricle a narrow channel passes downwards and backwards to the *fourth ventricle* which is situated just in front of the cerebellum, after which the system is continued downwards as the central canal

of the spinal cord. The cerebro-spinal fluid is produced by a number of highly vascular structures called the *choroid plexuses* which are situated in each of the ventricles we have mentioned. It escapes from the ventricular system into the sub-arachnoid space through three small holes in the fourth ventricle and thereafter it circulates over the whole surface of the brain and spinal cord where it is subsequently absorbed (Fig. 85). This process of production, circulation and absorption is a con-

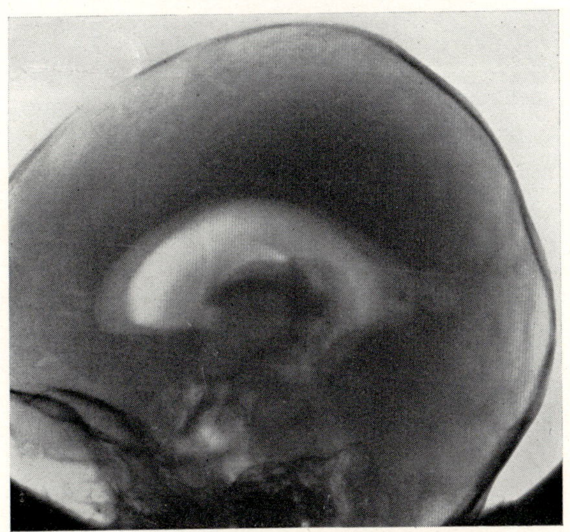

FIG. 86
A normal ventriculogram. Compare with Fig. 85.

tinuous one and several hundred cubic centimetres of cerebro-spinal fluid are produced and reabsorbed each day.

The ventricular system of the living child may be readily visualized on X-ray examination by substituting air or pure oxygen (which are relatively radio-opaque) in the place of the cerebro-spinal fluid and this may be carried out in one of two ways. In a *ventriculogram* a needle is introduced direct into the lateral ventricle, a few cubic centimetres of cerebro-spinal fluid aspirated and equal quantities of air or oxygen are then replaced. This is repeated until about 40 cubic centimetres have been exchanged. As a rule the use of oxygen is preferable to that of air in that it is less irritant to the ventricular lining. In an *encephalogram* oxygen and cerebro-spinal fluid are

exchanged through the sub-arachnoid space around the lumbar portion of the spinal cord, after which the gas ascends upwards to fill the ventricular system. X-ray examination is performed immediately following either procedure (Fig. 86), and readily demonstrates any abnormalities in the size or the shape of the ventricles.

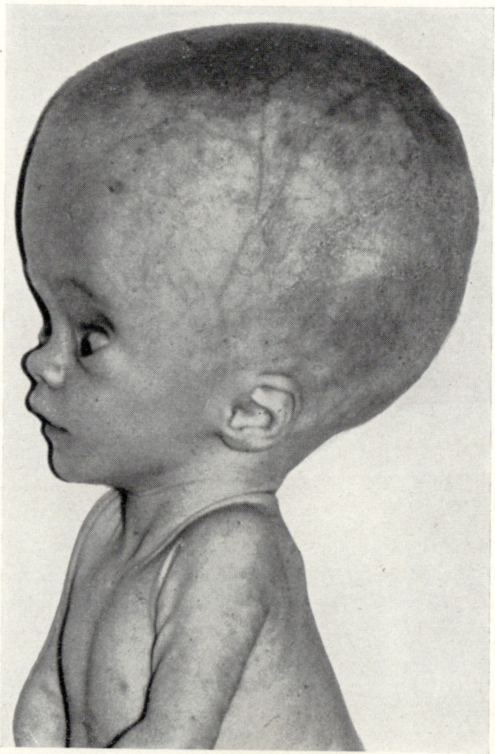

FIG. 87
Hydrocephalus.

The condition of *hydrocephalus* results from an obstruction to the normal route of escape of the cerebro-spinal fluid from the ventricular system, and as the cerebro-spinal fluid continues to be formed above the site of the obstruction, the resulting back-pressure causes gross distension of the ventricles and compression of the surrounding brain. Hydrocephalus is usually revealed during the first few months of life by a rapid increase in the size of the head, but by the time that this is

apparent, considerable distension of the ventricles and compression of the brain has already occurred. It is commonly due, either to a congenital block in the lower reaches of the ventricular system, or adhesions subsequent either to a sub-arachnoid haemorrhage at birth or to a previous attack of meningitis blocking up the 'exit' foramina in the fourth ventricle. As the ventricles continue to distend, the skull bones begin to separate from each other and the size and the tension of the anterior fontanelle is increased. Due to the rapid increase in the size of the head, the eyes are depressed downwards and forwards and the scalp veins become widely

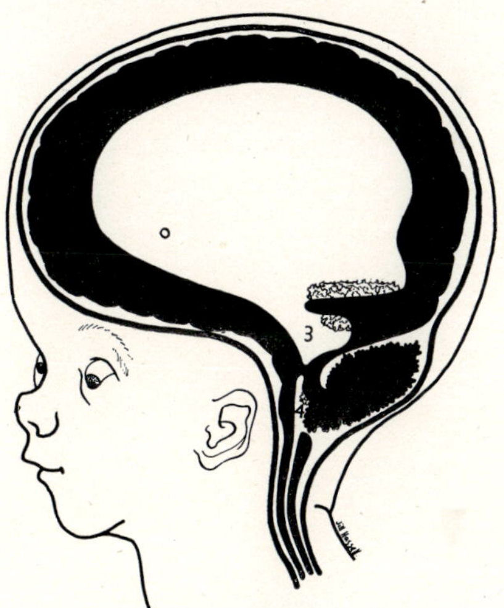

FIG. 88
A diagram to illustrate the state of affairs
shown in Fig. 87.

distended (Fig. 87). Although the brain is compressed to about a third or a quarter of its normal thickness (Fig. 88) the child's normal behaviour and progress frequently remain unaltered for some weeks or months. There comes a time, however, when the base of the brain becomes so compressed and distorted that it causes continual and uncontrollable attacks of screaming and vomiting, increasing spasticity of the limbs and back arching (opisthotonos) together with high temperatures (which are not due to infection but to distortion of the temperature regulating centre in the brain stem).

The treatment of hydrocephalus at the present time is most

unsatisfactory in that only a temporary benefit is usually conferred by surgical procedures. Since the introduction of plastic tubing a number of operations have been devised to drain the cerebro-spinal fluid away from the dilated ventricles and to conduct it to some situation where it will either be reabsorbed or be passed to the exterior. One end of a piece of polythene tubing is introduced through the substance of the cerebral hemisphere into one or other lateral ventricle and the other end is either tucked into the subarachnoid space, implanted into an adjacent vein, threaded beneath the skin and down to the peritoneal cavity, introduced into the Eustachian tube so that the cerebro-spinal fluid drains into the throat, or conducted downwards beneath the skin and implanted into the ureter so that the cerebro-spinal fluid drains into the bladder. Irrespective of the site to which the cerebro-spinal fluid is drained the immediate result of all operations is invariably beneficial in that the size of the head decreases and attacks of screaming and vomiting are alleviated. In almost all cases, however, the drainage ceases to work after a few months and the condition once again becomes progressive in character. Similar results also follow attempts to cut down the production of cerebro-spinal fluid by diathermy coagulation of the choroid plexuses in the lateral ventricles. Although a few long-term survivals have been recorded the child as a rule, despite further operative drainage procedures, dies within a year of the onset of the condition.

In older children the onset of hydrocephalus is somewhat different to that in infancy in view of the fact that the fontanelle has closed and expansion of the head cannot therefore occur. For this reason the signs of increased intracranial tension are usually the first manifestations of the condition (see below, Brain Tumours). It is very much less common than in infancy, and is due either to blockage of the foramina in the fourth ventricle by adhesions following meningitis or to occlusion of some part of the ventricular system by a tumour. Treatment is along the same lines as for hydrocephalus in infancy except in the rare instance where a causative tumour can be removed.

Hydrocephalus is, without doubt, one of the most distressing and disappointing conditions with which the nurse will ever have to deal. When feeding the child, the attacks of

screaming and vomiting will tax her patience and her ingenuity, and when interviewing the parents their questions and anxieties will equally tax her composure and her diplomacy.

SPINA BIFIDA

The term spina bifida describes a congenital malformation of a vertebra in which a part or the whole of its neural arch is missing (Fig. 89). It most commonly occurs in the lower

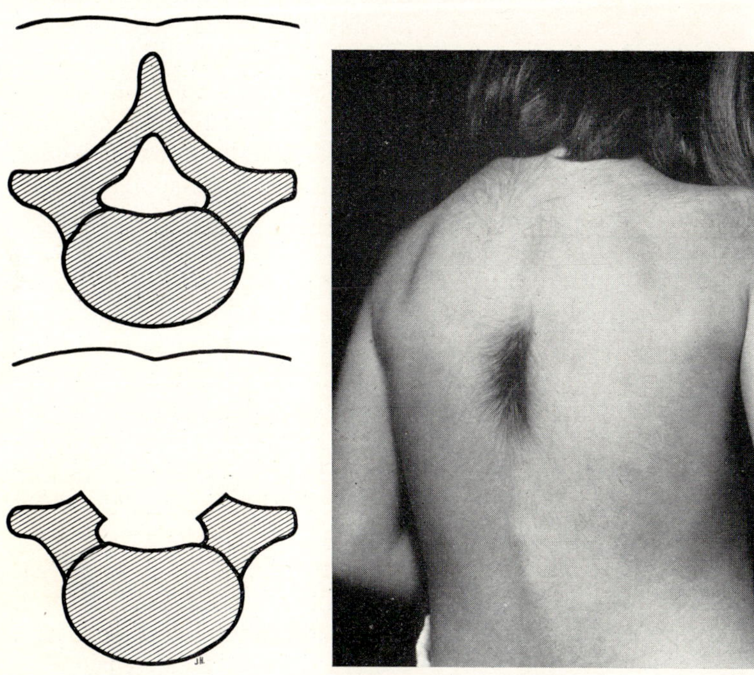

FIG. 89
To demonstrate the absent neural arch in spina bifida.

FIG. 90
A tuft of hair growing over a spina bifida.

thoracic and lumbar regions of the vertebral column and is frequently accompanied by a tuft of hair growing on the skin over the affected vertebra (Fig. 90). Spina bifida may be present in one or in several consecutive vertebrae and in this latter event one of two associated deformities of the spinal cord or the meninges may also be present.

1. MENINGOCELE.—A meningocele is a herniation of the arachnoid and the dura mater through the bony deficiency

of a spina bifida. It forms a soft cystic swelling in the midline of the back (Fig. 91) which contains cerebro-spinal fluid and which becomes increasingly tense when the child cries. A meningocele is most commonly situated in the lower lumbar or sacral regions (Fig. 92) but very occasionally it may occur in the upper thoracic or cervical region (Fig. 93). The skin overlying the swelling is usually normal in appearance but occasionally it has a mottled appearance similar to that of a meningomyelocele (see below). Treatment consists of excision of the herniated membranes but, for reasons which are not fully understood, this is sometimes followed by the onset of hydrocephalus.

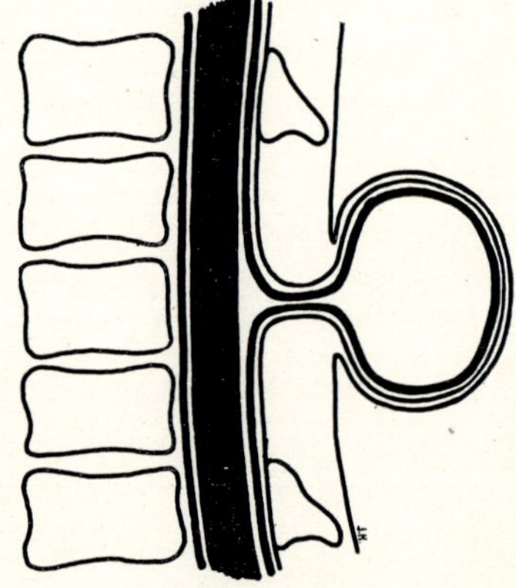

FIG. 91

A meningocele. Note the spina bifida and the herniation of the meninges.

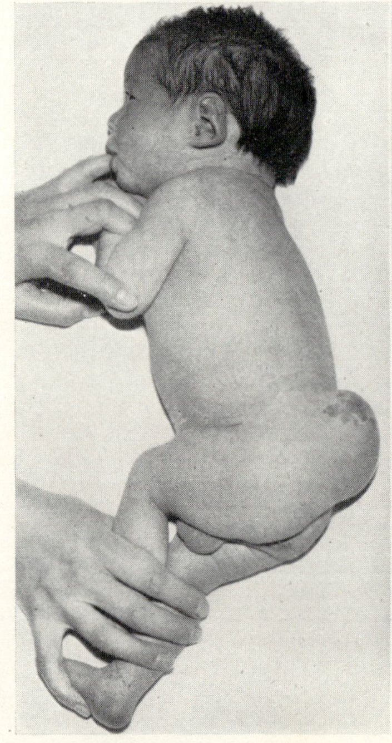

FIG. 92
A sacral meningocele.

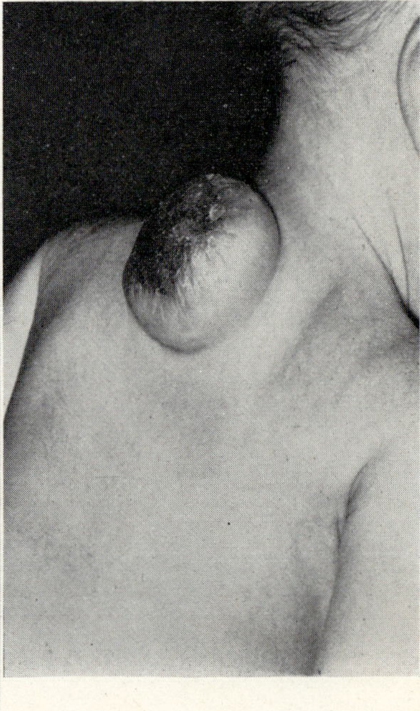

FIG. 93
An upper thoracic meningocele.

2. MENINGOMYELOCELE.—This condition is characterized by the herniation through the bony defect of the *spinal cord* as well as the meninges (Fig. 94). The spinal cord, together with the peripheral nerves that issue from it, are adherent to the inside of the swelling and the overlying skin is extremely thin and of a red and blue mottled discoloration (Fig. 95). Various degrees of paralysis and paralytic deformities of the lower limbs

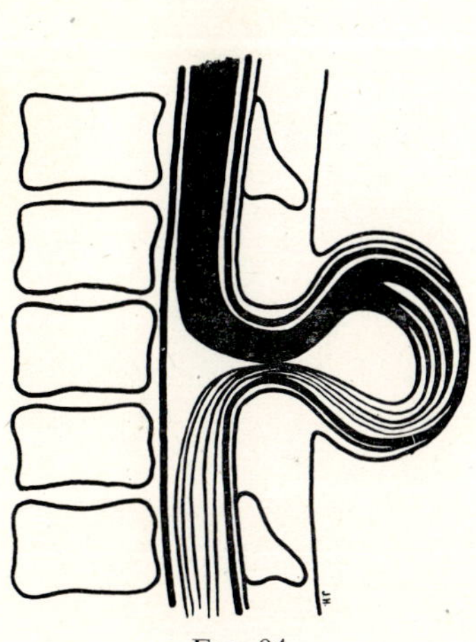

FIG. 94

A meningomyelocele. Note the adherence of the spinal cord and the peripheral nerves to the dome of the sac.

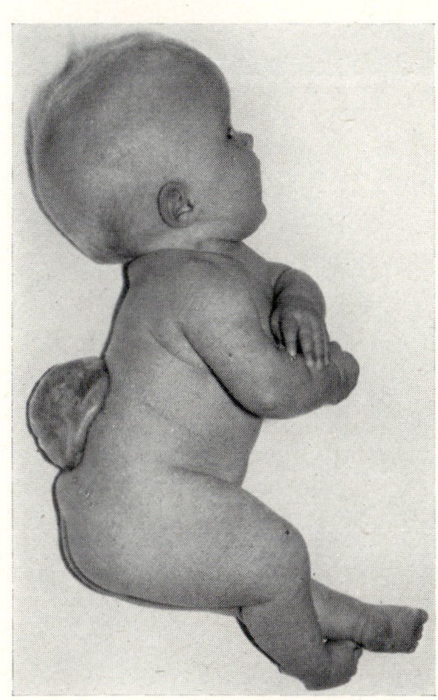

FIG. 95

A lumbar meningomyelocele.

together with paralysis of the bladder and the anal sphincters are frequently present. In order to prevent rupture of the sac and leakage of cerebro-spinal fluid to the exterior, the swelling should be covered with a rigid protector (usually made of plastic material) which is kept in place by several turns of crêpe bandaging around the infant's trunk. Although some authorities prefer to deal with this condition as soon as possible after birth, operation is usually delayed until about one year of age and then an attempt is made to remove the sac and replace the spinal cord and the nerves in the normal position.

HEAD INJURIES

Head injuries in children are most commonly sustained as the result of a fall and although such injuries may be conveniently divided into those affecting the scalp, the skull or the brain, it is most important for you to realize that in any one case all three layers may be involved to a greater or lesser degree.

INJURIES TO THE SCALP

HAEMATOMA.—A haematoma of the scalp is unlike a haematoma elsewhere in that around the soft, fluid swelling of the haematoma itself, the scalp becomes firm and slightly raised

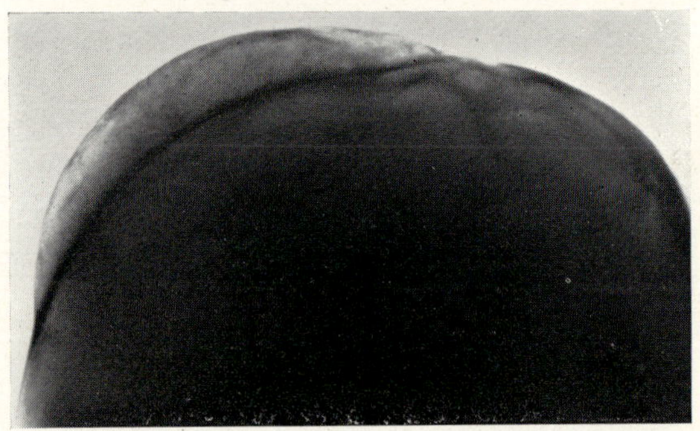

FIG. 96

A cephalhaematoma which has become ossified.

so that on palpation, one gets the impression that the soft centre of the haematoma is lying at a lower level than its circumference. It is this characteristic of a scalp haematoma that may cause confusion in differentiating it from a depressed fracture (see below).

CEPHALHAEMATOMA.—A cephalhaematoma is most commonly encountered in the newly born infant and it is believed to be due to birth trauma. It consists of a collection of blood lying beneath the pericranium (the periosteum) of one of the skull bones, and as the pericranium is securely attached to the skull suture lines the swelling of a cephalhaematoma is therefore localized in extent to the cranial bone over which it lies. As a rule most cephalhaematomas are slowly and completely absorbed, but occasionally they fail to do so and remain

stationary in size for long periods of time and may even become ossified (Fig. 96). As there is no way of telling at the outset which cephalhaematoma will absorb and which one will not, most authorities advise that the collection of blood should be expressed through a small ' stab ' incision.

LACERATIONS OF THE SCALP.—The scalp is one of the most vascular tissues in the body and for this reason no matter how ragged or extensive a laceration may be, healing is invariably prompt and complete. As lacerations of the scalp are frequently the result of falls or accidents out of doors, a sensitivity and a prophylactic dose of anti-tetanus serum should always be administered before the wound is dealt with. The hair should be gently shaved for about 1 inch on either side of the laceration and after the scalp has been carefully and thoroughly cleaned, the edges of the wound are cleanly excised. All blood clot and foreign material should be removed and the floor of the wound inspected (but not probed) for the presence of a fracture of the skull. The wound is united with non-absorbable sutures and if it is extensive, a small rubber drain should be left at one end of the wound in order to prevent the accumulation of a haematoma. The drain is removed after twenty-four hours and the stitches are taken out on the fifth post-operative day. Large wounds should be covered with a gauze and wool dressing and held in place by bandaging, but small wounds are best left without any dressing at all and merely covered with either Mastisol or Whitehead's varnish.

INJURIES TO THE SKULL

FISSURE FRACTURE.—This is by far the commonest fracture of the skull that you will come across and it consists of one or more long cracks or fissures passing across the vault of the skull (Fig. 97). As a rule there is little or no displacement of the bone on either side of the fracture, and the length of the fracture is seldom a true indication of the violence that has caused it. A temporary loss of consciousness for a few minutes following the accident is quite common but is by no means always present. Fissure fractures of the vault of the skull seldom, if ever, require surgical intervention. The child should be kept under careful observation in a quiet and darkened room (see below—Management of Head Injuries) until he or

she no longer complains of a headache. After this the child is allowed to sit up in bed and a few days later full ambulation should be attained.

DEPRESSED FRACTURE.—A depressed fracture is one in which the injury has reversed the normal convexity of the skull so that a 'saucer-shaped' depression is formed. In newly born infants such a depression is usually the result of trauma to the skull during the course of delivery and may indeed be so extensive that it merits the description of a *pond* fracture. Alarming though such a deformity may look it seldom needs surgical treatment, for in view of the fact that the anterior

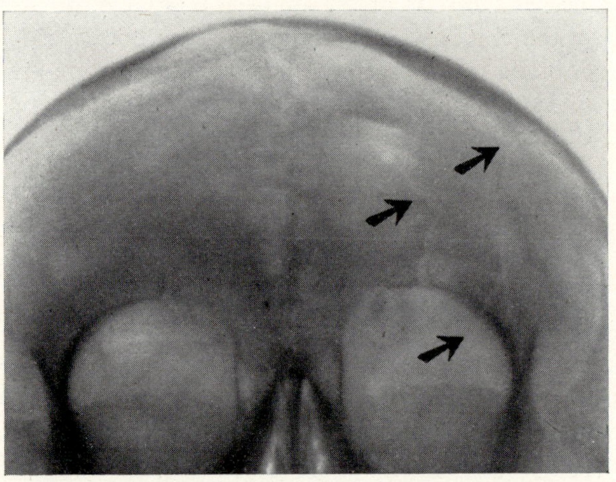

FIG. 97

Two fissure fractures of the frontal bone. Note that one of them has passed into the roof of the orbit.

fontanelle is still widely patent compression of the brain does not occur, and as the bone at this age is of about the same consistency as stiff cardboard it shortly resumes its normal contour of its own accord. Depressed fractures in older children, however, *must* be elevated by surgical operation in order to relieve pressure on the underlying brain.

COMPOUND FRACTURE.—Compound fractures of the vault of the skull are uncommon in childhood and are invariably the result of gross violence. Anti-tetanus serum should be administered and systemic penicillin should be commenced as soon as possible after the accident in order to prevent infection of the bone. When the child's general condition allows it a

careful toilette of the wound and closure of the scalp should be carried out under a general anaesthetic. A less obvious form of compound fracture of the skull occurs when a simple fissure fracture passes either across the frontal or ethmoid air sinuses or across the mastoid air cells, all three of which are in communication with the exterior through the nasopharynx (see Chapter V). The true compound nature of these fractures is only revealed on X-ray examination. Systemic penicillin should be commenced as soon as the diagnosis is revealed and continued for a week, after which, if no evidence of infection has occurred it may be discontinued. Similarly a fissure fracture passing across the base of the skull may involve the bone surrounding the middle ear and if the tympanic membrane is ruptured, blood will be seen to issue from the external auditory meatus. As in the previous instances, systemic penicillin should be commenced at once, the external auditory meatus cleared out with sterile swabs and a sterile wick of ribbon gauze wrung out in spirit placed in the meatus in order to prevent the entrance of infection.

INJURIES TO THE BRAIN

CONCUSSION.—Not infrequently the term concussion is used in rather a loose fashion and is often incorrectly applied. Concussion is a state of unconsciousness immediately consequent upon a head injury and is best regarded as a state of primary (neurogenic) shock. The level of unconsciousness may vary between a momentary loss and a prolonged state of unconsciousness for several hours associated with widely dilated pupils, shallow respirations, a faint pulse and sometimes double incontinence; but complete recovery is always the rule. In the more severe cases of concussion the child, having regained consciousness may pass through the stage of *cerebral irritation.* The child lies curled up on his side, his arm shielding his eyes from the light, and shows great resentment and frequently uncontrollable fits of rage when attempts are made to move him or talk to him. This stage seldom lasts more than a day or so and is followed by complete recovery of his faculties and demeanour. Headache is an invariable sequel to concussion but it seldom lasts for more than a few days. A good rule is to keep the child in bed for two days after the last appearance of a headache and then to allow him up and about.

CEREBRAL CONTUSION AND CEREBRAL LACERATION.
—These are usually associated with more severe injuries and the
unconscious state is deep and long-lasting. Damage to the
brain may be revealed by paralysis in the extremities, but as a
rule such cases show no signs of increased intra-cranial tension
but only a slow, and often incomplete, return to consciousness
over a period of many days.

EXTRA-DURAL HAEMATOMA.—This is a rare complica-
tion of head injuries in childhood and is usually associated with
a fissure fracture of the parietal bone which has ruptured the
middle meningeal artery (which lies between the inside of the
cranium and the dura mater). After a brief loss of consciousness the child may appear to recover completely but, after a few
hours, due to reactionary haemorrhage from the ruptured
vessel and consequent pressure on the brain, there is a steadily
progressive drowsiness which shortly passes into complete loss
of consciousness, deepens into coma and finally ends in death.
Treatment consists of making small trephine holes through the
skull over the middle meningeal vessel, evacuating the blood
and sealing the ruptured artery.

SUB-DURAL HAEMATOMA.—This is also an uncommon
complication of head injuries and whereas extra-dural haematoma occurs in older children, sub-dural haematoma is commonest in the first six months of life and is most frequently due
to birth trauma. There is an effusion of blood into the space
between the dura mater and the arachnoid (the sub-dural space)
and the gradually increasing pressure that it exerts on the brain
is responsible for the early signs of lethargy, irritability,
vomiting and a failure to gain in weight. As the condition
progresses the temperature becomes slightly elevated, the
reflexes are increased, the fontanelle begins to bulge and
generalized convulsions may follow. Treatment consists of
passing a needle into the haematoma through the anterior
fontanelle and aspiration of its contents. Very occasionally
it may be necessary to turn down a flap of bone in order to
evacuate the haematoma completely.

THE MANAGEMENT OF HEAD INJURIES

From what we have already said regarding the complications
of head injuries, it will be obvious that a correct diagnosis

may not be made for some time after the child has been admitted to hospital. Thus, the management of such cases consists for the most part of careful and continuous observation of the child so that the first sign of any of the complications we have mentioned may be recognized at the earliest moment. In other words, it is upon the changes that have occurred that decisions are made, and if these changes have not been observed mistakes in diagnosis are liable to be made. The child should be received into a quiet and darkened room and a full clinical examination carried out at once in order to establish a ' base-line ' with which to compare future examinations. Thereafter a half-hourly or hourly pulse chart should be instituted according to the severity of the case, the temperature and blood-pressure should be taken at four-hourly intervals and a careful watch kept on the size and the shape of the pupils, together with their reaction to light. The nurse must also endeavour to estimate the level of the child's consciousness—whether it is lighter or deeper than on admission—and the degree of restlessness and the quality and rate of the respirations should also be recorded. The level of consciousness is best assessed according to the following terms and criteria:

> Conscious—The child is alert and orientated in time and place.
> Confusion—The child is alert but disorientated and either restless or excited.
> Semi-coma—The child exhibits no spontaneous movements but responds to painful stimuli.
> Coma—There is no response to any form of stimulus.

All these observations are of the utmost importance to the surgeon in trying to arrive at a comprehensive diagnosis. A fall in the respiration and pulse rates, together with a rise in the blood-pressure is an indication of a progressive increase in intra-cranial tension, and a failure of one or other pupil to react to light and its subsequent dilatation are signs of urgent and cardinal importance. Except on the express orders of the surgeon in charge no sedation should be given to the child, for sedative drugs tend to decrease the degree of restlessness and the level of consciousness, both of which are important signs of great prognostic significance. After twenty-four hours (if it has not been done on admission) the skull should be X-rayed,

and some surgeons advocate performing a lumbar puncture about this time in order to discover whether or not the cerebro-spinal fluid is blood-stained. In cases where a return to consciousness has been delayed for a day or so, some authorities endeavour to reduce the size of the brain by decreasing its fluid content, thus lessening the degree of intra-cranial tension. This may be performed either by reducing the fluid intake to about 30 ounces a day, by the instillation of 2 ounces of 50 per cent magnesium sulphate solution into the rectum, or by the intravenous injection of 20 to 40 cubic centimetres of 5 per cent sucrose solution. If the child remains unconscious for twenty-four hours then the fluid requirements should be given by the rectal route. If unconsciousness persists after this, intravenous fluid administration should be commenced and, if in the rare instance where the child remains unconscious for more than two days, a fluid diet containing the full calorific requirements of the child should be administered into the stomach through a Ryle's tube; and if the child is not incontinent then catheterization will have to be employed in order to prevent distension of the bladder. The patient should be nursed on his side and turned at four-hourly intervals in order to permit attention to pressure areas and ensure equal ventilation of both lungs. A clear airway must be maintained at all times and frequent swabbing out of the mouth and aspiration of the pharynx may be necessary in order to remove excessive secretions. If vomiting is present then the foot of the bed should be raised and the child nursed in the semi-prone position with the head turned to one side.

BRAIN ABSCESS

An abscess within the substance of the brain is an uncommon condition in childhood and is most frequently due to the extension of an acute mastoiditis into the adjacent cerebral tissue. Less commonly it may result from metastatic spread of infection from the lungs in bronchiectasis and lung abscess and, very occasionally, multiple brain abscesses may be formed in a septicaemic or pyaemic condition. Now the nerve cells within the brain are surrounded by a supportive framework of cells called the neuroglia and these cells react to the presence of infection by forming a thick protective wall around it, much

15

in the same way as fibrous tissue is laid down around a focus of infection elsewhere in the body. This method of defence against infection is called *encapsulation* and it is upon the ability of the neuroglia to discharge this function that the treatment of brain abscess so largely depends. In the early stages of the condition general malaise, anorexia, and irregular fever, a rapid pulse, attacks of vomiting and profuse sweating are in evidence and intensive antibiotic therapy should be instituted in an endeavour to prevent the extension of the infection and to assist the process of encapsulation. Once encapsulation is complete, as evidenced by an improvement in the child's general condition, a small trephine hole is made through the skull over the abscess and a needle is introduced into it. Pus is then aspirated in order to decompress the abscess and before the needle is withdrawn 1 cubic centimetre of a radio-opaque dye is injected into the cavity so that subsequent X-ray examinations will reveal its size and its shape. Aspiration should be repeated when necessary and if the infecting organism is shown to be penicillin sensitive the aspirate may be replaced by a small volume of penicillin solution. This treatment should be continued for a week or so in order to allow the encapsulating layer to thicken and then, depending on its situation, the abscess is either removed intact or a portion of its wall is excised so that the pus may drain to the exterior and allow the abscess cavity to collapse completely.

BRAIN TUMOURS

Brain tumours are most uncommon in childhood and occur with equal frequency in boys and girls. They may be either benign or malignant, and the majority of them occur in the vicinity of the cerebellum and the lower regions of the brain. The diagnosis and accurate localization of a brain tumour depends upon intricate and highly specialized forms of investigation. *All* brain tumours first call attention to themselves by headache, attacks of vomiting, increasing lassitude and sometimes fits due to the increased intra-cranial tension that they produce. Providing a tumour is benign and close to the surface of the brain, a flap of bone may be removed from the vault of the skull and an attempt made to remove the tumour. Malignant brain tumours are impossible to remove and

although they may temporarily be shrunk by the effects of X-irradiation they invariably recur and terminate fatally.

SPASTIC AND FLACCID PARALYSIS

In order to understand the difference between spastic and flaccid forms of paralysis (a matter which the student nurse often finds difficult and perplexing) we must first consider the two fundamental components of the motor nervous pathway.

The basic unit of nervous conduction within the central nervous system is called the *neurone* and it consists of a single nerve cell and a long conducting filament, known as its axon. All the multitude of motor nerve pathways that connect the brain to the muscles are made up of *two* such neurones which are called the *upper motor neurone* and the *lower motor neurone*.

THE UPPER MOTOR NEURONE.—The nerve cell of the upper motor neurone is situated in that part of the brain where all the motor impulses concerned with voluntary movement originate (the motor cortex). Its axon passes downwards through the substance of the brain and enters the spinal cord where, at the appropriate level, it forms a synaptic junction with the nerve cell of the lower motor neurone.

THE LOWER MOTOR NEURONE.—The nerve cell of the lower motor neurone is situated in the anterior half of the grey matter of the spinal cord and its axon passes outwards within the substance of a peripheral nerve in order to reach the particular muscle that it is destined to supply.

All normal voluntary muscle movement is dependent upon the integrity of these two components of the nervous pathway. Without the lower motor neurone the upper motor neurone is unable to transmit to the required destination the impulse that it carries, and without the upper motor neurone the lower motor neurone is isolated from ‘ instruction ’ and receives no impulse to transmit to the muscles.

Depending upon which component of this pathway is interrupted, one of two widely differing forms of *paralysis* will result.

Spastic Paralysis

In this state of affairs the lower motor neurone is *intact* but the upper motor neurone has been interrupted somewhere along

its course either in the brain or the spinal cord.   In the absence of the information and restraint that is usually exerted upon it by the upper motor neurone, the lower motor neurone now acts independently and this produces an increase in the tone of the muscles that it supplies (that is to say, the muscles become more *spastic* than normal) and an increase in their reflex reactions. Voluntary movement is largely or completely absent and it is in this respect that the muscles are paralysed, but we must recall that reflex movement can still take place. Spastic paralysis due to interference with the upper motor neurone in the brain may occur in a variety of conditions, such as intra-cerebral damage, birth injuries and infective processes. Similarly, congenital abnormalities of the spinal cord (such as meningomyelocele) may produce the same effect by interfering with the axon of the upper motor neurone at a lower level.

Flaccid Paralysis

In flaccid paralysis, the upper motor neurone is *intact* but the nerve cell or the axon of the lower motor neurone has been destroyed.   The muscles normally supplied by the lower motor neurone lose their tone and rapidly waste to a shadow of their normal dimensions.   All reflex and voluntary movements are lost and the affected muscles become inert and useless structures. Flaccid paralysis may result from section or injury of a peripheral nerve but it is most commonly seen as an accompaniment of the disease of anterior poliomyelitis.

To summarize therefore, we may say that *spastic* paralysis is characterized by:

>The absence of wasting.
>Increase of tone.
>Increase of reflex reactions.
>Loss of voluntary movement.

and that *flaccid* paralysis is characterized by:

>The presence of wasting.
>Loss of tone.
>Loss of reflex reactions.
>Loss of voluntary movement.

ANTERIOR POLIOMYELITIS

(Infantile Paralysis)

Anterior poliomyelitis is a virus infection of the central nervous systems which is characterized by a brief generalized illness and which, as a rule, is followed by the appearance of flaccid paralysis in skeletal muscles. Though rare in infancy it may affect children of any age and from time to time its incidence may assume epidemic proportions, usually occurring in the late summer and autumn. The precise route by which the causative virus reaches the nervous system is as yet still undetermined, but there is good evidence to support the contention that it is absorbed from the nasopharynx or the intestinal canal (or both), following which it may either travel centrally along the course of the peripheral nerves or may reach the central nervous system via the blood-stream. After a generalized but transient infection of the meninges and the whole nervous system, the virus becomes concentrated in the motor nerve cells in the anterior half of the grey matter of the spinal cord, that is to say, around the nerve cells of the lower motor neurones. The local oedema which this produces compresses the nerve cells to such an extent that they lose their function and this causes a *flaccid paralysis* of the muscles that they supply. A proportion of the nerve cells are often irrevocably destroyed by this process so that permanent paralysis of some muscles is nearly always the sequel to the disease, but as the infection regresses and the oedema subsides some of the least affected nerve cells recover their function with the result that some degree of restoration of muscle movement and power can be expected during the convalescent period.

In its early stages, anterior poliomyelitis is liable to be a most unpredictable disease, for the mode of onset, the clinical course, the amount of paralysis and the degree of subsequent recovery all tend to differ considerably from case to case. The majority of cases, however, usually exhibit three well defined stages.

1. THE PRODROMAL STAGE.—This stage, which is not always present, consists of little more than a brief ' illness ' lasting but a few days and in some cases it may be so slight as to

warrant a no more dramatic diagnosis than being a ' bit off colour '. A sore throat, a mild pyrexia and a headache are the common symptoms.

2. The Preparalytic Stage.—This stage, which coincides with the invasion and generalized infection of the meninges and the nervous system, is revealed by the sudden onset of acute pains in the back, the trunks and the limbs. They are accompanied by a fever (up to 103° F.), nausea or vomiting and cerebral irritation with severe headache and neck stiffness is also present in a number of cases. The severity of these symptoms and signs, however, is liable to considerable variation. If a lumbar puncture is performed at this time the cerebro-spinal fluid is usually under a slightly increased pressure, the protein content is increased and the cells (both polymorphs and lymphocytes) number up to 200 per cubic millimetre (normal 0-3 per cubic millimetre).

3. The Paralytic Stage.—The onset of paralysis, which coincides with the concentration of the virus in one particular portion of the spinal cord is sometimes accompanied by a dramatic improvement in the child's general condition— so much so, in fact, that one may, at first, be tempted to think that the illness is passing off. The distribution of muscle paralysis depends upon which portion of the spinal cord is affected by the disease. Most commonly the lumbar portion of the cord is predominantly affected with consequent paralysis of a varying amount of the musculature of one or both lower limbs. Higher regions of the spinal cord are affected less commonly and result in corresponding paralysis of the trunk muscles or those of the upper limbs. If the disease extends above the origin of the phrenic nerve (the fourth cervical segment of the spinal cord) then *respiratory paralysis* due to paralysis of the diaphragm will supervene and if higher than this, paralysis of the pharyngeal and laryngeal muscles will occur (bulbar poliomyelitis).

Variations of the Clinical Picture.—In addition to these three stages the disease may make its appearance in several atypical forms. Firstly, an overwhelming infection may result in rapid paralysis of the cardiac and respiratory centres in the medulla oblongata and cause a relatively sudden death, unheralded by any premonitory symptoms. Secondly, para-lysis of certain muscles may also appear without any general

disturbance at all (silent paralysis). Finally, no true paralysis may be evident, the disease merely causing a temporary weakening (paresis) of certain muscles, from which full recovery occurs in a comparatively short while.

Treatment

We may conveniently divide the treatment of paralysis due to anterior poliomyelitis into four principal categories:

(1) The care of paralysed muscles.
(2) The management of pharyngeal paralysis.
(3) The management of respiratory paralysis.
(4) The management of combined respiratory and pharyngeal paralysis.

(1) THE CARE OF PARALYSED MUSCLES

Early Treatment

RELIEF OF PAIN AND SWELLING.—For the first few weeks after the appearance of the paralytic stage there is often pain, tenderness and swelling of the affected muscles and although this is not always severe, it frequently interferes with the child's rest and comfort. Providing there is no weakness of respiration analgesic drugs may be given to relieve the pain, but the application of heat by the use of hot packs is often more effective. A thick layer of cotton-wool is soaked in very hot water, wrung out as rapidly as possible, wrapped around the affected limb and covered with a layer of thin mackintosh and a few turns of a crêpe bandage (the Kenny Pack). These applications should be repeated four or five times a day. The relief of swelling is best treated by elevation of the affected part. In the case of the lower limbs the foot of the bed should be elevated a few inches, and in the case of the upper limbs the affected arm should be supported on pillows or in padded slings suspended from above the bed. If these measures are insufficient, *very gentle* massage from the extremity of the limb towards the heart will succeed in reducing any swelling that remains.

PREVENTION OF JOINT STIFFNESS.—Joints which are surrounded by paralysed muscles are prone to become increasingly stiff due to inactivity. In order to prevent such

stiffness, all the joints in the paralysed area should be *gently* manipulated through a full range of movements at least twice a day and this is usually most conveniently and satisfactorily carried out immediately after removal of the packs.

PREVENTION OF DEFORMITY.—In order to understand this aspect of early treatment we must first consider one of the fundamental principles of muscular movement. Every joint in the body is surrounded by at least *two groups of muscles* which perform opposite movements at the joint itself. For instance, whereas the anterior tibial group of muscles in the lower legs produce the movement of dorsiflexion at the ankle joint, the posterior tibial and calf muscles produce the opposite movement of plantar flexion. On contraction of the dorsiflexors the plantar flexors must necessarily relax in order to allow the movement of dorsiflexion to take place, and vice versa. When at rest, however, both groups of muscles exert a minimal but equal and opposite pull against each other in order to maintain the foot in a constant position, and this state of continuous minimal contraction within the muscles is known as *tone*. Now anterior poliomyelitis causes a flaccid paralysis not so much of individual muscles but rather of groups of muscles, and as we have already seen flaccid paralysis is accompanied by a loss of voluntary movement and of muscle tone. Thus, in the instance we have cited above, if the group of dorsiflexing muscles is paralysed, then the normal tone in the unparalysed group of plantar flexors will exert a constant and relentless pull against its old antagonists; in this way a gross plantar flexion deformity will be produced at the ankle joint together with shortening of the unparalysed muscles and stretching and lengthening of the paralysed ones. Should recovery from the paralysis subsequently occur during the convalescent months, any deformity that has become established in the meantime will prevent the restoration of normal movement and it is therefore of paramount importance that such deformities should be prevented at all costs. It is for this reason that, from the onset of the paralysis, the limb should be maintained in a position that effectively prevents over stretching of the paralysed muscles. Light removable plaster of Paris, plastic or metal splints are used for this purpose and they should be removed at least twice a day so that toilette of the skin and passive movements of the paralysed joints may be performed.

Restoration of Function

EXERCISE.—About four to six weeks after the appearance of the paralysis, exercises designed to encourage movements in the paralysed muscles should be commenced. About two months later the child should be encouraged to use the limb as a whole and this is most effectively carried out in a specially built water-pool in which the support of the water reduces the 'weight' of the limb and thus allows the most feeble attempts at movement to be performed with greater ease. As the child becomes steadily more accomplished, walking exercises outside the pool should be allowed but appliances designed to prevent over-stretching of the recovering muscles should be fitted to the limb(s) for use during this form of activity.

RECONSTRUCTIVE SURGERY.—After a year to eighteen months following the onset of paralysis, it may be assumed that no further recovery will take place and surgical measures designed to stabilize paralysed joints, to improve function and to prevent further deformity will have to be undertaken. One of the commonest surgical procedure used in this respect is that of *tendon transplantation*. Although the details of this form of treatment need not concern you it is important that you should understand the principles involved. The tendon of a functional muscle is cut across close to its insertion and then implanted into the cut end of the tendon of a paralysed muscle. The limb is then enclosed in plaster of Paris for four to six weeks in order to allow healing to take place. After this time the muscle and tendon that have been transplanted are encouraged in their new duties by exercises and electrical stimulation in order to restore the 'balance of power' around the appropriate joint, to improve the sense of balance and to prevent the subsequent occurrence of deformity. If there is no muscle control whatsoever around a joint, then a splint designed to maintain the join in the optimum position may have to be worn permanently. In certain situations such as the ankle joint and the joints of the foot, operative fixation (arthrodesis) of the joint may sometimes be employed in order to increase stability and to obviate the necessity of wearing an external appliance. Arthrodesis involves removal of the articular surfaces of the joint so that the underlying raw bony surfaces may heal together in a solid block and thus replace the hitherto uncontrollable joint.

SCHOOLING.—Throughout the country there are a number of schools which are devoted entirely to the education and care of children who have been crippled either from anterior poliomyelitis or from other causes. These schools are intended primarily for children with severe degrees of residual paralysis, so that graduated activity and due care and attention of the paralysed limbs may proceed hand in hand with the child's education. In *borderline* cases, however, every effort should be made to have the child accepted at a school for normal children. For such a child to enter into the competitive atmosphere provided by association with normal children is a far greater incentive to him than the comparative ease with which he may become ' top-dog ' among children considerably more handicapped than himself.

(2) THE MANAGEMENT OF PHARYNGEAL PARALYSIS

Paralysis of the pharyngeal and laryngeal musculature results from an attack of bulbar poliomyelitis and in the majority of cases it is unaccompanied by paralytic effects elsewhere in the body. The duration of the paralysis is normally between a few days and two to three weeks, but during this time the ability to swallow is completely abolished. Apart from the obvious necessity of artificial feeding, pharyngeal paralysis is attended by two great dangers—firstly, the likelihood of the aspiration into the lungs of vomit, and secondly, the aspiration into the lungs of collections of mucus in the pharynx and the upper reaches of the trachea. In order to prevent these serious complications the child should be nursed in the semi-prone position, and the foot of the bed should be raised about 18 inches from the floor so that collections of vomit or mucus tend to gravitate to the exterior. (*On no account* should any child suffering from this condition be nursed in the supine position.) If, owing to the tilt of the bed, there is a tendency for the child to slip downwards this can easily be prevented by fitting a simple harness over the shoulders and securing it to the foot of the bed. The child should be turned every two hours and particular attention should be paid to the care of the skin over the shoulders, as pressure sores are liable to develop in this situation when the semi-prone position is adopted. In no circumstances, whatsoever, should the child

be left unattended, for if he or she should sit up and inhale vomit a rapidly fatal collapse may ensue. The accumulation of mucus in the throat is most easily revealed by strapping a small throat microphone over the child's larynx. The microphone is connected to a loud speaker placed on the bedside table and is *never* switched off. The nurse should listen carefully to each breath so that she may detect the sounds of bubbling and rattling due to the accumulation of mucus and in order that she may estimate the depth of each inspiratory effort, for in some cases serious weakening of respiratory function is liable to supervene. Mucus should be aspirated by the ward sucking apparatus as soon as it is revealed by the loud speaker, and if necessary the degree of tilt should also be increased. In this latter respect a ' tipping-bed ' if available, is more easily managed than propping the foot of the bed on trestles and chairs. Four-hourly feeds starting with 4 ounces of milk per feed should be administered through a polythene tube passed through the nose into the stomach and, providing there is no vomiting, feeding should thereafter be continued at two-hourly intervals and increased in amount until the full fluid, calorific, and vitamin requirements of the child are met.

(3) THE MANAGEMENT OF RESPIRATORY PARALYSIS

All cases of anterior poliomyelitis which show either weakening of respiration or frank respiratory paralysis should be nursed in a respirator. There is a wide variety of such apparatuses but essentially they all consist of an airtight cabinet which is connected to an automatic motor bellows. The head-piece of the cabinet is detachable and is mounted on a sliding tray on which the child is laid. The head and neck protrude through an aperture in the head-piece and a rubber diaphragm forms an airtight junction between the child's neck and the margin of the aperture (Fig. 98). When the head-piece is locked into position, the mechanical bellows suck air out of the cabinet and the consequent lowering of pressure that this produces causes the chest to expand and air to be sucked into the lungs through the exposed mouth and nose. Immediately following this, the suction of the bellows is released and the elastic recoil of the chest causes the air to be driven out of the lungs. The bellows can be adjusted so that this process

is repeated from between twenty to thirty times per minute according to the respiratory needs of the child, but a pair of hand bellows for emergency use should always be at hand in case the motor fails. Along the sides and the top of the cabinet are port-holes covered with thin rubber diaphragms through which the hand may be introduced in order to move the child within. The whole apparatus is mounted on a pivot so that it may be tipped as required.

The child is clad only in a simple nightdress and it is usually advisable for bed socks to be worn in order to protect the feet from the draught of the bellows. Particular attention should be paid to the skin of the neck which should be covered with

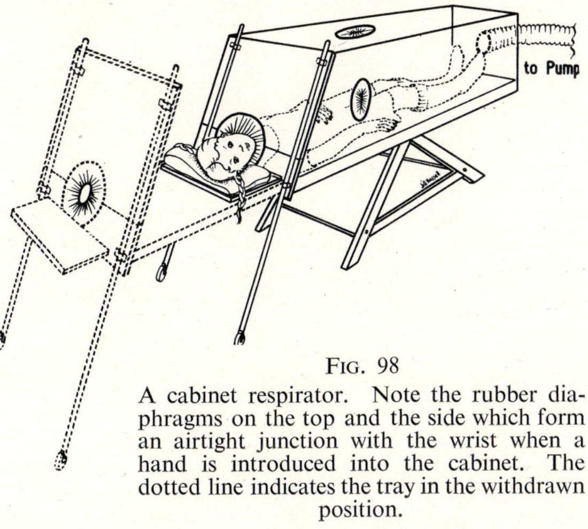

FIG. 98

A cabinet respirator. Note the rubber diaphragms on the top and the side which form an airtight junction with the wrist when a hand is introduced into the cabinet. The dotted line indicates the tray in the withdrawn position.

thick vaseline and a light padded bandage so that the slight 'to and fro' movement of the rubber diaphragm during the working of the bellows does not cause excoriation. Unnecessarily repetitive though it may seem, it is most important for you to keep uppermost in your mind the obvious fact that the child can not control her own respirations. For this reason, mouth feeding must be most carefully timed and be given only at the end of the inspiratory phase otherwise particles of food are liable to be aspirated into the lungs, and for the same reason both the mouth and pharynx must be meticulously cleaned after a meal. Should vomiting or sudden aspiration of food occur, the apparatus must immediately be tipped head downwards and the larynx and trachea thoroughly sucked out.

In the majority of cases the child may be brought out of the respirator for a few minutes at a time without incurring respiratory embarrassment so that she may have her pressure areas treated and have an opportunity to void her urine and empty her bowels.   Owing to the lack of voluntary respiratory effort, constipation is a frequent accompaniment of respiratory paralysis and a low glycerine enema (1 ounce glycerine in 4 ounces of water) may, if necessary, be given every second or third day.   Respiratory infections and pulmonary collapse are common complications and for this reason the child should be turned every two hours, the nurse and all visitors should always wear protective gauze masks, 500,000 units of penicillin should be given by intramuscular injection daily and a chest X-ray should be taken every other day.   A good indication of the beginnings of recovery in respiratory function is to ask the child to count as far as she can each time she is out of the respirator.   Once she can count up to ten without taking a breath she may be allowed out of the respirator for progressively longer periods each day until such time as she no longer needs the assistance of the apparatus, but during this time a most careful watch must be kept for any signs of respiratory fatigue or distress.

(4) THE MANAGEMENT OF COMBINED RESPIRATORY AND PHARYNGEAL PARALYSIS

In cases suffering from both respiratory *and* pharyngeal paralysis further considerable difficulties are encountered, for due to the paralysis of the pharynx the likelihood of aspiration into the lungs is greatly increased, even when the patient is nursed in a cabinet respirator with a high degree of tilt.   In order, therefore, to by-pass the mouth and the pharynx it invariably becomes necessary to perform a tracheotomy, but even so this provides added nursing difficulties both in the care of the tracheotomy tube and in the turning of the patient. Unsatisfactory though this method may be, it was until recently the only procedure available for combined respiratory and pharyngeal paralysis.   It was not until the widespread epidemic in Denmark in 1952, however, that a new method was evolved. This has now become known as the *Copenhagen method* of treatment and it consists of passing through the tracheotomy a rubber endotracheal tube with an inflatable cuff around it,

after which the cuff is inflated so that it forms an air-tight junction with the walls of the trachea, and thus effectively prevents aspiration of foreign material into the lungs. The endotracheal tube is then connected to a mechanical pump which delivers humidified air or oxygen into the lungs under a positive pressure. It is of interest to note that during the Danish epidemic, as no suitable mechanical apparatus was then available the pump consisted solely of a medical student who, working in shifts with his colleagues, continually compressed and released a rubber bag connected to the endotracheal tube in order to ventilate the patient's lungs. The paralysed pharynx is cared for in exactly the same way as we have previously described.

CHAPTER XIII

THE BONES AND JOINTS

The Anatomy of Bone

FROM the outset it is most important that you should get out of your minds the conception that apart from its shape, living bone is in any way similar to the brittle and dessicated specimens upon which you perform your studies. Whereas dead bone is made up of an inert collection of inorganic mineral substances, living bone is composed of a richly vascular, ever changing framework of living cells arranged in such a manner as to confer not only strength but also *resilience* upon the bone as a whole. In addition, during the period of growth the bone is in a constant state of reabsorption and replacement (*remodelling*) so that the shape and contour will remain the same while the dimensions increase in both length and girth.

Bony tissue may be either *compact* or *cancellous* in structure, the former making up the hard outer surface of the bone (the *cortex*) which provides the chief source of strength, and the latter consisting of an intricate bony network within the medulla, the architecture of which is designed to furnish additional support against the predominant stresses and strains to which the bone is most commonly subjected during activity.

For the purposes of description all growing bones (with the exception of the skull bones) may be divided into the following principal components :

1. **The Shaft or Diaphysis.**—The shaft of a bone is made up for the most part of a thick cylinder of cortical bone. In the region of the mid-shaft there is little or no cancellous bone, the medulla being occupied by a collection of fatty material but at each end of the diaphysis (*the metaphysis*) there is a dense collection of cancellous bone.

2. **The Epiphysis.**—The epiphysis caps each end of the shaft of the bone (Fig. 99) and is composed of a thin layer of cortical bone and a dense network of cancellous

bone. Separating the epiphysis from the metaphysis is a thick layer of cartilage (the *epiphyseal plate of cartilage*) and it is at this structure that active growth takes place. Not being radio opaque it is easily recognized in X-ray

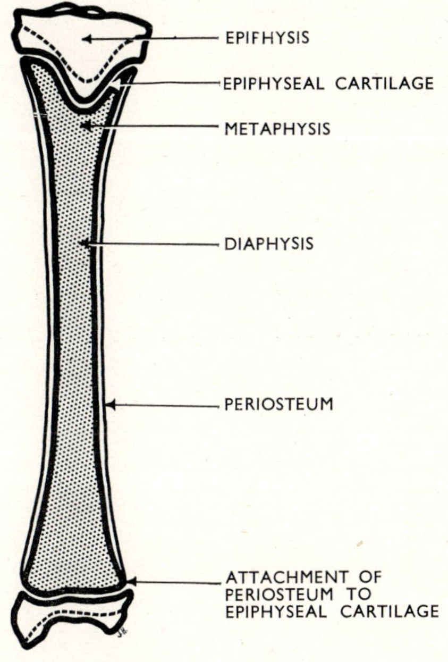

Fig. 99

To show the principal components of a typical
bone. The dotted lines indicate the attachment
of the joint capsule.

photographs as a gap between the epiphysis and meta-physis, but when growth has ceased so the plate of cartilage disappears and the epiphysis and metaphysis become fused together.

Closely investing the whole bone with the exception of the articular surfaces is a tough membrane (the *periosteum*) which is firmly attached to each epiphyseal plate of cartilage. It carries minute blood-vessels for the nourishment of the cortex, and when lifted from the surface of the bone either by a fracture or by the formation of pus beneath it (see osteomyelitis), it has the property of laying down new bone (sub-periosteal new bone) in the space that has been formed.

CONGENITAL ABNORMALITIES

CONGENITAL DISLOCATION OF THE HIP

Congenital dislocation of the hip may be either unilateral or bilateral and occurs about five times more commonly in girls than it does in boys. The precise cause of the dislocation is as yet undetermined, but as it is a painless condition there is a strong tendency for it to pass unrecognized until the child begins to walk when the instability of the affected hip produces an obvious abnormality in the child's gait; and as the success of treatment depends to a large extent upon how soon it is commenced after birth, you must appreciate that early recognition of the condition is of the first importance.

Clinical Features

Due to the fact that the head of the femur has failed to enter the cavity of the acetabulum but resides outside it instead, the whole limb on the affected side is consequently displaced a corresponding distance away from the mid-line of the body. This produces a visible widening of the perineum which, although it is not always obvious in unilateral dislocation, is easily recognized in cases of bilateral dislocation. With increased muscular activity and especially with the assumption of the erect position, the head of the femur becomes displaced in an upwards direction and this causes an obvious *shortening* of the affected limb. This in turn causes a secondary shortening of the hamstring and adductor groups of muscles and often

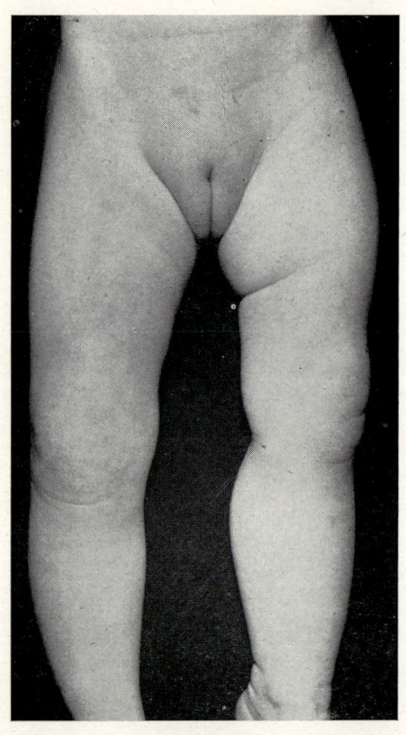

Fig. 100

Congenital dislocation of the left hip. Note the obvious shortening and the extra thigh skin crease.

16

produces a deep extra crease in the skin on the adductor surface of the thigh. These outward manifestations of the condition, namely, widening of the perineum, shortening of the leg and an extra thigh crease are the predominant visible signs all of which are well illustrated in Fig. 100, and the nurse is well advised to keep them to the forepart of her mind. It is not uncommon for a sharp-eyed nurse to detect an hitherto unrecognized congenital dislocation of the hip in an infant or

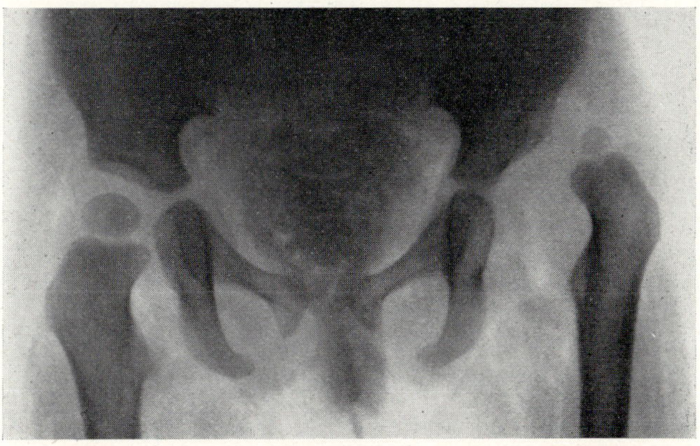

Fig. 101

Note the obvious dislocation, the small femoral epiphysis and the shallow acetabulum.

young child whom she is nursing for an altogether unrelated condition. Once the child begins to walk the presence of a dislocated hip becomes obvious at a glance by the pronounced, painless and persistent limp that it produces. This limp is due to the fact that when weight is taken on the affected limb the head of the femur instead of supporting the pelvis, rides up and down on the lateral pelvic wall (*telescoping*) and acts more as a vertical piston than as a prop. X-ray examination reveals the obvious dislocation and, in addition, demonstrates two principal associated abnormalities, namely, a smaller upper femoral epiphysis on the affected side and an abnormal shallowness of the acetabulum (Fig. 101).

Treatment

The principles of treatment are firstly to obtain reduction of the dislocation and thereafter to maintain the reduced position until such time as it has become sufficiently stable to

prevent redislocation. Prior to reduction the shortening of the limb should be overcome by skin traction combined with a gradually increasing divarication of the legs. This may be carried out in a variety of ways but it is most easily effected on a Robert Jones abduction frame (Fig. 102). X-ray photographs are taken at weekly intervals in order to demonstrate the position of the head of the femur and in certain instances the combination of traction and abduction may be sufficient to effect reduction of the dislocation. As a general rule, however, once there is X-ray evidence that the upward displacement of the head of the femur has been overcome (usually after about

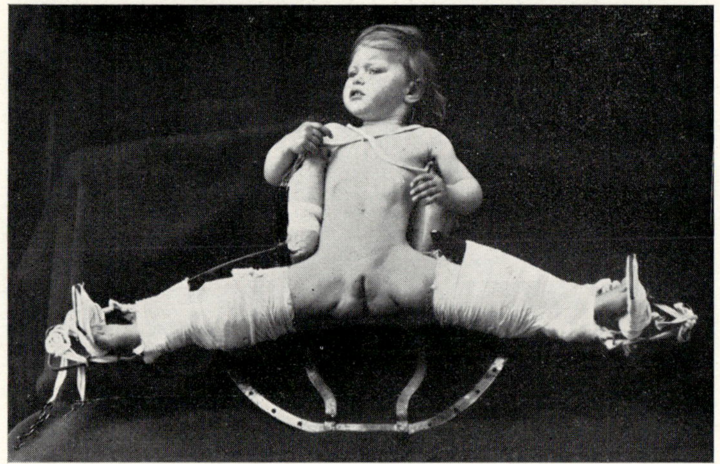

FIG. 102
Traction and divarication on a Robert Jones abduction frame.

four to six weeks of traction), manipulative reduction is carried out under a general anaesthetic. The success of the reduction is immediately verified by an X-ray examination performed in the operating theatre. Following this *both* hips (irrespective of whether the condition is unilateral or bilateral) are immobilized in plaster of Paris in one of two principal positions.

THE LORENZ PLASTER.—This position which is illustrated in Fig. 103 is sometimes also known as the ' frog plaster ' or the 90—90—0 position (that is to say, 90° of flexion, 90° of abduction and 0° of rotation at each hip joint). As a rule two canvas braces are incorporated in the plaster so that the child may be secured in the upright position during the daytime, supported

on a modified lavatory seat so that the excreta are voided directly into the receiver placed beneath the perineum.

THE BATCHELOR PLASTER.—Due to the fact that the head and neck of the dislocated femur usually incline forwards at a greater angle than in the normal bone (the angle of anteversion), a more secure reduction is often obtained if the limb is fully internally rotated. Both limbs are therefore placed in the position of 45° of abduction and full internal rotation; plaster

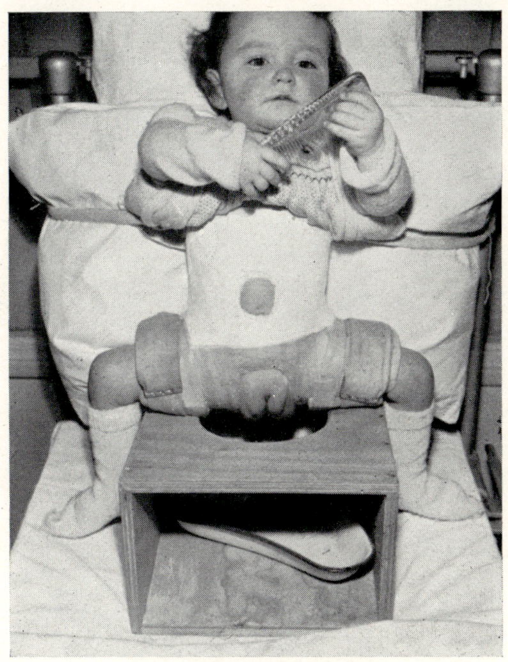

FIG. 103
The Lorenz plaster.

of Paris is applied from mid-thigh to mid-calf on each limb and the two casts joined together at the knee by a metal bar which is incorporated in the plaster (Fig. 104). Providing the reduction is satisfactory this type of plaster, though not immobilizing the hips, none the less secures the reduction by maintaining a constant degree of internal rotation and abduction. The obvious advantages of this method are firstly, that there is no plaster in the region of the groins and perineum and thus the liability of discomfort due to soiling with faeces and

urine does not arise; secondly, it allows active contractions of the muscles around the hip joint (particularly the flexors) to take place and thus prevents the muscle wasting and weakening that always accompanies total immobilization.

Once reduction of the dislocation has been obtained and a comfortable plaster has been applied, the child may be returned to her home but the parents must be instructed that should the plaster become cracked or softened they must bring her back

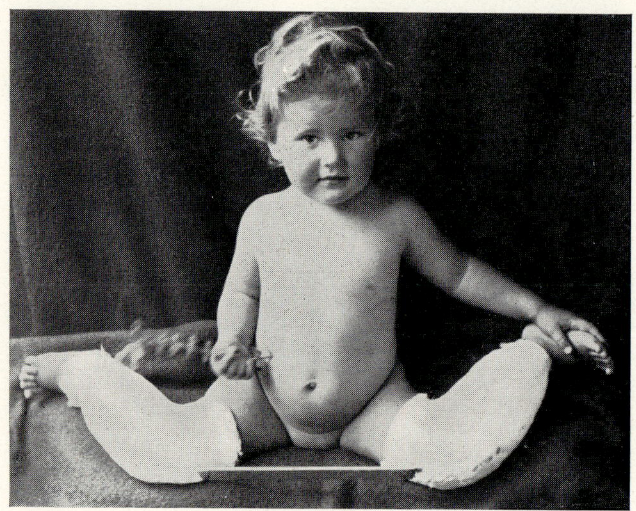

FIG. 104
The Batchelor plaster.

to hospital at once. About three months after the original reduction the child should be re-admitted to hospital and the plaster removed under a general anaesthetic. Both clinical and radiological examinations are then carried out in order to confirm the reduced position and to estimate its stability after which a new plaster is applied and the child returned to her home for a further period of three months. This routine is continued at three monthly intervals until X-ray examination reveals deepening of the acetabulum and an upper femoral epiphysis equal in size to that on the normal side (Fig. 105). Once these criteria are satisfied no further immobilization is necessary and although some authorities prefer to keep the legs abducted by a removable leather and metal splint for a further three months or so, as a general rule it is

safe to allow the child to commence walking without any form of appliance.

However satisfactory the final function of the hip may appear to be, it is most important for you to realize that its capability to withstand the stresses and strains of everyday life is less than a normal hip, and it is for this reason that osteo-arthritic changes are prone to develop in the reduced hip by the age of twenty-five to thirty years.

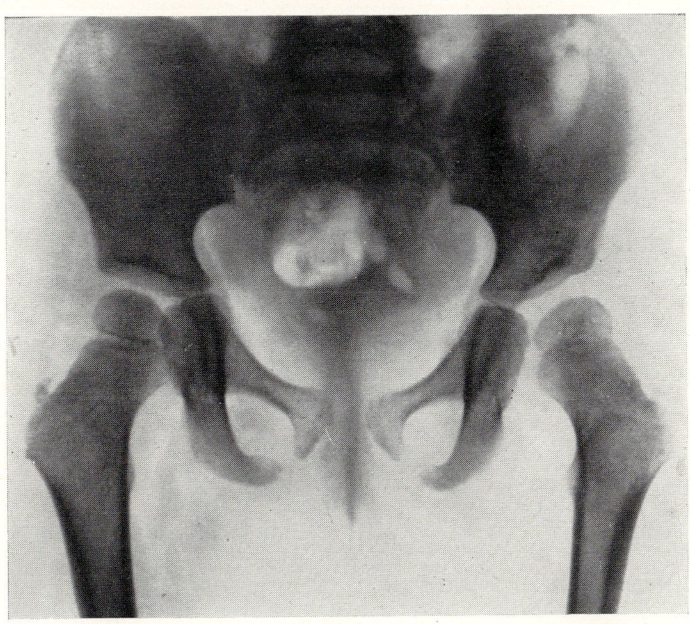

FIG. 105

Eighteen months after the original reduction. Note the increase in depth of the acetabulum and the equal size of the femoral epiphysis. (Compare with Fig. 101).

Complications

In the majority of children of up to two to three years of age a stable hip is usually obtained by the methods we have just considered. Occasionally, however, in spite of expert reduction and management, redislocation of the hip may occur each time the plaster is changed. This may be due to one of two main causes. Firstly, the cavity of the acetabulum may be occupied by a tough plug of tissue (a limbus) which effectively prevents the entry of the head of the femur, and stable reduction

will therefore be impossible until the limbus has been removed by open operation. Secondly, the acetabulum may not deepen sufficiently and thus fail to provide a socket deep enough to contain the head of the femur. If the acetabulum remains in this state for more than a year without any evidence of deepening, then an operation designed to increase the size of its upper margin (a *shelf* operation) may have to be carried out in order to prevent redislocation.

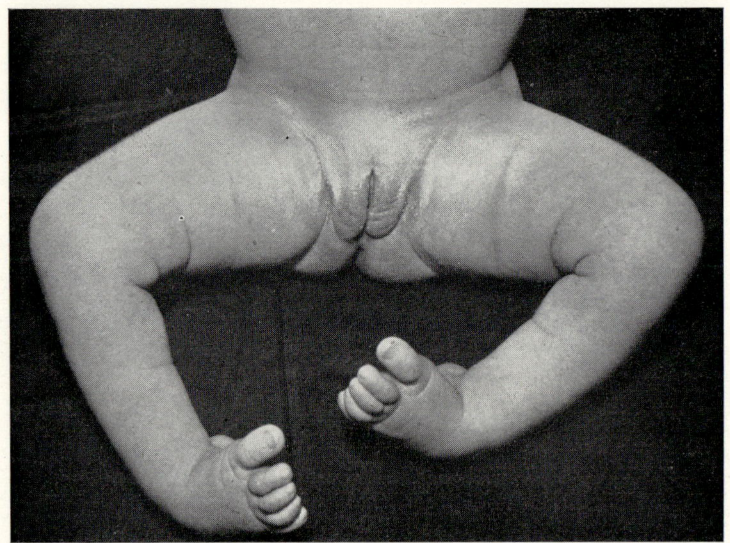
Fig. 106
Bilateral talipes equinovarus.

Finally, we must again stress the importance of early recognition of this condition, for the longer it remains untreated the less satisfactory the final result is liable to be. Up to about two years of age the immediate results of treatment are almost invariably successful but after this age the likelihood of success falls rapidly, and in children over six years old reduction is usually impossible, the only hope of obtaining a stable hip being by makeshift reconstructive operations.

CLUB FOOT (TALIPES)

There are two principal varieties of congenital club foot:

(1) Talipes Equinovarus.   (2) Talipes Calcaneus.

(1) **Talipes Equinovarus**

Formidable though this term may at first appear it is easily split up into its descriptive components. The word *talipes* merely means a deformity of the ankle and foot; *equinus* denotes a hoof or horse-like appearance (that is to say, an abnormal degree of plantar flexion at the ankle joint) and *varus* refers to the inversion of the foot and the bending inwards (adduction) of the forefoot towards the mid-line (Fig. 106).

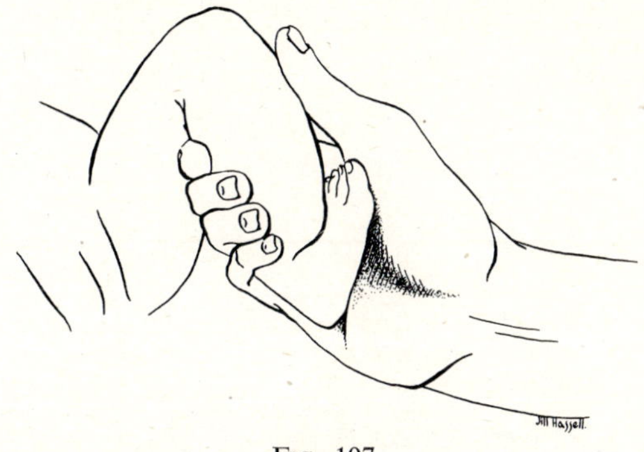

FIG. 107
The position of full overcorrection.

The condition may be either unilateral or bilateral and although there is still albeit a dying controversy as to the precise cause of the deformity, it is now generally agreed that it is due to an abnormal degree of compression and moulding of the infants feet whilst ' in utero '.

The deformity is always present at birth and as the subsequent treatment and general management is liable to be a long and tedious business, it is most important that it should be commenced in the first week or so of life while the feet are still sufficiently pliable to be remoulded into the normal position. Each day after birth the feet and ankles should be gently but firmly manipulated towards the position of *over-correction*, and each time that this has been done a few lengths of adhesive strapping may be applied in order to maintain the improvement that has been gained. After about a week of this procedure the position of full overcorrection of the deformity is usually obtained (Fig. 107), and thereafter (but on no account beforehand) this position should be maintained by the application of

a suitable appliance. Some authorities still favour the use of a plaster of Paris cast applied from above the knee with the knee joint in 90° of flexion and continued downwards to include the ankle and foot in the overcorrected position. Although this is an eminently satisfactory method of maintaining the over-correction it has the great disadvantage of preventing movement at the knee joint and thus restricting the natural and necessary exercise of the infant's feet by the inborn expedient of kicking.

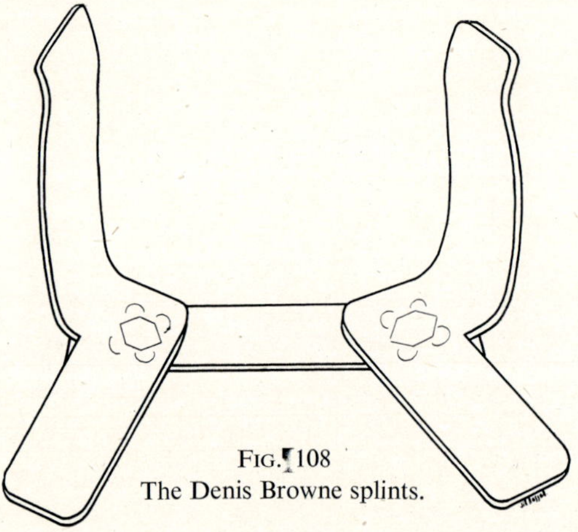

FIG. 108
The Denis Browne splints.

It was expressly to overcome these disadvantages that the Denis Browne splints were originally designed and their use has now become a widely accepted and popular method of treatment. The use of the word ' splint ' in describing the Denis Browne contrivance is misleading, for as we shall see they are in fact a composite system of levers. Each ' splint ' consists of a footplate and an upright component which is connected to its fellow by a detachable metal bar (Fig. 108). In order to prevent friction between the metal and the infant's skin a length of adhesive orthopaedic felt should be stuck to the sole of the infant's foot and to the outer aspect of the lower leg so that when the splints are applied, any friction that takes place will do so between the felt and the metal. If, as is so commonly done, the felt is stuck to the metal then friction will take place between the *felt* and the *skin* and pressure sores will be the inevitable result. The foot is secured to the footplate by adhesive strapping and when this has been done you will see by reference to Fig. 109 that, due to the resumption of the

inversion deformity, the upright arm of the splint will now project outwards at an angle to the long axis of the limb. It is by bringing this component into line with the limb and by securing it there with a few turns of strapping that the inversion deformity is *levered* into the position of eversion, a manoeuvre that is addedly effective if the outside margin of the foot is built up with a greater thickness of orthopaedic felt. Irrespective

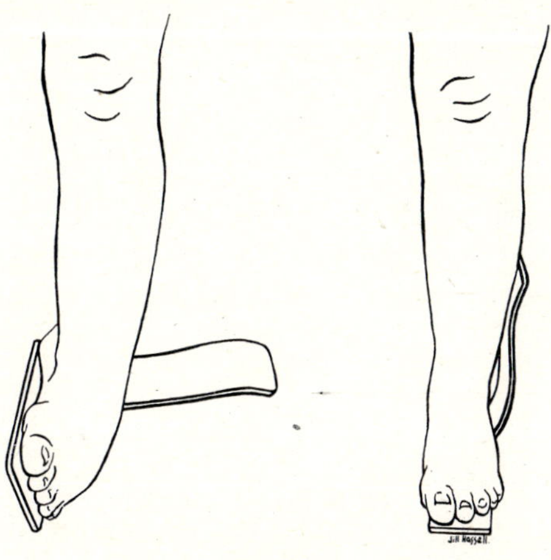

FIG. 109

The application of the Denis Browne splints. The strapping has not been shown for the sake of clarity.

of whether the deformity is unilateral or bilateral both feet are dealt with in this manner, after which both ' splints ' are bolted on to the metal bar (Fig. 110). In this way the knee movements remain unrestricted, the infant is free to kick and exercise the limbs and any attempt to resume the position of inversion on the part of one foot will, through the medium of the metal bar, cause increased eversion of the other foot, and vice versa. Quite often the toes become blanched after the splints have first been applied, but, as a rule, the circulation is re-established within them after an hour or so. However, a close watch should always be kept on the colour of the toes and if they are still white two or three hours after the splints have been applied, the strapping should be removed and re-applied. At three weekly intervals the splints should be removed and before re-application a manual manipulation of the foot and ankle into

the fully overcorrected position should always be performed. This regime should be continued from three to four months or longer until, with the splints removed, the infant's feet assume the normal position. If, as all too frequently occurs, the splints are now discarded, a recurrence of the deformity is

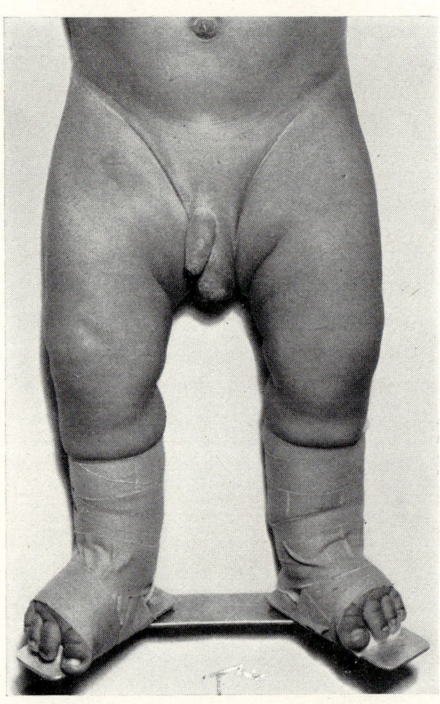

FIG. 110

The splints applied.

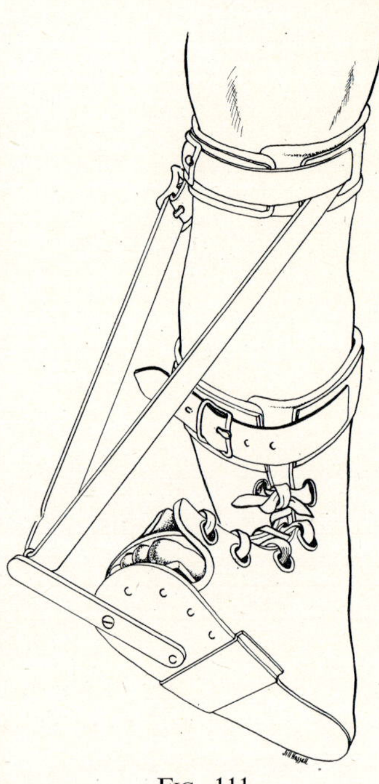

FIG. 111

The Denis Browne night boot. Note that the metal lever protruding from the sole can be adjusted in order to alter the degree of eversion.

bound to occur and it is for this reason that a Denis Browne night boot (Fig. 111) should always be applied to the foot or feet in place of the splints until the child begins to walk, when each step the child takes is itself a corrective manipulation. Even so the night boot should still be worn during the hours of sleep until the child is three to four years old, in order to prevent any tendency of the deformity to recur.

(2) Talipes Calcaneus

This is a very much less severe deformity than talipes equinovarus and one which is infinitely easier to treat. The

child is born with one or both feet in an abnormal degree of dorsiflexion and in addition there may also be a degree of inversion (talipes calcaneovarus) or eversion (talipes calcaneovalgus) of the feet (Fig. 112). Treatment merely consists of repeated gentle manipulation of the foot into the normal position. This should be performed several times after each feed and may be quite easily and satisfactorily carried out by a conscientious mother. After two or three weeks of this treatment the foot assumes the normal position and thereafter causes no concern or disability, nor is there any tendency for the deformity to recur. In cases of very severe deformity it may be necessary to maintain the foot in the corrected position for a few weeks in plaster of Paris but, as a general rule, this is seldom necessary.

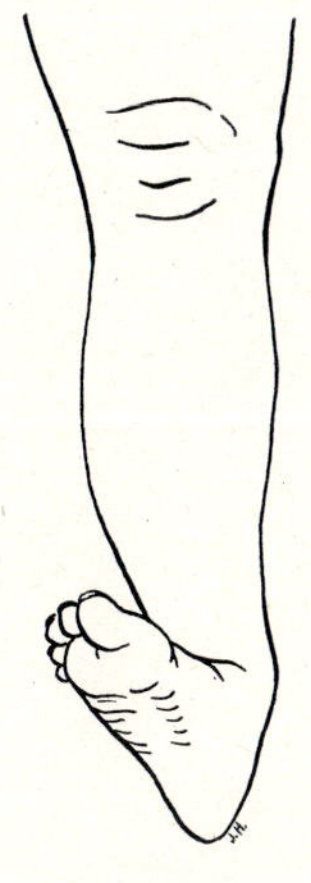

Fig. 112
Talipes calcaneovalgus.

ABNORMAL POSTURE

Abnormalities in posture are frequently attributed to a wide variety of causes, some of which are obvious in their significance and others of which are largely conjectural. For this reason we shall consider here only the essential features of those postural abnormalities that you will most commonly encounter.

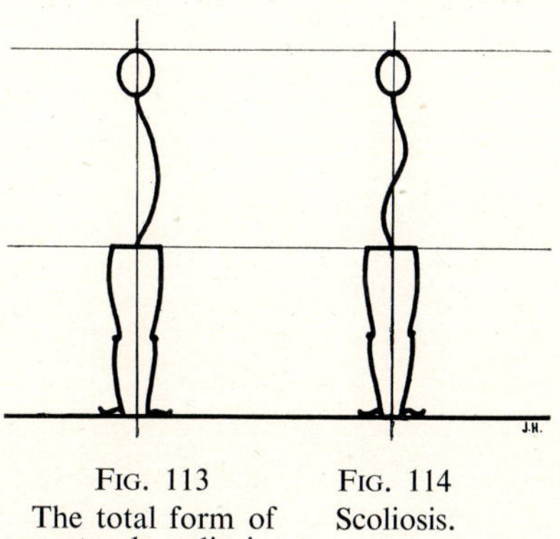

Fig. 113
The total form of postural scoliosis.

Fig. 114
Scoliosis.

Scoliosis

The term scoliosis refers to a lateral curvature of the spine of which there are two main varieties.

Postural Scoliosis.—The form most commonly occurs in girls, usually about eight to twelve years in age and usually

takes the shape either of a single curve of the whole spine to one side or the other of the mid-line (a total scoliosis) or a curve to each side (Figs. 113 and 114). Whichever form it takes, the curve is completely obliterated on full flexion of the spine. There

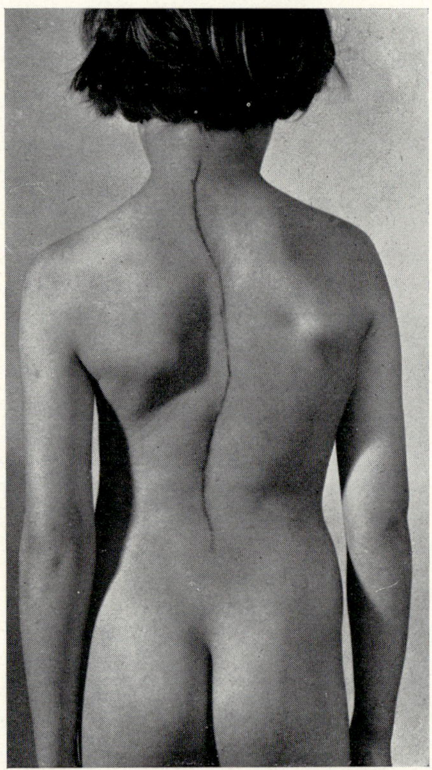

FIG. 115

Scoliosis. Note the prominence of the ribs on the convex side of the curve and the prominence of the scapula on the other.

is no demonstrable organic cause of the condition and it is generally considered to be due to rapid skeletal growth which is unaccompanied by a corresponding increase in strength of the spinal musculature. Correction of the deformity is obtained by back extension exercises designed to improve the tone and strength of the paravertebral muscles; but it is most important that the exercises should be rigorously supervised and, in order

to make the child ' posture conscious ', the parents should be instructed to supervise the exercises at home and continually to draw their child's attention to any tendency on her part to resume the abnormal position.

STRUCTURAL SCOLIOSIS.—Structural scoliosis consists of at least two lateral curves, a primary curve in one direction and a compensatory curve to the other (Fig. 114), which are not as a rule obliterated by full spine flexion.   Usually it is due to a demonstrable organic lesion such as a congenital absence of the lateral half of a vertebra (which produces a lateral kink in the line of the spine), though there are a number of cases for which no cause can be found (idiopathic scoliosis).   The ribs on the convex aspect of the curve bulge backwards in a prominent manner and there is usually an undue prominence of the scapula on the opposite side (Fig. 115).   Treatment is designed to lessen the degree of curvature and maintain the improvement by back strengthening exercises, but if in spite of these measures the degree of curvature continues to increase, operative fixation of the spine at the point of maximum curvature may have to be undertaken.

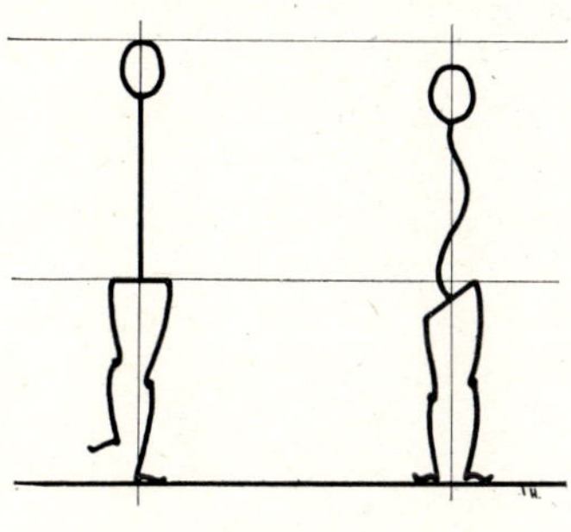

FIG. 116
Scoliosis due to a short leg.

Congenital shortening of one leg is not an uncommon cause of a mild scoliosis, the mechanism of the curvature being demonstrated in Fig. 116.   Treatment is simply directed to building up the sole of the shoe on the affected side until the pelvis is level when both legs are held straight.

TORTICOLLIS

True torticollis is a deformity of the neck in which the head is tilted to one side and it is due to a contracture of one or the other sternomastoid muscles (Fig. 117).   The condition seldom becomes apparent until the neck begins to elongate at about four to five years of age, and as it is both insidious in onset and slow in progression it is frequently first noticed by persons other

than members of the child's family.   In a proportion of cases
the features of the face on the same side as the contracted
sternomastoid muscle are smaller than those of the opposite
side, and this *facial asymmetry* (as it is called) is likely to persist
for several years after the torticollis has been cured and may,

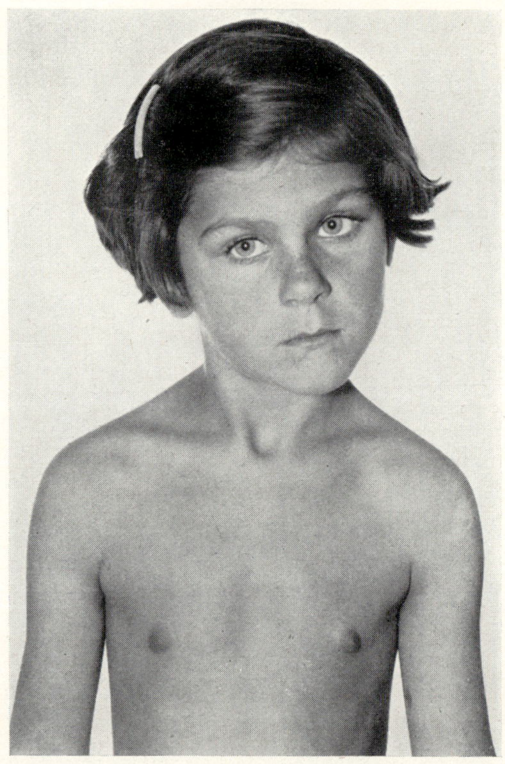

FIG. 117

Torticollis.

in certain instances, remain as a permanent feature throughout
life.   The precise cause of the contracture of the sternomastoid
muscle is not known but it is believed to be associated in a
number of cases with a *sternomastoid tumour of infancy*.   This
is a swelling which appears in the lower third of the sternomastoid muscle at or shortly after birth, and which usually
disappears within the first few months of life.   Its true nature is

as yet undetermined and, although it was at one time thought to be due to rupture of the sternomastoid muscle during labour with subsequent fibrosis and contracture, it is now generally considered to be due to an interference with the blood-supply of the muscle during the course of a difficult delivery; but whether the contracture is in any way due to the tumour is not known. None the less, while the tumour is still present, full passive movements of the infant's neck should be performed by its mother after each feed, and this procedure should be continued for some months after the disappearance of the tumour in order to prevent the possibility of the subsequent development of a contracture.

Congenital torticollis is treated in a number of different ways but all methods are based upon the same principles, namely, division of the contracted muscle and over-correction of the deformity. One of the simplest ways of treating this condition is known as a *closed tenotomy* or *Elmslie's* operation. Under a general anaesthetic a tenotome is introduced underneath the skin just where the sternomastoid tendon joins the sternum. The tendon is then cut through, and the neck forcibly manipulated into an over-corrected position. Only a very small dressing is required to cover the wound made by the tenotome and the child is then returned to bed where the head and neck are maintained in the over-corrected position by sandbags. Some surgeons, however, consider that in addition to the sternomastoid tendon the deep fascia should also be divided, and for this reason they advocate an *open operation*. Under a general anaesthetic a long incision is made $\frac{1}{2}$ an inch above and parallel to the clavicle. The sternomastoid tendon, together with all the deep fascia on the affected side are cut across and the neck manipulated into the over-corrected position before the wound is closed, after which the neck is maintained in the over-corrected position for a period of several weeks by the application of plaster of Paris. Whichever method of operative treatment is carried out, it is the *after care* and training that are of the greatest importance. Each morning and night the child should sit in front of a full length mirror and, for at least twenty minutes, should carry out full active movements of the cervical spine. The mirror allows the child to observe her progress and also any tendency on her part to revert to the original deformity. This daily stretching and

exercising of the neck should be continued for a period of six months to one year.

Torticollis may result from causes other than contracture of the sternomastoid muscle. It may be due to a congenital malformation of a cervical vertebra (a hemi-vertebra) which produces a lateral 'kink' in the cervical spine; it may be associated with the compensatory curve of a scoliosis, or it may temporarily be due to acute cervical lymphadenitis—the child holding the head to one side in order to relieve the discomfort caused by the inflamed glands. It goes without saying that in such instances there is no contracture of the sternomastoid muscle and that treatment is directed to the parent condition. In infants who are as yet not old enough to hold up their heads of their own accord, torticollis frequently results from the mother's habit of continually carrying the infant on the same arm so that the head always tilts over to the same side. This is merely a postural form of torticollis without any organic contracture and it is easily remedied by advising the mother to carry the infant on the other arm for a change.

Genu Valgum

(Knock Knee)

Genu valgum is a very common condition in the first eight years of life and occurs with equal frequency in both boys and girls. Whereas in the normal erect position both knees and both ankles may be easily approximated, in genu valgum the ankles are separated when the knees are placed together. In that the shafts of the femora, which are widely separated at their upper ends, incline inwards toward the mid-line and meet the tibiae at an angle, there is a natural tendency to an increase in this angulation in all children (i.e. the production of genu valgum). Apart from this skeletal predisposition to the condition, it is liable to be accentuated by early walking, insufficient rest in the twenty-four-hour period and overweight—in other words—overloading of the legs.

The treatment of genu valgum has undergone considerable changes and mollification in the last few years. Whereas it was previously the custom to apply metal calipers to the limbs both day and night, the tendency nowadays is to pay more

attention to 'reducing the load' on the limbs—that is to say, dieting when the child is overweight and securing sufficient rest during the day, especially in rapidly growing children. In mild cases, when the distance between the malleoli is less than 2 inches, it is customary to build up the *inside* of the heel of the shoes in order to relieve the strain on the stretched internal ligament of the knee joint, and daily corrective manipulations, massage and exercise are also valuable in reducing the degree of deformity and promoting the strength of the supporting musculature. When the inter-malleolar separation is more than 2 inches, some authorities in addition to the above measures, advise the wearing of padded night splints to which the limbs are secured in a corrective position during the hours of sleep. It is important, however, for you to realize that, beneficial though all these measures may be, there is a strong tendency for the legs to grow quite straight of their own accord and that the success attributed to the various methods of treatment must be balanced against this natural ability of the limbs to correct their temporary deformity in the early years of life.

Genu Varum

(Bow Leg)

Unlike genu valgum, genu varum is frequently a manifestation of rickets and usually becomes more obvious and pronounced when the child begins to walk. The bowing may affect the whole limb or it may affect the tibiae alone. Treatment is directed firstly to the general treatment of rickets by ultra-violet light and vitamin D, and secondly, to the straightening of the limbs by the application of corrective night splints. In severe cases of bowing of the tibias that are not improved by these measures, it may become necessary to produce an incomplete fracture at the mid-shaft of the bone (osteoclasis) following which the limb is manually straightened and the limb immobilized in an above knee plaster of Paris cast until union has occurred in the corrected position.

Bowed tibiae in newly born infants are very common findings and only very rarely are they associated with rickets. No treatment is necessary, for the tibiae invariably grow quite straight before the child is old enough to stand.

INJURIES TO BONES—FRACTURES

The term *fracture* denotes a break in the continuity of a bone. Such a break may be either *complete*, in that the whole thickness of the bone is broken across (Fig. 118) or it may be *incomplete*, that is to say, the bone is bent and only part of it may be broken. As the bones of children are far more elastic and resilient than adult bones, the incomplete variety of fracture is by far the commonest type that you will encounter. This latter form of fracture is usually referred to as a *greenstick* fracture and as such it is well named, for just as a growing twig or branch of a tree only breaks on one side of the wood when it is angulated (Fig. 119) so the pliable growing bones of children exhibit the same tendency to break only at the cortex on one side of the bone (Fig. 120).

The Effects of Fracture

The principal effects produced by a fracture are *pain, swelling* and *deformity* of the limb. The swelling usually takes several hours to develop and is produced by haemorrhage from the broken bone ends together with the haemorrhage and traumatic oedema occurring in the adjacent soft tissues. The deformity is due either to the alteration in the line of the bone or to the over-lapping of the broken ends of the bone (displacement) or to a combination of both factors. Generally speaking, the degree of pain and swelling is very much less in the case of greenstick fractures than it is in complete and displaced fractures, but deformity may be of a major or minor degree in both varieties.

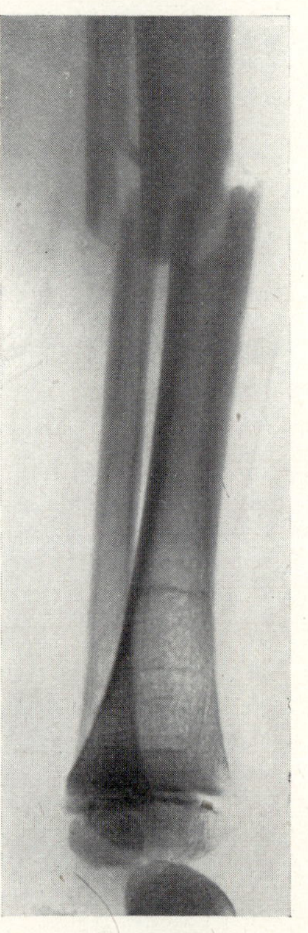

FIG. 118

A complete fracture of the tibia and fibula.

The Healing of Fractures

Following a fracture the space created between the bone ends and beneath the raised periosteum is occupied by haematoma

and inflammatory exudate resulting from the causative trauma. Thus the first stage in healing is similar in all respects to the repair of any other tissue in the body, irrespective of

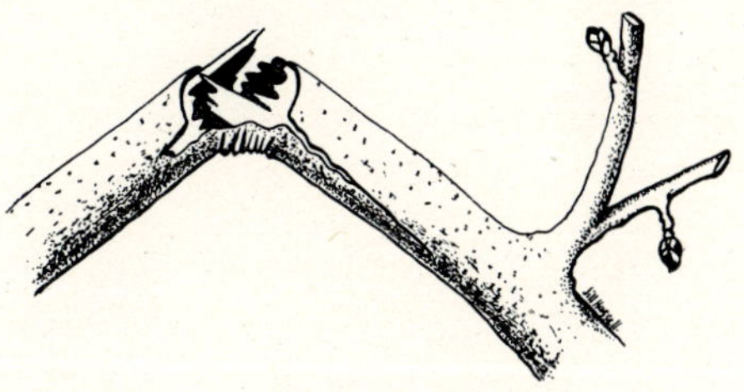

FIG. 119

A drawing of a fractured green stick. Note how only one side of the wood has given way and how the bark has buckled on the opposite side.

whether the inflammatory state has been caused by trauma or infection (see Chapter I). A few days after the fracture has been sustained granulation tissue begins to invade the haematoma, firstly, in order to absorb and remove the clotted blood, and secondly, in order to lay down a delicate connective tissue

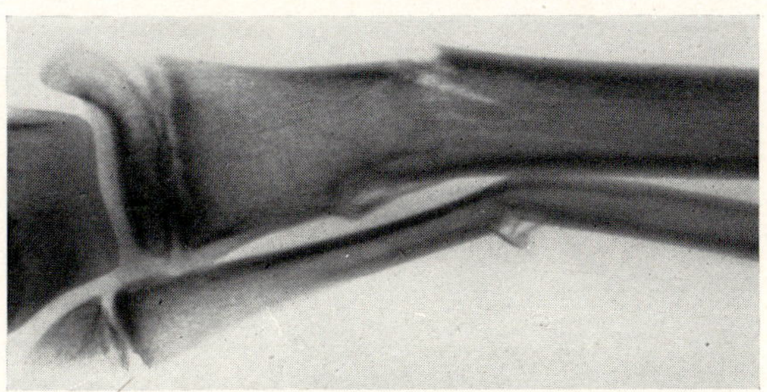

FIG. 120

A greenstick fracture of the tibia and fibula. Note how the cortex has broken on one side only and how it has buckled on the other. (Compare with Fig. 119).

network between the two bone ends. After a short while cartilage cells appear within this network and come to occupy the interval between the bone ends and beneath the raised periosteum. Within about two weeks after the fracture, bone cells and calcium salts are laid down in the vicinity of these cartilage cells and this combination of connective tissue, cartilage, bone cells and calcium is known as *primary callus* which, because of its bone and calcium content becomes readily

visible in X-ray photographs taken about this time, and this constitutes the first radiological sign of healing. The formation of the primary callus proceeds for about eight to ten weeks, but in the majority of fractures it is essential that during this time complete immobilization of the broken bone ends should be maintained so that no movement shall interfere with its consolidation. Once the formation of the primary callus is complete, the fracture becomes sufficiently well ' buttressed ' and thus strong enough to allow a return to the normal use and activity of the injured limb. Over the succeeding months the collection of primary callus, which has effected union between the bone ends, is slowly reabsorbed and replaced by mature bone which is laid down in the usual lines of stress and strain. The subperiosteal new bone is absorbed and the normal contour of the bone restored so that about a year after the fracture has been sustained there is usually little or no radiological evidence of the original break.

In the case of a greenstick fracture (in which only one cortex of the bone is broken), the formation of primary callus is very much less in evidence and is revealed only as a deposition of new bone beneath that portion of the periosteum that has been raised from the bone as a result of the break. Immobilization, therefore, is seldom required for more than two to three weeks after which the resumption of full activity may be allowed.

The Principles of Treatment

Irrespective of the site of a fracture the treatment may be divided into three clear-cut stages:

1. Correction of any angulation or displacement or overlap of the two broken bone ends that may be present (*reduction*).
2. Maintenance of the reduced position until such time as union has taken place (*immobilization*).
3. Restoration of the function of the previously immobilized joints and muscles (*rehabilitation*).

1. REDUCTION.—Immediately consequent upon a fracture, the surrounding muscles enter into a state of involuntary contraction (known as reflex *spasm*) in an attempt to reduce movement at the fracture site and thus minimize the degree of pain and the likelihood of further damage to the bone and the

adjacent tissues. In order to manipulate the two ends of the broken bone into apposition, it is essential that this protective spasm should first be overcome, and it is for this reason that a general anaesthetic is always necessary. Once any significant degree of shock has been overcome by the appropriate treatment (see Chapter III) reduction of the fracture should be carried out under a general anaesthetic at the earliest opportunity.

2. IMMOBILIZATION.—In view of the fact that a bone is used primarily as a lever through which movement is effected at the associated joints, it is essential that in order to secure complete immobilization, the joint above and the joint below the fracture site should also be prevented from movement. A plaster of Paris cast is the most popular and effective method of immobilization and we shall consider its use together with other forms of splintage when dealing with the various individual fractures. Suffice it therefore at this point for us to consider one very important aspect of plaster of Paris technique. However expert the application of plaster of Paris may be, a small irregularity on the inside of the cast may often be present and by pressure on the skin cause a certain amount of discomfort. Complaint on the part of your patient of any such discomfort must always be regarded as of the greatest importance and *never* be lightly dismissed. If it is disregarded you may feel yourself to have been justified in a day or so when all discomfort has disappeared, but you must never lose sight of the fact that the subsequent absence of discomfort is not due to a more comfortable accommodation of the limb within the plaster but to actual *death* of the affected piece of skin and the sensory nerve endings. Thus when the cast is eventually removed you may be faced with a deep, ragged and ulcerating *plaster sore* which will require weeks of treatment before it can be persuaded to heal. It is for this reason that any discomfort beneath a newly applied plaster of Paris cast which lasts for more than a few hours, should be reported *at once* and a ' window ' cut in the plaster in order to inspect the skin. In addition a careful watch should always be maintained on the colour of the skin at the distal extremity of the plaster, for if the plaster is too tight or if there is increased swelling at the fracture site following manipulative reduction, then the venous return from the extremity will be impeded and the foot or hand (as the case

may be) will become increasingly blue and swollen. In such an eventuality the plaster should be split from end to end and its margins gently separated in order to increase the capacity of the cast.

In very rare instances when repeated manipulations have failed to secure a satisfactory reduction of the fracture it may become necessary to effect reduction by an open operation at the fracture site (open reduction), and occasionally it may become necessary to maintain the reduced position by the application of a non-corrosive metal plate secured to each component of the fracture by non-corrosive metal screws (internal fixation).

3. REHABILITATION.—As a result of immobilization the joints are liable to stiffen and the muscles are liable to waste and weaken from disuse, but as a rule these two legacies of immobilization are soon overcome by the child's natural ebullience following resumed activity. In certain instances, however, it may be necessary for additional assistance to be given in the form of supervised exercises and faradic stimulation of muscle groups before full restoration of function and power is achieved. Occasionally, and especially is this so following fractures of the lower limb, you will come across children who are extremely chary and at times desperately afraid of using the limb again. This is not altogether surprising when you remember that the last time the child used the affected limb was at the time the fracture was sustained, and therefore considerable patience may need to be exercised before the child's confidence in his or her previously injured member is fully restored.

Compound Fractures

A compound fracture is one in which the skin over the fracture site has been broken and a communication established between the fracture and the exterior. The most important aspect in the management of these fractures is the *prevention of infection*. As soon as possible after the injury, large doses of intramuscular penicillin should be administered and a prophylactic dose of anti-tetanus serum (and in certain instances antigas gangrene serum) should also be given. Once any significant degree of shock has been overcome, the wound edges should be excised under a general anaesthetic and all dead and dying tissue together with any foreign material should be gently

removed. Following this the wound edges are loosely approximated with non-absorbable sutures and thereafter the fracture should be treated along the lines we have already indicated. Penicillin should be administered for at least five days, after which it may be discontinued if no evidence of infection such as an increased pulse rate, elevation of the temperature or an increase in local pain has occurred.

INDIVIDUAL FRACTURES

The following are the commonest fractures that you will encounter.

The Clavicle

The fracture site is usually situated in the mid-shaft of the bone and there may or may not be some overlap of the fragments. In order to secure absolute immobilization of the fracture it would be necessary to enclose the whole arm, the shoulder and the upper chest, in plaster of Paris but as the clavicle fortunately heals satisfactorily without such rigid immobilization, all that is necessary is that the arm should be rested in a sling or a 'collar and cuff' and that the shoulders should be braced back in order to prevent overlap of the fracture. This may be accomplished either by a 'figure-of-eight' bandage applied to include both shoulders or by placing a soft padded ring around each shoulder and tying them tightly together across the child's back. In either case the bandage or rings should be removed at least once a day in order to attend to the toilette of the skin of the armpit which is especially prone to become sore and excoriated. After two to three weeks the figure-of-eight bandage (or the rings) may be discarded and the arm merely rested in a sling for a further week, after which no further treatment is necessary. Greenstick fractures of the clavicle do not require the shoulders to be braced back as the fracture is an incomplete one. All that is necessary is that the arm on the affected side should be rested in a sling for about two weeks after which full activity may be resumed.

The Shaft of the Humerus

Fractures of the mid-shaft of the humerus also heal remarkably well in spite of inadequate immobilization. Two slabs

of plaster of Paris should be applied to each side of the upper arm and held in place by a cotton bandage, and the lower arm should be suspended in a collar and cuff (*not* in a sling) so that any overlap of the fragments will slowly be reduced by the weight of the elbow and forearm hanging from the collar and cuff. The fracture is usually sufficiently stable after four to five weeks to allow the resumption of normal use.

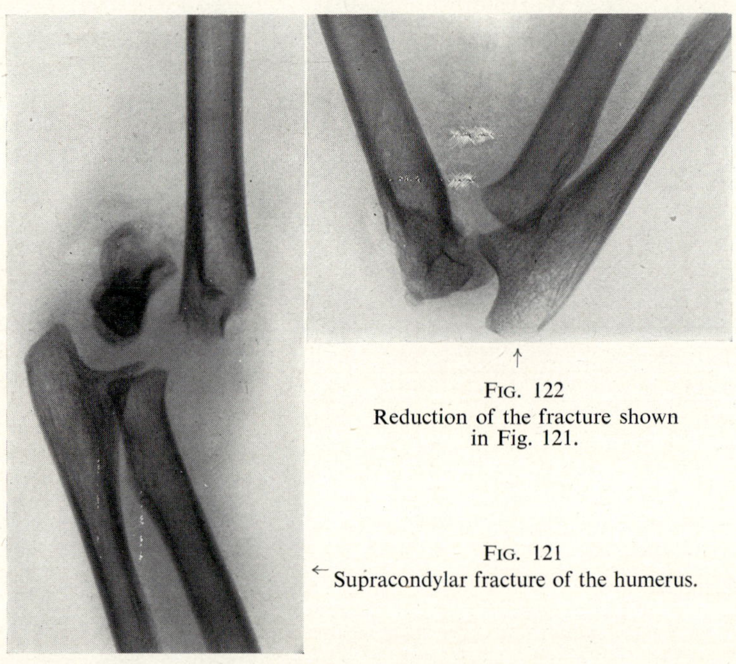

Fig. 122
Reduction of the fracture shown
in Fig. 121.

Fig. 121
Supracondylar fracture of the humerus.

Supracondylar Fracture of the Humerus

This is one of the most important and potentially one of the most dangerous fractures with which you will ever have to deal. It is attended by gross swelling and deformity in the region of the elbow, the fracture site being situated at the lower end of the humerus just above the condyles which are displaced backwards and upwards (Fig. 121). Reduction should be carried out as soon as possible after the injury and, in order that full function of the elbow may ultimately be obtained, accurate reposition of the fragments is essential. Once reduction has been effected the arm should be slung in a collar and cuff with the elbow flexed to an angle less than 90° (Fig. 122). Although some

authorities prefer to place a plaster of Paris slab from the upper arm to the knuckles this expedient is not necessary, as with the elbow in the flexed position the triceps muscle behind the fracture is put on the stretch and thus effectively prevents redisplacement of the fracture. Active finger and shoulder exercises should be practised each day and when after about three weeks all traces of swelling have disappeared, active movements of the elbow joint may then be commenced. A full range of movement is seldom obtained at the elbow joint before two to three months after the injury and may at times be delayed even longer; but in those cases where accurate reposition of the fragments has not been obtained or when elbow movements have been allowed before the swelling at the elbow has disappeared, then a permanent limitation of elbow movement is the inevitable result.

COMPLICATIONS.—In a small percentage of supracondylar fractures, the brachial artery may also be damaged by the broken bone ends and as a result enter into a state of *spasm*. This spasm not only obliterates the lumen of the brachial vessel itself so that the blood-flow within it is stopped but it also extends into the branches of the artery both above and below the site of the fracture (the collateral circulation), with the result that the whole of the forearm and the hand is deprived of its arterial blood supply. Such a complication is liable to arise up to forty-eight hours after the injury and most commonly occurs within the first twelve to twenty-four hours. It is revealed by a deathly pallor of the hand and forearm and a complete absence of arterial pulsation. In a very short while (as little as ten to twelve hours) both the extensor and flexor muscles of the forearm and hand begin to die and are rapidly replaced by fibrous tissue which shortly but inexorably contracts to produce a hideous, rigid, functionless, claw-like deformity of the hand known as Volkmann's Ischaemic Contracture. Treatment of such a contracture, once established, is of little or no avail; it is the rigid and almost ceaseless observation of the hand and radial pulse during the forty-eight hours following reduction of the fracture that is the only sure method of preventing the onset of this irreversible complication. It is therefore in this respect that the nurse carries a very high degree of responsibility. Once spasm has occurred a true surgical emergency is at hand and the surgeon in charge of the

case must be summoned *at once*. The arm should be taken down out of the collar and cuff and warm compresses applied to the antecubital fossa. This only very occasionally has any beneficial effect and if the colour of the skin of the hand does not improve, and there is no return of pulsation in the radial artery, open operation at the site of the fracture should at once be performed under a general anaesthetic. The artery in spasm is laid bare and a local application of an anti-spasmodic drug such as papaverine, should be applied to its walls. In the vast majority of cases this is sufficient to relieve the spasm within two to three minutes; if, however, this is without effect then that portion of the artery in spasm must be excised between ligatures. This has the effect of releasing the other arteries in the vicinity (the collateral circulation) from their spasm and will allow arterial blood to flow into the forearm and hand once more. The wound is then closed and thereafter treatment is precisely the same as in the uncomplicated fracture.

The Radius and Ulna

Greenstick fracture of the shafts of the radius and ulna are among the commonest fractures of childhood. Under a general anaesthetic the bones are bent back into normal alignment and immobilized in a plaster of Paris cast reaching from the upper arm down to the knuckles, with the elbow flexed to a right angle. This should be worn in a sling for four to six weeks after which it is removed and exercises instituted in order to restore full movements in the previously immobilized elbow and wrist joints. Fractures of the shafts of both bones complicated by displacement and overlap are less common than the greenstick variety and are much more difficult to reduce. If manipulative reduction fails to secure a normal alignment, then open reduction may become necessary and, in certain instances, internal fixation may also be indicated. Following such procedures the limb is immobilized in precisely the same manner as we have already outlined, but the period of immobilization in these cases depends upon the degree of callus formation revealed in X-ray photographs which may be longer delayed than in the closed type of fracture.

The Femur

In childhood, fracture of the femur occurs most commonly

at or about the mid-shaft of the bone. The thigh is grossly swollen, deformed and shortened, and the limb distal to the fracture is always rotated outwards. As the mid-shaft is impalpable due to the thickness of the surrounding muscles, accurate alignment of the two bone ends by manipulative means is usually difficult or impossible, and it is for this reason that

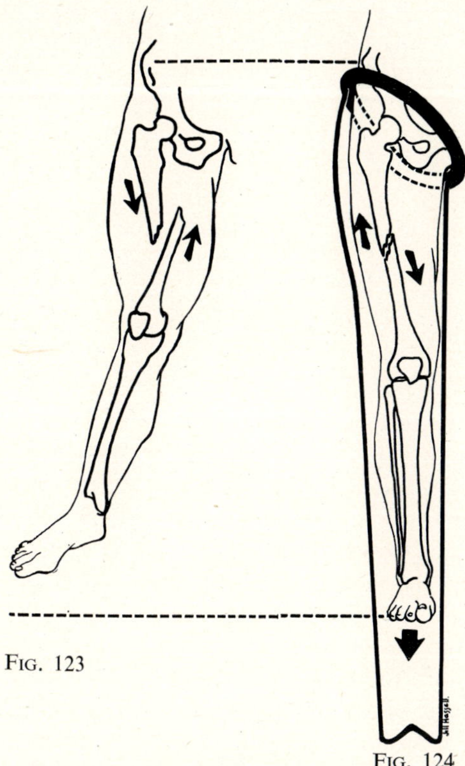

Fig. 123

Fig. 124

Fig. 123.—Fracture of the femur. Note the deformity, shortening and external rotation of the limb. Fig. 124.— Reduction of the fracture effected by the skin traction pulling the lower fragment away from the steadied pelvis.

fractures of the femur are most satisfactorily treated by skin traction in a Thomas splint. For some reason the mechanism and application of a Thomas splint invariably causes the nurse an unnecessary amount of difficulty to understand, and it will be as well to digress at this point in order to stress the simplicity of its use and its effectiveness in the treatment of fractures of the femur. As we have already mentioned, the basic features

of successful reduction of a displaced fracture is firstly to overcome the spasm of the surrounding muscles and secondly to maintain the corrected position until union has occurred. By reference to Figs. 123 and 124 you will see how this is effected by the use of the Thomas splint. Fig. 123 illustrates

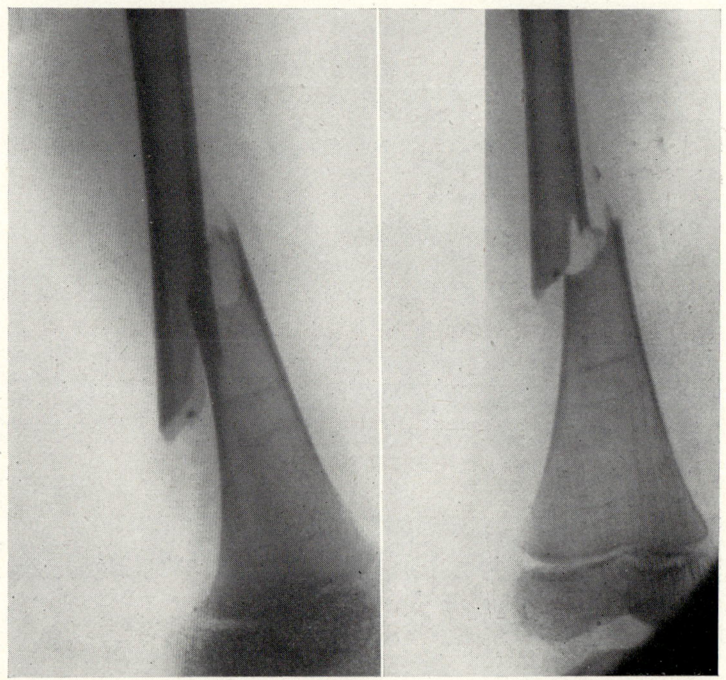

<table>
<tr><td>FIG. 125</td><td>FIG. 126</td></tr>
<tr><td>Fracture of the mid-shaft of the femur. Note the degree of overlap and the rotation of the lower fragment.</td><td>Reduction of the fracture by skin traction.</td></tr>
</table>

the typical position of the limb following the injury and the arrows indicate the pull and the effect of the surrounding muscle spasm. In order to overcome this spasm, the pelvis is held steady by the engagement of the ring of the splint against the rim of the pelvis and the ischial tuberosity (see Fig. 124) and skin traction applied to the limb distal to the fracture site overcomes the pull of the muscle spasm and effects reduction of the fracture with restitution of the normal length of the limb. Once a satisfactory reduction of the fracture has been obtained in this manner (Figs. 125 and 126), the limb is supported between

the shafts of the splint by canvas or felt 'stretchers' and is lightly bandaged on to the splint in order to prevent any rotation. The splint is then suspended from an overhead beam (Fig. 127) and thereafter the child should be encouraged to move about in the bed as much as possible so that, with the exception of the fractured limb, all the other muscles in the body are kept in active use. X-ray examination of the fracture site

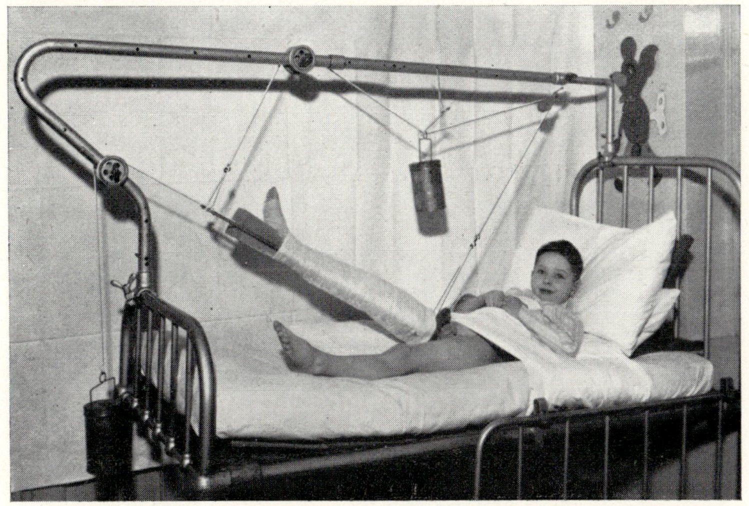

FIG. 127
The suspended Thomas splint.

should be carried out in the ward by a portable X-ray apparatus at weekly intervals in order to reveal any overdistraction or overlap of the fragments that may occur, in which case the weights attached to the skin traction should be adjusted accordingly and the correction verified by further X-ray examination. Union usually occurs within about eight weeks after which the splint and traction may be discontinued. The child should then be instructed in exercises designed to restore the movements in the previously immobilized hip and knee joints, and after a week of these exercises carried out in bed the child may be allowed to walk for increasing periods each day until full ambulation is achieved.

Children under two to three years of age are not easily nursed in a Thomas splint and are best treated by the method

known as 'gallows traction'. Skin traction is applied to both lower limbs and the attached cords led over pulleys, as shown in Fig. 128, to weights which are just sufficiently heavy to lift the child's buttocks off the bed. In this way the counter-traction of the body-weight acting against the pull of the skin

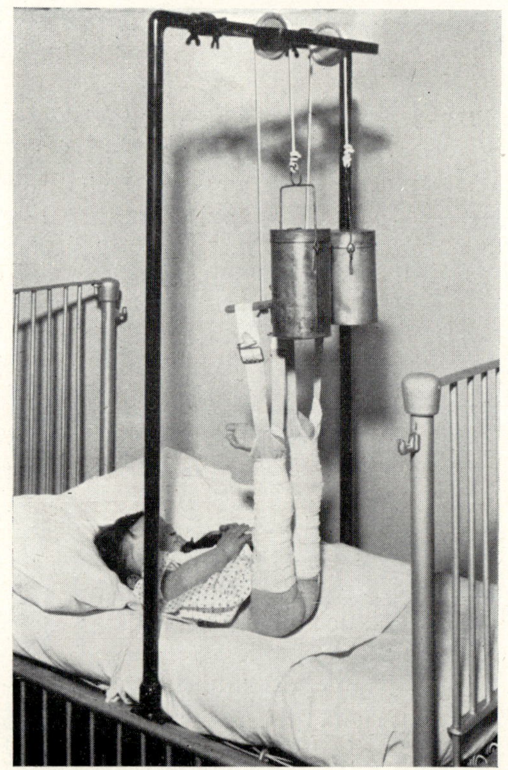

FIG. 128

Gallows traction. Note that the buttocks are just lifted off the bed.

traction is sufficient to effect and maintain a satisfactory reduction of the fracture. Union is usually complete within four to five weeks after which the traction may be discontinued.

The Tibia and Fibula

Fracture of the tibia and fibula may be complete or green-stick. In either case the fracture should be reduced under a general anaesthetic and a plaster of Paris cast applied from the

upper thigh to the heads of the metatarsal bones, with the knee joint in 5° of flexion and the ankle joint at 90° of dorsiflexion. A heel may be applied to the plaster and walking allowed after a few days. If, however, the fracture is oblique rather than transverse, weight bearing on the limb should be postponed until X-ray examination shows healing to be well advanced.

Displacement of the Epiphyses

Although almost any epiphysis in the body may be displaced as a result of injury, the two most common situations are the lower radial epiphysis and the lower tibial epiphysis. Treatment in either case merely consists of manipulation of the displaced epiphysis into the normal position and subsequent immobilization for a period of two to three weeks. Very occasionally displacement of either of these epiphyses may be complicated by premature fusion between the epiphysis and the metaphysis with consequent cessation of growth. This may cause local deformity due to the continued growth of the unaffected bone (i.e. the ulna or the fibula) and if severe the deformity may have to be rectified by a reconstructive operation.

INJURIES TO JOINTS

Joint injuries may be classified as being *penetrating* or *non-penetrating*, the former term implying that a communication has been established between the joint cavity and the exterior. Although either type of injury may conceivably occur in any joint in the body, they are most commonly encountered in the knee joint because of its superficial and exposed situation.

Non-penetrating Injuries

These are usually due either to a blow or a fall on to the knee and as a result of the state of inflammation that is produced by the trauma, the synovial membrane lining the joint cavity exudes a large quantity of fluid (an effusion, or ' water on the knee ') which may or may not contain a proportion of blood. The joint becomes obviously distended and movements are painful and limited. The limb should be rested (preferably by bed rest) and the joint covered with a thick layer of wool and a firmly applied crepe bandage followed by another layer of

wool and bandaging (a Robert Jones type of bandage) in order to compress the joint and thus restrict as far as possible the production of fluid within it. After a few days when the distension of the joint begins to decrease and movements become less painful, graduated exercises and increasing periods of walking may be allowed. Full activity should not be resumed until all traces of the effusion have disappeared.

HAEMOPHILIA.—This is a rare form of inherited abnormality which only occurs in the male members of succeeding generations. It is characterized by a considerable increase in the clotting time of the blood (normally about three minutes) with the result that minor injuries such as cuts and abrasions fail to seal themselves by the formation of a blood clot but instead continue to bleed. For this reason children with haemophilia who sustain a seemingly trivial blow to the knee are prone to develop profuse bleeding within the joint cavity. The same treatment that we have already mentioned should be employed but the period of rest is necessarily much longer in order to reduce to a minimum the chances of renewed bleeding.

Penetrating Injuries

Penetrating injuries usually result from a fall on to a sharp object such as a piece of glass. The wound is usually quite small and apparently insignificant but if the tissues immediately around it are gently compressed a few bubbles of air and one or two drops of thick yellow synovial fluid may escape from it thus revealing the true nature and extent of the injury. Sometimes it may be difficult or impossible to decide whether a wound is in fact penetrating or non-penetrating and, in such an instance, in view of the great dangers associated with the establishment of an infection within a joint cavity (see below— Suppurative Arthritis), it is essential that the wound should be treated as a penetrating injury. As soon as the diagnosis of an obvious or possible penetrating injury has been made, intramuscular penicillin should be commenced at once and under a general anaesthetic the wound should be cleanly excised and sutured. In addition, some authorities advise the instillation of 30 to 50,000 units of penicillin directly into the joint cavity. Following these measures the whole limb should be lightly secured to a plaster of Paris back slab. Thereafter an hourly record of the pulse and a four-hourly temperature

18

chart should be maintained and the joint inspected daily in order to determine whether further intra-articular injections of penicillin are necessary. The intra-muscular penicillin injections should be continued for at least five days or until the temperature has been normal for forty-eight hours or more.

Providing this form of treatment is instituted within eight to twelve hours following injury, a full recovery of function at the affected knee joint may be confidently expected. Treatment commenced after this time interval, however, is likely to be complicated by the establishment of infection within the joint cavity and the possibility of a suppurative arthritis and ultimate ankylosis of the joint.

INFECTIONS OF BONES

Acute Osteomyelitis

Acute osteomyelitis is an acute suppurative infection of bone which always commences in the metaphysis; the commonest situations being the upper end of the tibia, the lower end of the femur, the upper end of the femur and the upper end of the humerus, in that order of frequency. The commonest infecting organism is the Staphylococcus aureus which is generally considered to gain access to the bone by blood-stream spread from a distant septic focus such as a boil or infected skin abrasion. It is for this reason that the condition is sometimes referred to as acute haematogenous osteomyelitis. The reason why the metaphysis is always the site of the disease is thought to be due to blood-stream infection of a small metaphyseal haematoma in which the organisms thrive with the rapid production of an abscess. As the metaphysis contains the thin-walled blood sinusoids of the richly vascular red bone marrow, the formation of a small haematoma due to rupture of these delicate vessels frequently follows minor trauma and this is thought to account for the fact that osteomyelitis is very much more common in boys (who are reputed to injure themselves more frequently than girls).

Once pus has been formed in the metaphysis it tracks through the Haversian system of the cortex to form a subperiosteal abscess (Fig. 129), and this abscess may in turn rupture the periosteum and allow the pus to enter the subcutaneous tissues.

Pus may also spread along the medulla of the bone or in the direction of the epiphyseal plate of cartilage, but this latter structure effectively prevents its entry into the adjacent joint.

Clinical Features

At first the child may complain of little more than a mild ache in the region of the affected metaphysis but within about twenty-four hours the pain becomes intense in character. The overlying skin becomes acutely inflamed and slightly swollen and the limb is held desperately still in order to prevent the excruciating pain that accompanies movement. The temperature is elevated to 103° to 104° F. and in fulminating cases may be even higher when the child's behaviour may border on delirium. Any attempt to examine the limb is met with screams of protest; the inflamed area is exquisitely tender and as a rule there is an effusion into the adjacent joint.

Treatment

As a large percentage of cases of acute osteomyelitis are accompanied by a septicaemia, a blood culture should always be performed before treatment is commenced in order to determine the nature of the causative organism and its sensitivity to the various antibiotic agents. As soon as this has been done intra-muscular penicillin in doses of two million units per day should

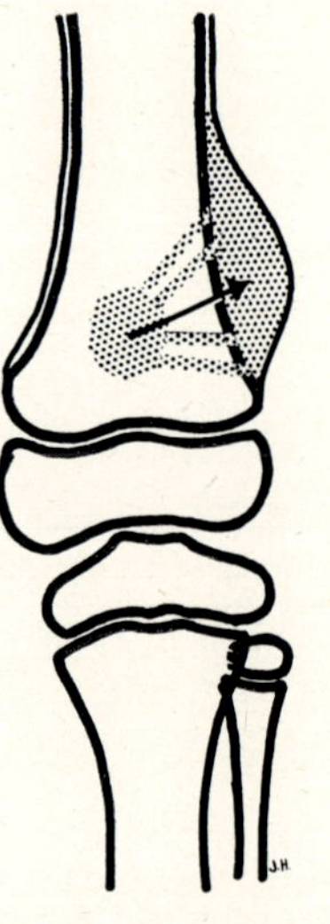

Fig. 129

To illustrate the origin and the spread of the pus in osteomyelitis of the lower end of the femur. Note the subperiosteal abscess.

be commenced and the affected limb put at rest in a plaster of Paris back slab. It is at this point that authorities are liable to diverge in their opinion as to the subsequent course of treatment. There is a strong tendency at the present time to withhold any form of operative treatment other than the aspiration of a subcutaneous abscess should it be formed, and to rely entirely upon rest of the limb and the bacteriocidal effect of penicillin or other antibiotics. Be that as it may, the commonest form of treatment that you will see carried out is incision over the affected bone, evacuation of

the sub-periosteal abscess and the drilling of a series of holes in the cortex in order to assist the drainage of pus, after which the wound is loosely approximated with non-absorbable sutures and the limb once more immobilized on a plaster of Paris back slab. In fulminating cases this form of treatment should obviously be carried out as soon as possible, but in less severe cases operation is often postponed for twenty-four hours in order to estimate the effect that penicillin has had upon the infection. If at the end of this period there is not a substantial improvement then operation is carried out forthwith. Irrespective of the particular course of treatment that is followed, penicillin should be continued for a minimum period of three weeks, but even so, it is a regrettable fact that the disease, however expertly treated, is particularly prone to enter into a chronic phase which is characterized by chronic bone abscess formation and periods of acute exacerbation of the infection, sometimes for many years to come.

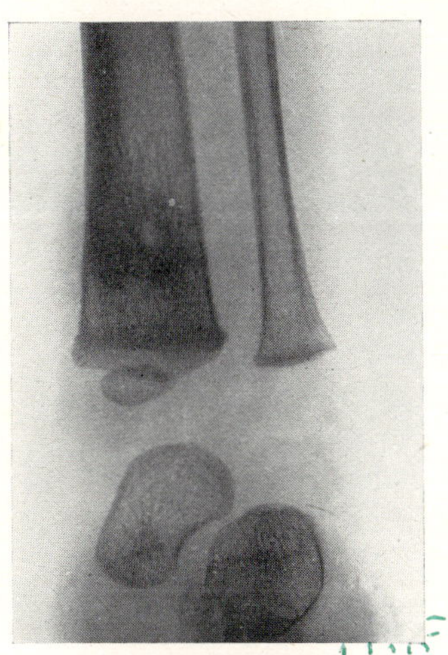

FIG. 130

A small bone abscess resulting from neonatal umbilical sepsis.

Osteomyelitis occurring within the first few weeks of life is invariably due to a metastatic spread of infection from an infected umbilical stump (Fig. 130). Operation is never indicated in these cases as the condition rapidly subsides following the administration of antibiotic drugs.

Chronic Osteomyelitis

Chronic osteomyelitis is invariably a legacy of the acute phase of the disease. The bone forms a thick wall of dense bone around the surviving focus of infection (a Brodie's abscess), which, in view of its liability to undergo exacerbations of acute inflammation, remains as a constant liability to the individual for many years. In addition fragments of bone, which died during the acute phase of the disease (sequestra), may take many months to separate from the living bone following which they slowly make their way to the surface

through which they eventually discharge themselves, leaving behind a chronic sinus which may discharge pus for many months to come. The treatment of chronic osteomyelitis is often a most disappointing undertaking and there are many diverse procedures used in an attempt to eradicate the infection, such as curettage, excision (when feasible) and saucerization of the Brodie's abscess.

Occasionally a chronic pyogenic bone infection may arise without a previous acute phase and, in order to distinguish this variety of abscess from the one we have just described, it is best referred to as a *chronic staphylococcal bone abscess*. As a rule the child complains of little more than a mild intermittent ache in the region of the abscess, the true diagnosis only being revealed on X-ray examination. According to its situation within the bone, the abscess may be excised intact or opened and curetted under a 'penicillin cover'. These measures are usually sufficient to eradicate this type of chronic bone abscess once and for all.

INFECTIONS OF JOINTS

Suppurative Arthritis

Suppurative arthritis is an acute pyogenic infection of a joint cavity and may result either from a neglected penetrating injury; from the extension of an acute osteomyelitis (when the metaphysis of the bone is within the joint cavity, such as the head of the femur or the head of the humerus), or it may be due to a metastatic infection from a pre-existing septic process elsewhere in the body. The joint becomes rapidly distended with pus, the capsule and ligaments become oedematous and softened, and may give way to allow pus to burst through them into the subcutaneous tissues. The articular cartilage is rapidly destroyed and the bone ends laid bare so that following recovery, bony ankylosis is an inevitable sequel. In addition there is always the possibility that the infected joint may itself be the origin of further metastatic infections to other parts of the body.

CLINICAL FEATURES.—Once pus has formed within the cavity of the joint the child rapidly becomes very ill and the temperature swings dramatically. The affected limb is held quite still and any attempt at moving the joint causes intense

pain. The joint itself becomes distended and acutely tender and the skin over it becomes acutely inflamed. In view of the possibility of subsequent ankylosis of the joint the limb should always be nursed in the position which will be most useful to the child should this complication finally occur (the position of function).

Treatment

The affected joint should be placed at rest, and then aspirated, firstly, in order to obtain a specimen of the pus for identification of the causative organism and its sensitivity to the various antibiotics, and secondly, to reduce the tension within the joint cavity. Before the aspirating needle is withdrawn, 100 to 150,000 units of penicillin should be introduced into the joint and intramuscular penicillin also commenced in doses of 2 million units per day. Aspiration and penicillin replacement should be continued each day or every other day until there is no evidence of infection within the joint. In view of the rapidity with which disintegration is liable to proceed within the joint structures, it cannot be stressed too frequently that treatment in this condition is of the utmost urgency.

Transient Arthritis

This condition, the precise nature of which is still undetermined, most frequently affects the hip joints in children usually between about five and ten years of age. As a rule the child complains of an aching pain in the region of the hip which is usually worse at the end of the day and which is often relieved by the night's rest. All movements at the hip joint are restricted and painful and the temperature may be elevated to 99° to 100° F., but apart from these features no other clinical or radiological abnormality can be discovered. Quite frequently there is a history of a sore throat a few weeks before the onset of the hip symptoms, and it is this fact that lends support to the theory that a transient arthritis is a very mild metastatic infection occurring in the head or neck of the femur, which causes a temporary effusion into the joint. Although some authorities advise the systemic adminstration of penicillin, it is doubtful if this is always necessary, for, as a general rule, the symptoms and signs usually disappear of their own accord after one to two weeks of rest. It is, however, important that

X-ray examination of the hip should always be repeated following recovery, for it is not unknown for an early atypical tuberculous infection of the hip to masquerade under the guise of a transient arthritis.

OSTEOCHONDRITIS

Osteochondritis is a disorder of the epiphysis of a growing bone. Although the precise nature of the condition is still undetermined, it is generally believed to be due, not to an inflammatory condition as its name implies, but rather to a temporary interference with the vascularity of the epiphyseal region which results in *degeneration* and *softening* of its bony structure (avascular necrosis). This is followed after a variable period of time by revascularization of the epiphysis, with subsequent *regeneration* and *hardening* of the bony structure. In the case of weight-bearing bones the period of epiphyseal softening is liable to result in its compression and deformity, and treatment is therefore directed to the relief of this squashing effect until such time as revascularization has occurred and the bony structure has once more become sufficiently strong to withstand the effects of weight-bearing without compression of its substance.

The condition commonly affects boys more than girls and usually occurs between about five and twelve years of age. Although almost any epiphysis in the body may be affected it is the upper femoral epiphysis, the navicular bone, the epiphyses of the tibial tubercle, the calcaneum and the vertebrae that are affected sufficiently frequently to merit individual mention.

The Upper Femoral Epiphysis (Perthes' Disease)

The commonest mode of onset of Perthes' disease is by the gradual appearance of an unexplained limp. Pain, which may occasionally be severe, is not as a rule a predominant feature of the condition nor is there any significant wasting of the thigh muscles (see Chapter XIV, Tuberculosis of the Hip). Most movements at the hip-joint itself may be present to a greater or lesser degree, but it is the rotatory movements that are always absent. The true diagnosis is only revealed by the X-ray appearances which show a patchy, increased density of the

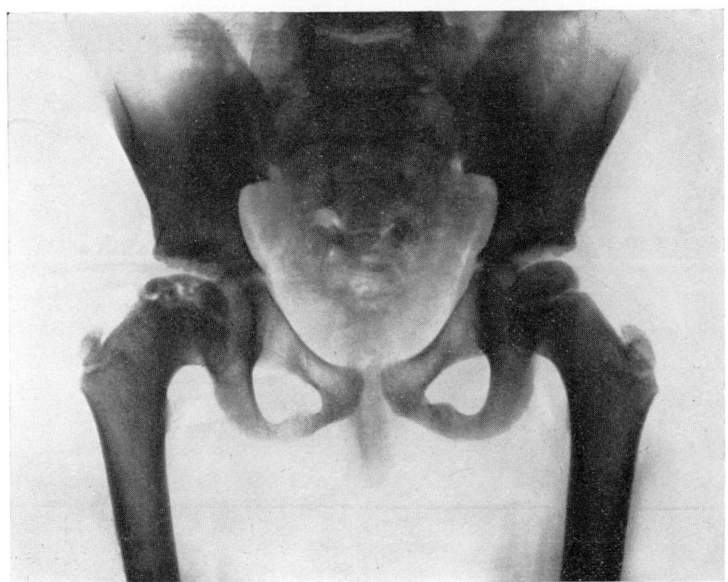

Fig. 131

Perthes' disease of the right hip.

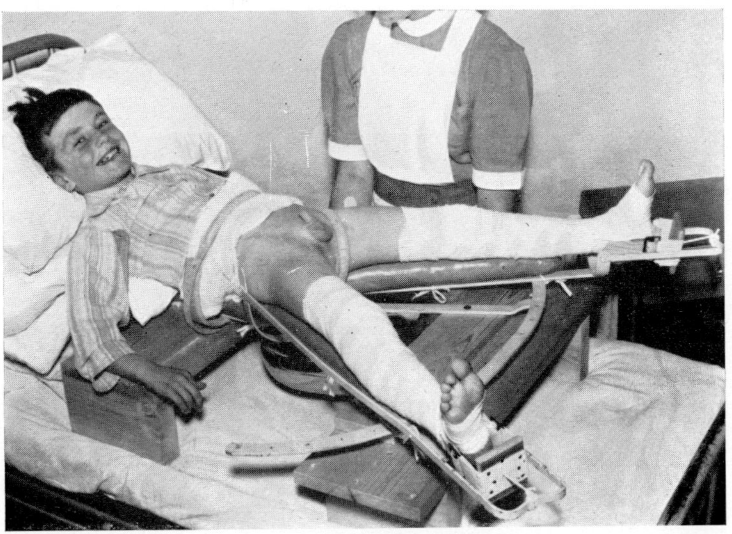

Fig. 132

Perthes' disease of the right hip treated on a Robert Jones abduction frame.

epiphysis (apparent fragmentation) together with a diminution of its depth, and deformity of its outline (Fig. 131).

Treatment is designed both to put the joint at rest and to effect a distraction of the head of the femur away from the acetabulum in order to prevent compression and deformity of the softened epiphysis, and this is most satisfactorily carried out on a Robert Jones abduction frame (Fig. 132). As the period of epiphyseal softening in Perthes' disease usually lasts about a year to eighteen months it is essential that the child should remain on the frame for the whole of this period until X-ray examination reveals evidence of recalcification of the epiphysis. For this reason it is preferable that treatment should be carried out at a 'long-term' ortho-paedic hospital where educa-tional facilities are available. Once there is evidence that revascularization of the epiphysis is well advanced, the child may be removed from the frame and allowed to become ambulant in a weight-relieving caliper until such time as the epiphysis is considered to be strong enough to withstand the compressional strains of normal activity.

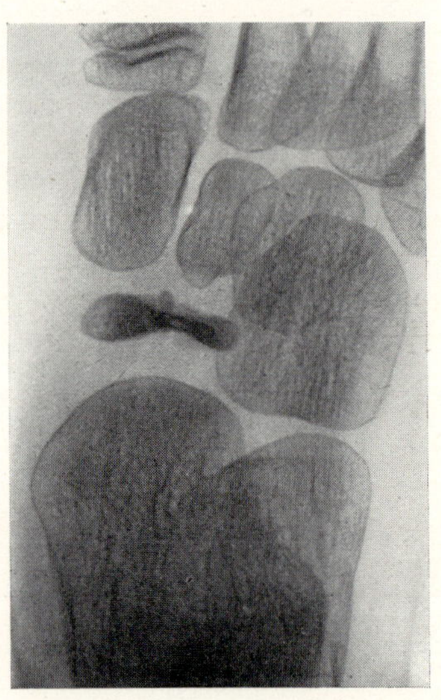

FIG. 133

Kohler's disease of the navicular bone. Note the compression and the apparently increased density of the bone due to its collapse.

The Navicular Bone (Köhler's Disease)

Osteochondritis in this situation (Fig. 133) commonly presents with a slight limp in the affected limb and a mild degree of pain over the medial aspect of the foot. Rest in bed for a few days is usually sufficient to relieve the symptoms, after which the child may be allowed to resume full activity. Some authorities prefer to incorporate a support in the shoe for the longitudinal arch of the foot but it is doubtful if this measure supplies sufficient benefit to be worth-while.

The Tibial Tubercle (Osgood-Schlatter's Disease)

In this form of the condition the child usually complains of pain in one or both limbs in the vicinity of the tibial tubercle, which is accentuated by exercise. In very mild cases restricted activity and the forbidding of organized games is usually sufficient to procure relief of the symptoms. In more severe cases bed rest for a few weeks is indicated and occasionally it may be necessary to immobilize the affected limb or limbs in a plaster of Paris cast for a month before the symptoms disappear.

The Calcaneum

The posterior epiphysis of the calcaneum when affected by osteochondritis, causes the child a pain in the heel which is usually made worse by exercise. In severe cases it may be necessary to rest the affected foot completely either by bed rest or by immobilization in a walking plaster of Paris cast, but as a general rule the symptoms may be relieved by a soft sorbo pad worn immediately beneath the heel and by the avoidance of organized games.

The Vertebral Epiphyses (Scheuermann's Disease)

Osteochondritis of the epiphyses of the upper thoracic vertebrae is most commonly encountered at about sixteen to seventeen years of age, and produces a kyphotic curve in the region of the upper thoracic spine. An aching pain is usually present in the back especially towards the end of the day and treatment is directed to improvement of the tone and strength of the paravertebral muscles by back extension exercises. In very severe cases it may, first of all, be necessary to overcome the deformity by a period of recumbency in the corrected position.

TUMOURS OF THE BONE

Osteoma

An osteoma is a small benign tumour which is usually situated towards one end of a long bone. It consists for the most part of cancellous tissue, its most prominent portion being capped by a small plaque of cartilage. Although the tumour

may commence growing in early childhood it usually remains undetected until adolescence or early adult life when it may cause some mild discomfort. It is readily visualized on X-ray examination and, if causing symptoms, it may be easily removed by surgical excision.

The presence of multiple osteomas, each arising from the metaphysis of the long bones, is indicative of an uncommon familial condition known as *diaphyseal aclasis*. The tumours seldom grow to a large size and treatment is confined to removal of those that become troublesome.

Osteogenic Sarcoma

This is one of the most malignant tumours that you will ever encounter. Although fortunately rare in incidence, it is most frequently situated at the lower end of the femur in children of about ten years of age and upwards, and it invariably draws attention to itself by the onset of pain in the vicinity of

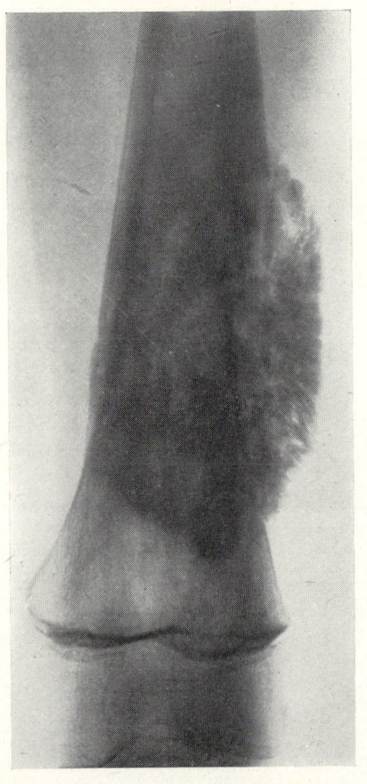

Fig. 134

Osteogenic sarcoma of the lower end of the femur.

growth. This is later followed by the appearance of an obvious swelling, the skin over which is frequently warmer than that of the rest of the limb. X-ray examination shows a mass of new bone arranged in radiating layers (the sun-ray appearance) growing outwards from the cortex (Fig. 134).

The treatment of osteogenic sarcoma is still depressingly disappointing. Some authorities favour immediate amputation of the limb well above the site of the growth, whereas others advise a pre-operative course of X-irradiation. In the majority of cases, however, irrespective of the method of treatment employed, metastases shortly appear in the lungs and death is the inevitable outcome.

Ewing's Tumour

This is a very rare tumour of bone which, unlike the others that we have mentioned, always occurs in the diaphysis. The predominant symptom is pain in the mid-shaft of a long bone, usually the tibia and X-ray examination reveals a number of layers of sub-periosteal new bone arranged around the sides of the cortex (the ' onion peel ' appearance). The tumour is acutely sensitive to X-irradiation and rapidly disappears following a course of treatment. Subsequent recurrence of the growth is, however, likely to occur, each recurrence showing a progressively increased resistance to X-irradiation. Some authorities prefer to amputate the limb whereas others rely upon the effects of irradiation. In either case, however, the prognosis is extremely poor.

CHAPTER XIV

THE SURGICAL ASPECTS OF TUBERCULOSIS

FOR a full survey and description of the vast subject of tuberculosis the reader should consult suitable works of medical reference. Our present concern in this chapter is to consider only those aspects of the disease that are amenable to surgical treatment; that is to say, tuberculous infections of the cervical lymph glands, the genito-urinary system and bones and joints—manifestations of the disease which are often grouped together under the collective and somewhat proprietary term of Surgical Tuberculosis. It is most important for you to realize, however, that although surgery is of value in these conditions, it still remains a subsidiary adjuvant to the long term medical management of the disease. In order to place our considerations in the correct perspective we must first make a brief summary of the mode of onset and subsequent spread of tuberculous infection together with the tests that are commonly employed to confirm its presence, the drugs that are used to treat it and the methods of prevention that are in current use.

There are two types of the tubercle bacillus that produce the disease in mankind, the human type and the bovine type. They are indistinguishable both in their microscopic appearance and in their clinical effects, and can only be differentiated from each other by their individual growth characteristics on culture media. The incidence of the bovine as opposed to the human type of infection, varies from district to district and country to country and depends largely upon the number of tuberculous cattle in a given community and the number of persons who habitually consume the milk from such cattle without the precaution of previous sterilization or pasteurization. In Scotland, for instance, the incidence of the bovine type of infection is still unusually high compared with other areas of the British Isles and in 1944 it amounted to 77 per cent of all cases of abdominal tuberculosis and tuberculosis of the cervical glands.

In order of frequency, the portal of entry of the tubercle bacillus into the body is through the lungs, the intestines, the nasopharynx and more rarely the skin. Once within the body the causative organism sets up the characteristic changes that we discussed in Chapter I, namely, tubercle formation, caseation, liquefaction (i.e. cold abscess formation) and in cases

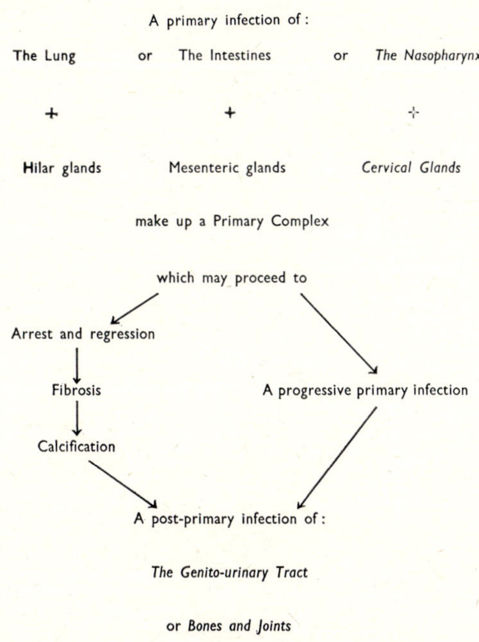

Fig. 135

The fate of the primary complex. (Italic letters denote " Surgical Tuberculosis ".)

where the infection is successfully resisted—fibrosis and subsequent calcification. From the primary site of infection wherever it may be, secondary involvement of the regional lymph glands invariably occurs and this association of the primary focus and secondary glandular involvement is known as the *primary complex*, the three principal examples being the lung and the hilar lymph glands, the intestines and the mesenteric lymph glands and the nasopharynx and the cervical lymph glands. The fate of the primary complex largely depends upon the success with which the resistance of the body can overcome the virulence of the infecting organisms. If this is completely

successful the primary complex undergoes arrest, regression and subsequent calcification (though you must recall that active organisms may lie dormant in centres of calcification for many years).   If it is less successful, then local advance of the disease will occur and the lesion become a *progressive primary infection*. The risk of dissemination of the infecting organisms by the blood-stream (haematogenous dissemination) is always present and although it is more likely to happen in the presence of a progressive primary lesion, it may also occur quite ' silently ' in cases where a primary focus is difficult or impossible to demonstrate by clinical or radiological means.   Such foci of infection occurring as the result of haematogenous spread are known as *postprimary* infections, the most important examples, from the *surgical point of view*, being tuberculosis of the genito-urinary tract and of bones and joints.

This sequence of events concerning the establishment of the tubercle bacillus within the body and the possibility of its subsequent dissemination is summarily depicted in Fig. 135.

AIDS TO DIAGNOSIS

Not infrequently it is difficult to differentiate the presenting symptoms and signs of a tuberculous infection from those of other pathological processes and it is for this reason that the following ancillary procedures are commonly employed in order to clarify the diagnosis.

(1) Tuberculin Testing

The substance used in these tests is a specially prepared extract of dead tubercle bacilli known as *old tuberculin* which, when applied to the skin of a child who has previously suffered a tuberculous infection causes an allergic reaction at the site of application.   Positive results, however, are not necessarily a direct indication either of the duration of the infection nor of its activity.   There are two forms of tuberculin testing in common use today:

(*a*) THE JELLY TEST.—Although not as reliable as the Mantoux test, this method is much easier to perform and is commonly used in mass surveys in order to discover an otherwise yet unrecognizable tuberculous infection, and in some Children's Hospitals it is performed as a routine on all children,

both in-patients and out-patients. The skin is thoroughly cleansed with acetone and when dry it is given five or six gentle strokes with abrasive ' Flourpaper '. After this, tuberculin jelly is applied to the skin and covered with a piece of dry lint which is secured with a strip of adhesive plaster. This is removed after forty-eight hours and the result read twenty-four hours later. So that the child shall not interfere with the dressing, the test is usually performed on the skin between the shoulder blades. A positive reaction is revealed by the presence of at least four vesicles at the site of application.

(*b*) THE MANTOUX TEST.—In this test either a solution of old tuberculin or the purified active principle of it (purified protein derivative—P.P.D.) is introduced into the superficial layers of the skin, 0·1 cubic centimetre of a 1 : 10,000 solution of old tuberculin or of 0·00002 P.P.D. being injected *intradermally* to raise a small weal on the flexor surface of the forearm. The test should be read seventy-two hours later, a positive result being an area of induration not less than 5 millimetres in diameter. If negative the test may be repeated using gradually increasing concentrations of the solution, up to 1 : 100.

(2) **Radiology**

As the primary focus of tuberculous infection is most commonly situated in the lungs, an X-ray of the chest should always be taken in all cases of suspected tuberculosis in order to detect either a ' healed ' primary focus or an active lesion. This should be followed by X-ray examination of the presenting situation of the disease. Very occasionally in tuberculosis of bones a plain X-ray photograph may fail to reveal any evidence of the disease, although its presence is clinically suspect. In this event a specialized form of X-ray examination known as a *tomogram* may be of great value. This consists of taking a series of X-ray photographs which are focused on to the bone at varying depths so that any minute focus of infection that is present will be revealed in one or more of the films.

(3) **Culture and Animal Inoculation**

The tubercle bacillus is notorious for its reluctance to grow on culture media and great difficulty is always experienced in persuading it to do so. For this reason the failure of growth

to occur is not sufficient evidence on which to exclude a tuberculous infection, but none the less when tuberculous material is available, culture of it should always be carried out for, should a positive growth occur, it is irrefutable evidence of the disease. In order to overcome the possibility of a misleading negative culture an emulsion of suspected tuberculous material should always be injected into the peritoneal cavity of a guinea-pig (an animal which is acutely susceptible to tuberculous infection). After a few weeks the animal is killed and if there were any tubercle bacilli (however few) in the injected material, the peritoneum will show the appearances of gross tuberculous peritonitis. This test is a far more reliable one than culture, and should always be employed when the diagnosis is in doubt and when suspected material is at hand.

(4) Biopsy

This procedure is of particular value in cases of enlarged cervical lymph glands when reasonable doubt exists as to the true cause of the enlargement. Under a general or local anaesthetic an easily accessible gland is excised after which the skin wound should be united by primary suture. Having been placed in a sterile container, it is sent *at once* to the pathological laboratory where half of it is used for culture and guinea-pig inoculation and the other half is prepared for microscopic examination. Biopsy is also occasionally carried out in suspected tuberculosis of the knee joint, when a portion of the synovial membrane or one of the regional lymph nodes may be excised and subjected to the same investigations we have just mentioned.

(5) The Examination of Fluids

The examination of fluids is carried out in order to discover the presence of the tubercle bacillus, for without its identification the diagnosis of early tuberculosis can never be considered to be proven. The same examination that we have already mentioned, namely, microscopic inspection, culture and guinea-pig inoculation are applied to the suspected fluid be it urine or aspirated fluid from an abscess or distended joint. In the case of urine it is customary to obtain the first specimen of the day, for it is in this specimen that the tubercle bacilli are most likely to be present in the greatest numbers. Some pathologists,

19

however, prefer to perform their examinations on *all* the urine that has been voided over a twenty-four hour period. If tubercle bacilli cannot be demonstrated in three separate specimens (either early morning or twenty-four hour specimens) taken on alternate days then, although a tuberculous infection cannot be definitely excluded, it renders the diagnosis extremely unlikely.

(6) **The Erythrocyte Sedimentation Rate (E.S.R.)**

As in many other conditions the value of the E.S.R. is commonly, though not always, raised in tuberculous disease. This investigation is not therefore of great value as a diagnostic aid but in repeated estimations it is extremely useful in indicating the *progress* of the condition—an increase in its rate being indicative of an increasing activity of the disease and a decrease being indicative of regression and arrest.

ANTI-TUBERCULOUS DRUGS

Streptomycin was the first and most powerful anti-tuberculous drug to be discovered, but although it has been used in the treatment of tuberculous disease for the last nine to ten years it is still early to make an accurate assessment of its long-term effects. It is of the most value in the treatment of tuberculous arthritis but its therapeutic efficacy in tuberculosis of the cervical lymph glands and tuberculosis of the urinary tract is as yet not fully determined. As ' surgical tuberculosis ' is a disease of gradual development and of slow response, the drug should be administered over a minimum period of twelve weeks and, in order to combine the maximum therapeutic effect with the least liability to toxic manifestations, it should be given by intra-muscular injection in daily doses of $\frac{1}{2}$ gram in children under five years of age and $\frac{3}{4}$ gram in older children, there being nothing to gain by dividing the daily dose into two separate injections. Although often dramatically effective during the first few weeks of treatment, the chief drawback to its use is a strong tendency on the part of the drug to induce a resistance in the tubercle bacillus against its action. It is for this reason that streptomycin therapy is *always* combined with the oral administration of *para-amino salycilic acid* (P.A.S.), which effectively delays the emergence of resistant strains of the

organisms and occasionally prevents their occurrence altogether. P.A.S. should be given in doses of 8-16 grams per day (2-4 grams every six hours) according to age and as it has a most unpleasant taste it is usually dispensed in cachets or capsules. The most recently evolved anti-tuberculous drug, which has now been in use for two to three years, is known as *iso-nicotinic hydrazine* (*isoniazid*) and, given in conjunction with streptomycin and P.A.S., it has the properties of increasing the ' anti-tuberculous effect ' of the former and assisting the ' anti-resistance action ' of the latter. It should be given by the oral route in doses of up to 4 milligrams per kilo body-weight per day and divided into two daily doses.

As the precise value of each of the anti-tuberculous drugs that we have mentioned is still difficult to determine and assess, it is generally agreed that in the present state of our knowledge and experience all cases of tuberculous disease which are considered suitable for drug therapy should be given *all three* substances in the dosage we have laid down.

B.C.G. IMMUNIZATION

A form of immunization against tuberculosis has been the dream of medical men for generations, but it was not until Calmette and Guerin succeeded in depriving the tubercle bacillus of its natural virulence and subsequently used a suspension of the ' tame ' organisms as an agent for inoculation against the disease, that the dream began to take on the semblance of reality. The avirulent form of the bacillus that they evolved was called the *bacille Calmette Guerin* (B.C.G.), but like so many organisms that have been rendered avirulent, the original strain of B.C.G. showed a tendency to recover its virulence and produce the active form of the disease instead of inducing an immunity against it. It was this fact that caused B.C.G. inoculation originally to fall into disgrace and disrepute, but more recently a strain of B.C.G. has been evolved in which the likelihood of an increase in virulence has been reduced to a minimum, with the result that its use as an immunizing agent against tuberculosis is now generally accepted and widely practised throughout the United Kingdom. The degree of immunity conferred on the individual by B.C.G. inoculation is difficult to determine, but although it is less effective than a naturally acquired active immunity, it has been shown to

produce a very good protection against the immediate dangers of a primary infection and it is for this reason that it is primarily indicated in Mantoux negative children of tuberculous families.

The technique of B.C.G. immunization consists merely of an *intracutaneous* injection of 0·1 cubic centimetres of the inoculum into the skin of the flexor surface of the forearm. After a few weeks a small, painless nodule appears at the

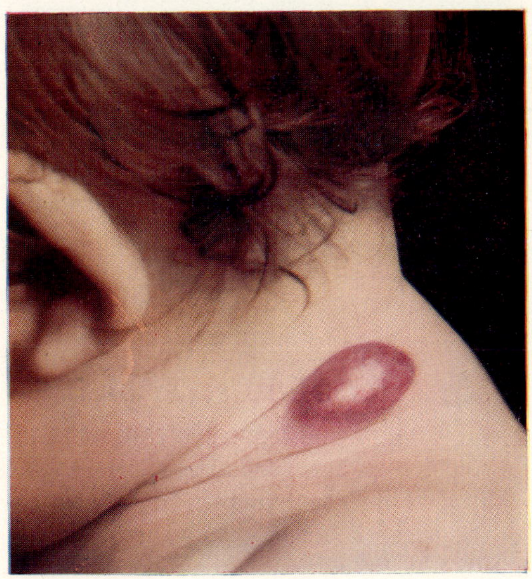

FIG. 136
A ' B.C.G.' abscess in danger of bursting through the skin.

site of the injection. This gradually undergoes softening and pustule formation and this change is frequently accompanied by a mild enlargement of the regional lymph glands. After a few months both the pustule and the lymph gland enlargement disappear without trace. The time taken for the immunity to develop (as demonstrated by a positive Mantoux reaction) is usually between six and eight weeks following the injection, though in infants it may take as long as three months.

Before leaving the subject of immunization it is important to stress the fact that the injection should be *intra*-cutaneous. If by mischance or misjudgment the injection should be *sub*-cutaneous then rapid enlargement of the regional lymph glands, followed by their breakdown and abscess formation within

them is especially prone to occur (Fig. 136). In such an eventuality it is often difficult to decide what is the best form of treatment. If the abscess is evacuated there is the possibility that this will interfere with the production of the intended immunity, whereas if it is left alone then there is the danger that it may rupture through the skin and become secondarily infected. Probably the best course to follow is to leave it alone until such time as it threatens to burst, when it should be cleanly incised and evacuated. If after a few months the Mantoux reaction is still negative then a further injection may then be made.

TUBERCULOSIS OF THE CERVICAL LYMPH GLANDS

Tuberculous lymphadenitis may appear in one of two distinct and widely different forms. They differ both in the situation of the glands involved, in the origin and subsequent spread of the infection and also in the treatment and prognosis. For the purpose of description the two forms of the disease may be classified as tuberculous lymphadenitis of:

(1) The upper cervical glands.

(2) The lower cervical glands.

(1) Tuberculous Lymphadenitis of the Upper Cervical Glands

In this condition the tuberculous process is invariably limited to the upper cervical glands on one side of the neck only. It occurs with equal frequency in both boys and girls and is always secondary to a primary focus of tuberculous infection within the mouth or pharynx, the most common situation being the tonsil. As the primary focus is both symptomless and invisible, the condition is not revealed until the tonsillar gland and its immediate neighbours undergo a painless enlargement, due to their involvement in the disease process (i.e. the establishment of a primary complex). Once the glands have become enlarged the Mantoux reaction becomes positive, there may be a slight elevation of the evening temperature and the E.S.R. may also be increased. The skin over the affected glands is normal in appearance and is freely movable over the swellings beneath it.

As in most tuberculous infections the subsequent progress of the condition depends upon the balance between the resistance of the child and the virulence of the organisms. A swing in favour of the tuberculous infection is followed by an increased elevation of the evening temperature, an increase in the value of E.S.R. and by an extension of the inflammatory process into the tissues surrounding the individual glands. This *periadenitis* as it is called, causes the glands to feel as if they are ' matted ' together and is a sure indication of the predominence of the infective process over the defences of the child's body. As the child's resistance increases so the pyrexia and the E.S.R. return to normal and the shape and identity of the individual glands again become discernible as the periadenitis regresses and finally disappears. Providing this swing of the balance in favour of the child's resistance is maintained, the infection is slowly overcome with the result that the glands steadily diminish in size and finally become impalpable, after which calcium salts may be deposited in the glands (which renders them readily visible in an X-ray picture of the neck). This calcification may be regarded as an attempt on the part of the body to imprison any stray tubercle bacilli which may still be lurking in the substance of the gland and so decrease the likelihood of an exacerbation of the infection.

COMPLICATIONS.—The simple course of events that we have outlined above is all too frequently interrupted by various complications. In the early stage of the infection, before the child's resistance has had a chance to increase, the affected glands may break down with the production of caseous material and tuberculous pus. Such a collection is known as a *cold abscess* and if left untreated it is likely to approach the skin, through which it may subsequently burst and discharge its contents to the exterior. This results in a permanent track or *tuberculous sinus* which connects the skin with the infected glands and through which there is a constant discharge of tuberculous pus. Such a sinus may take weeks or months before it can be persuaded to close and even when healing has taken place there is the ever present danger of its re-opening. In order to prevent a sinus occurring the cold abscess should be opened through a small skin incision and its contents gently but thoroughly scooped out, after which the incision should be accurately sutured and the wound allowed to heal. Secondary

infection of a cold abscess resulting from an incidental infection of the oropharynx, is revealed by redness of the overlying skin and the appearance of local pain and tenderness (Fig. 137). In other words, the cold abscess has been converted into a ' hot abscess ' and large doses of intramuscular penicillin should be administered in an attempt to prevent it bursting through the skin.   If resolution of the acute infection follows this treatment, the cold abscess should later be treated in the manner we have already described. If, however, the ' hot abscess ' should burst through the skin, penicillin should be continued until the acute infection has been overcome and then the contents of the gland should be scooped out and the skin closed over it.

Treatment

Apart from the complications we have already described the treatment of tuberculous lymphadenitis is concerned, firstly, with increasing the child's resistance to the infection, and secondly, with the prevention of secondary pyogenic infection of the tuberculous glands.   If at the onset of the disease, or indeed at any time during its course, the evening temperature is elevated or the E.S.R. is increased, then the child should be confined to bed until they have both returned to normal.   The tonsils and the adenoids should be removed in order to eradicate any focus of infection that they may contain and the teeth inspected regularly every two months.   Particular attention should be paid to the child's surroundings, and a high calorie, properly balanced diet which should be rich in vitamins is one of the first essentials.   Children living in a densely populated city area should be transferred to a convalescent home in the country where they may enjoy happy and stimulating

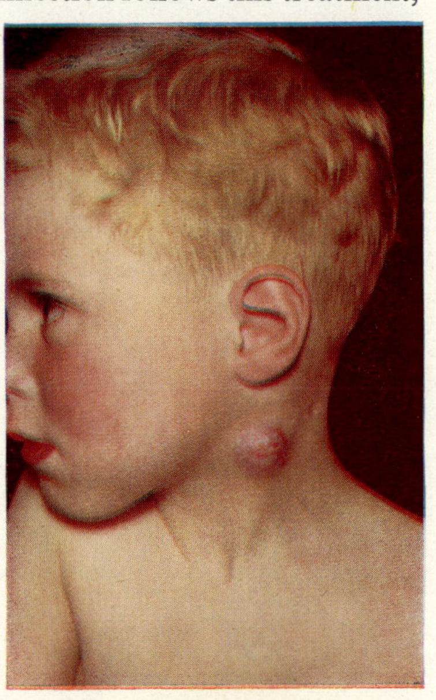

FIG. 137

Secondary infection of a cold abscess following an incidental attack of tonsillitis.

surroundings and an abundance of fresh air. When all traces of periadenitis have disappeared and the size of the glands has remained unchanged for a minimum period of six months, then and only then may surgical removal of the affected glands be undertaken.

The value of anti-tuberculous drugs in this condition is still not fully determined. Some surgeons advise their use during the stage of periadenitis and also employ them as a ' cover ' before, during and immediately after an operation for the removal of the glands. Other authorities discourage their use as a routine measure on the grounds that they may prevent the child from obtaining the fullest degree of resistance against the infection.

Tuberculous Lymphadenitis of the Lower Cervical Glands

Whereas tuberculosis of the upper cervical glands is always secondary to a primary focus of infection in the mouth or pharynx, is unilateral in distribution and is commonly characterized by caseation and cold abscess formation (i.e. a manifestation of the primary complex), tuberculosis of the lower cervical glands is *not* associated with a primary infection of the mouth or pharynx, is usually *bilateral* in distribution and only very rarely proceeds to caseation. Tuberculosis of the lower cervical glands is always secondary to an established *pulmonary* form of tuberculosis, the infection reaching the glands either as an upward extension from tuberculous glands in the chest, or more rarely as a result of spread by the bloodstream. It is a very much less common form of tuberculous lymphadenitis and accounts for less than one-tenth of the whole number of cases. Periadenitis does not as a rule occur and the limits of each of the enlarged glands are clearly defined and are firm and sometimes even ' rubbery ' to the touch. Surgery is only very occasionally employed and then only in order to perform a biopsy of an easily accessible gland if the diagnosis is in doubt. Other than this, surgical removal of the enlarged glands is strongly contra-indicated and treatment is directed primarily to the pulmonary and not to the cervical aspect of the disease.

TUBERCULOSIS OF THE GENITO-URINARY SYSTEM

Tuberculosis of the genito-urinary system is an uncommon condition in childhood and one which does not enjoy such a

favourable prognosis as it does in the adult. It is always a blood-born post-primary infection and although the primary focus may be difficult and sometimes even impossible to discover, you must never lose sight of the fact that genito-urinary tuberculosis is an incident in an already established form of the disease. The condition commences as a small focus in the cortex of one or other kidney and until such time as it has enlarged sufficiently to ulcerate into the renal pelvis, the disease is symptomless. Once communication with the pelvis has been established pus cells and tubercle bacilli are recoverable in the urine, and secondary tuberculous ulceration and fibrosis of the ureter and the bladder follow in due course, causing thickening and shortening of the ureter and a fibrous contraction of the bladder with diminution of its capacity. In male children secondary infection of the epididymis by way of the vas deferens may appear at any stage and may even be the first manifestation of the disease.

Clinical Features

Even when communication between the cortical focus and the renal pelvis has been established the disease is not always at once apparent. The general health of the child seldom suffers appreciably until the condition is well advanced but occasional transient episodes of irregular fever, undue tiredness and a slight loss of weight may occur. The commonest presenting sign is *haematuria*, the bleeding usually being sporadic and slight in amount, so much so that it may be dismissed by the parent as a trivial happening. Once the ureter and bladder become involved then frequency of micturition, dysuria and supra-pubic pain make their appearance. Pus cells are present in the urine in profusion and the examinations that we have already mentioned for detecting the presence of the tubercle bacilli should be carried out on three separate early morning or twenty-four hour specimens which have been collected on alternate days. An intravenous pyelogram invariably reveals either distortion of the renal calyces or calcification of the renal substance, but for fear of disseminating the infection, the temptation to perform a retrograde pyelogram should be resisted unless it is absolutely essential for confirmation of the diagnosis. The cystoscopic appearance vary between a normal bladder (in spite of well marked radiographic

changes in the kidney), early involvement of the ureteric orifice or extensive ulceration and fibrous contraction of the bladder wall.

Treatment

The treatment of all cases of unilateral tuberculosis of the urinary tract, however early or advanced it may be, is by removal of the diseased kidney and ureter (nephro-ureterectomy). Anti-tuberculous drugs alone are insufficient as a curative measure but they provide a valuable and powerful adjuvant to surgical procedures and should always be given in the dosages we have already mentioned. At operation the kidney is approached through a loin incision and after the renal artery and vein have been ligated and the ureter has been mobilized as far down as possible, the kidney is withdrawn from the loin incision and the wound is closed around the intact ureter. The child is then placed in the supine position and through a mid-line abdominal incision the junction between the lower end of the ureter and the bladder is located and the ureter is then divided just above it. Once this has been done traction is applied to the exteriorized kidney and this pulls the whole length of the ureter out through the wound in the loin. As this operation is a somewhat extensive one, some authorities prefer to limit their surgical manoeuvres to simple nephrectomy trusting that the anti-tuberculous drugs will succeed in overcoming any infection left behind in the remaining portion of the ureter. Secondary involvement of the bladder is not a contra-indication to surgery for once the kidney and ureter have been removed the tuberculous infection of the bladder frequently subsides altogether. It goes without saying that prior to either operation being carried out, the presence of a normal functioning kidney on the opposite side should always be confirmed.

Bilateral tuberculous infection of the urinary tract is beyond the scope of surgery altogether. Anti-tuberculous drugs should always be given in the forlorn hope that they may be of benefit, but the outlook is invariably hopeless. Very occasionally you will come across a case in which there is gross tuberculous infection of one kidney and only a very early focus present in the other one. In such an instance there may be a case for removal of the more severely affected kidney in an attempt to relieve the defences of the body of the major part of

their burden and thus reinforce their effect on the small remaining focus of infection. Such an instance is, however, most uncommon.

TUBERCULOUS ARTHRITIS

Irrespective of the joint involved the course of tuberculous arthritis is always characterized by a slow and insidious onset, a long period of activity and progression, and finally a gradual regression of the infection and repair of the diseased tissues. It is always a post-primary manifestation of tuberculosis and, although no age group is exempt, the maximum incidence is between two and five years of age—the joints most commonly affected being the spine, the hip and the knee, in that order of frequency. Once established within the articular tissues, the tuberculous foci gradually increase in size and by encroaching upon the normal tissues come to replace them by tuberculous material. The substance of the bone is invaded and decalcified, the articular surfaces eroded, the capsule is softened and the cavity of the joint becomes distended with caseous material and tuberculous granulation tissue. As the disease progresses, the capsule of the joint is particularly prone to give way and allow the tuberculous material to enter the superficial tissues with the formation of a cold abscess. In this event it is of paramount importance that the cold abscess should at all costs be prevented from rupturing through the skin and forming a tuberculous sinus—a complication which materially worsens the prognosis of the disease due to the secondary pyogenic infection of the joint that will inevitably ensue.

As a result of treatment and a gradual increase of resistance in the child's body, the stage of activity and progression is followed after a variable period of one to three years by regression of the infection and the slow process of repair. What bony tissue that has not been destroyed is slowly re-calcified, cold abscesses are slowly absorbed and later calcified, and the tuberculous granulation tissue is replaced by fibrous tissue. In this way the interior of the affected joint becomes ' tethered ' by fibrous tissue (*fibrous ankylosis*) which, as a rule, effectively prevents the return of movement. If, as a result of sinus formation there has been a secondary pyogenic infection of the joint then fibrous ankylosis does not usually

occur and the diseased bone ends unite together in solid union (*bony ankylosis*).

Clinical Features

(1) MUSCLE SPASM.—This is usually one of the earliest manifestations of tuberculous arthritis and is invariably the most constant and predominant signs of the disease. It is caused by the irritation of the articular surface which initiates intense spasm of all the muscles surrounding the joint. It may be regarded as a protective phenomenon in that it automatically immobilizes the joint and thus prevents the pain that would accompany movement. Occasionally, during the hours of sleep, the spasm may relax sufficiently to allow some degree of passive movement to take place and, in consequence, the child may suddenly awake and cry out with pain. In the past great reliance has been placed on these 'night starts' as a diagnostic sign, but as they only occur in a small proportion of cases and then only when the course of the disease is well advanced, their diagnostic value is open to doubt.

(2) PAIN.—Pain is often an early symptom but it is important for you to remember that in some cases it may be absent altogether. Not infrequently, minor trauma is incriminated as a predisposing cause of tuberculous arthritis but it would seem more likely that trauma merely serves to call attention to the already existing disease by overstretching the protective muscle spasm and thus causing a degree of pain out of all proportion to the injury.

(3) DEFORMITY.—Sooner or later, deformity always becomes an accompaniment of the condition. It may be produced either as a result of the collapse of infected bone (as in the case of the spine) or due to the unequal pull exerted by spasm of a strong group of muscles against a weaker group (as in the case of the hip and the knee).

(4) LIMP.—A limp is often an early feature of the disease and is due to either pain or the onset of limitation of movement at the affected joint.

(5) SWELLING.—As a rule swelling of the joint only becomes apparent when a superficial joint such as the knee is affected.

(6) MUSCLE WASTING.—The precise cause of muscle wasting in tuberculous arthritis is still obscure, but none the less it is a pronounced feature of the condition and when the knee is affected the wasting of the thigh and calf muscles may often throw the swelling of the joint into exaggerated relief.

(7) COLD ABSCESSES AND SINUSES.—Cold abscesses arising from deep seated joints are notorious for their ability to track through the tissue planes for considerable distances before becoming apparent as a swelling beneath the skin. Treatment consists either of aspiration of the abscess or incision and evacuation of its contents in order to prevent its rupture through the skin, the latter procedure being followed by primary suture. Although both methods incur the risk of subsequent sinus formation, the modern usage of anti-tuberculous drugs has reduced the incidence of this complication to a minimum. Once established, it is exceptionally difficult to persuade a tuberculous sinus to heal. Success may sometimes be obtained by the local instillation of $\frac{1}{4}$ gram of streptomycin but all too often the temporary closure that this may effect is followed by its subsequent breakdown and re-opening.

The Principles of Treatment

The treatment of tuberculous arthritis is most satisfactorily carried out in a sanatorium where careful attention may be paid to the improvement of the child's resistance and where educational facilities are also available, but as our present concern is the treatment of the diseased joint itself the reader should consult medical works for a full consideration of sanatorium régime and management.

The local treatment of tuberculous arthritis may be summarized in one word—*rest*. Rest of the joint during the active phase of the disease, and rest of the joint either by external or internal splintage during the stage of regression until all signs of activity within the joint have disappeared and apparent healing has taken place. Irrespective of the situation of the diseased joint all methods of putting it at rest should obey the following principles:

(1) The joint must be *completely* immobilized.

(2) Immobilization should be maintained in a position that will allow the best possible function of the limb once ankylosis has taken place.

(3) Some form of light traction should always be applied in order to keep the softened bone ends slightly apart and thus prevent their distortion by mutual pressure.

(4) The form of splintage used should provide easy access to the joint so that a vigilant watch may be maintained for the appearance of a cold abscess.

During the stage of activity the anti-tuberculous drugs that we have mentioned should be administered in courses of between three and six months, but with the exception of evacuation of cold abscesses open operation during this phase is largely contra-indicated, though it is possible that with continual experience in the use of these drugs major operative interference may become an accepted and safe procedure in the future.

The stage of regression and repair is evidenced by the absence of pyrexia, a fall to a low and constant level in the E.S.R. and X-ray evidence of progressive recalcification and consolidation of the diseased bone. When these conditions are satisfied and repair is well advanced, then ambulation may be allowed but it is essential that the affected joint should still be protected either by a brace in the case of the spine, or a caliper in the case of the lower limb. These measures are necessary in view of the fact that tubercle bacilli are still imprisoned in the diseased joint and excessive movement may cause a reactivation of the disease. The decision as to when internal fixation of the joint should be substituted for external splintage is a difficult one to make, but generally speaking it is not undertaken for several years after apparent healing has taken place. The method of internal fixation varies according to the joint involved, but the principle of the procedure is to procure immobilization of the joint by bone grafts placed around it so that the diseased area itself is not disturbed (extra-articular arthrodesis). Once healing of the bone grafts has occurred the child is allowed to become fully ambulant and, as the diseased area is now protected from movement by the arthrodesis, external appliances become no longer necessary.

From what we have said you will appreciate that tuberculous arthritis is a long term disease in which the term ' cure ' is

replaced by ' apparent healing '—for the likelihood of reactivation of the infection is always at hand.   It is for this reason that all cases must undergo regular surveillance (including E.S.R. estimations and X-ray examinations) for a number of years after ' apparent healing ' has occurred.

TUBERCULOSIS OF THE SPINE (POTT'S DISEASE)

Tuberculosis of the spine occurs with equal frequency in both boys and girls and accounts for about 50 per cent of all cases of tuberculous arthritis.   In order of frequency it occurs in the lower dorsal, the lumbar, the upper dorsal and the cervical regions of the spine.   As a rule the infection commences in the vicinity of the upper or lower margin of a vertebral body and from there extends into one or more adjacent vertebrae.   As more and more bone is replaced by tuberculous material so the strength of the bone is impaired and its tendency to collapse is increased.

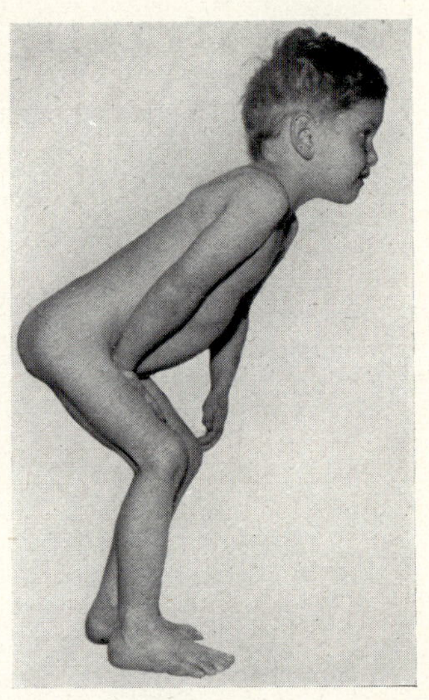

Fig. 138

Tuberculosis of the lower dorsal spine.   Note the characteristic crouch when attempting to bend down.

Clinical Features

In the early stages of the disease the only significant symptoms and signs may be nothing more than a gradually increasing tiredness on the part of the child and a disinclination to play as energetically as usual.   As the disease progresses the classical sign of muscle spasm makes its appearance in the back muscles and effectively prevents any form of movement occurring at or around the affected portion of the spine.   Any attempt at getting up or bending down is performed in a characteristic crouching fashion, the child moving the knees and hips while the back is held as rigid and as straight as a ramrod (Fig. 138).   Mild pain and tenderness are usually present in the region of the affected vertebrae and

occasionally there may be a slight limp. These facts should impress upon you the great importance of regarding the onset of unexplained backache or a limp in childhood with the respect that they both deserve. Deformity of the spine first appears as a gradual forward bend or kyphosis, but once destruction and collapse of one or more vertebrae has occurred the deformity becomes a sharp kyphotic *angulation* and X-ray examination reveals decalcification, erosion and collapse of the bone (Fig. 139). The E.S.R. is commonly raised to 20-30 millimetres per

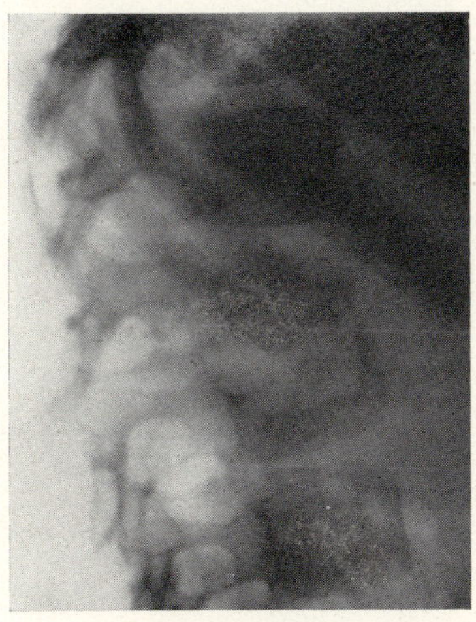

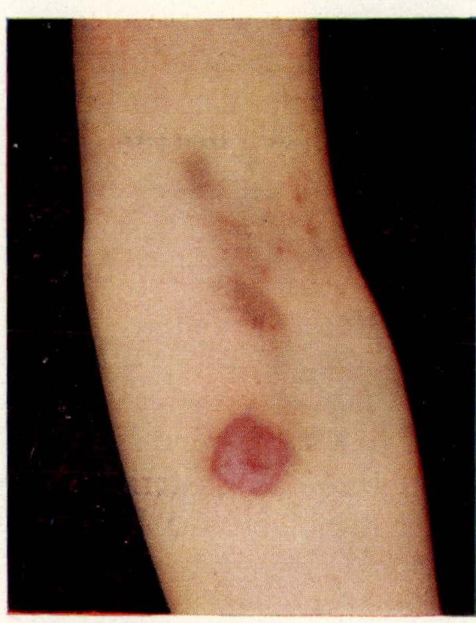

<table>
<tr><td align="center">Fig. 139</td><td align="center">Fig. 140</td></tr>
<tr><td align="center">An X-ray of the case shown in Fig. 138. Note the degree of bone destruction.</td><td align="center">The Mantoux reaction of the case illustrated in Figs. 138 and 139.</td></tr>
</table>

hour; a mild pyrexia of 99-101° F. is usually present particularly in the evening, and the Mantoux reaction is strongly positive to dilutions of 1 : 10,000 (Fig. 140).

Complications

COLD ABSCESS FORMATION.—Cold abscess formation is such a common happening in Pott's disease that it is usually regarded as a concomitant of the condition rather than a complication. In the dorsal spine, an abscess forms as a large, deep seated, rapidly expanding, thick walled swelling which extends on either side of the mid-line and which is clearly demarcated in an X-ray photograph (a paravertebral abscess). Aspiration

of the abscess should always be attempted but if this is insufficient to control its size, then the posterior ends of one or more ribs overlying the abscess together with the adjacent transverse processes of the vertebrae should be excised (the operation of costo-transversectomy). The abscess is then opened and completely evacuated and the wound closed by primary suture. In the lumbar spine the associated abscess often tracks through the tissue planes to present either in the loin (a lumbar abscess) or it may track along within the sheath of the psoas muscle and present as a soft swelling beneath the skin just below the inguinal ligament (a psoas abscess).

PARAPLEGIA.—The onset of paraplegia is a far more serious complication of the disease and although it is never associated with tuberculosis of the lumbar spine it occurs in about 10 per cent of cases of tuberculosis of the dorsal spine. It most commonly occurs some time during the first year of the disease and is due either to thrombosis within the blood-vessels supplying the neighbouring spinal cord, or to compression of the cord by a cold abscess or tuberculous granulation tissue. In the case of thrombosis, although surgical treatment is of no avail, recovery often takes place spontaneously within a month or so from the time of onset, but if the paraplegia is thought to be due to actual compression of the cord then costo-transversectomy should be carried out and the compression relieved. Very occasionally paraplegia may supervene some years after the disease has become quiescent and in such an instance it usually indicates reactivation of the infection.

Treatment

The stage of activity in Pott's disease usually lasts from one to two years and during this time the child should be immobilized, either on a frame or in a plaster of Paris bed. Some authorities advise immobilization with the back in the hyper-extended position in order to protect the diseased vertebrae from compression, but if this position is adopted it should be discontinued once healing begins to take place in order to allow the vertebrae to fall together and to consolidate in apposition with each other. Anti-tuberculous drugs should always be administered for a period of not less than six months and X-ray examinations should be carried out at regular

intervals in order to reveal the progress of the disease and to disclose the onset and course of the paravertebral abscess. The stage of regression and repair as evidenced by the absence of pain and pyrexia, a constantly low value of the E.S.R. and X-ray evidence of recalcification and consolidation, should be well advanced before immobilization is discontinued. Once ambulation has been obtained, a light metal brace, secured to the shoulders and hips, should be worn in order to prevent anything more than minimum mobility of the spine and when the child has worn such an appliance and remained in good health for a year or so, then the advisability of internal fixation of the diseased area of the spine by bone grafting may be considered. At this point it is as well to remember that experience in the treatment of Pott's disease with anti-tuberculous drugs is still comparatively recent and it may well be that in the future, operative fixation of the spine may be safely performed during the period of activity and thus obviate the necessity of wearing an external protective appliance.

TUBERCULOSIS OF THE HIP JOINT

Like all cases of tuberculous arthritis, tuberculosis of the hip joint is characterized by a long period of activity of the disease followed by slow regression of the infection and ultimately fibrous ankylosis of the joint. It occurs slightly more frequently in boys than in girls, and although the initial focus of infection is usually situated in the acetabulum or in the upper end of the femur, spread into the cavity of the joint and subsequent involvement of all the articular tissues invariably supervenes.

Clinical Features

Pain is a usual but not predominant feature of the disease and seldom amounts to little more than a mild ache coming on especially after exercise or towards the end of the day, and occasionally it may radiate into the knee. The constant and outstanding sign of tuberculosis of the hip, however, is the onset of a *limp* and here we must again emphasize the importance of regarding any otherwise unexplained limp as being the harbinger of tuberculous disease until such time as the opposite

has been proved. The limp is usually produced in this fashion; although the initial focus of infection is within the substance of the bone, it none the less causes a mild effusion of fluid in the cavity of the joint and in order to increase the volume of the joint and thus accommodate the effusion without discomfort, the limb is automatically held in the position of abduction and external rotation (Fig. 141 *a*) (that is to say the

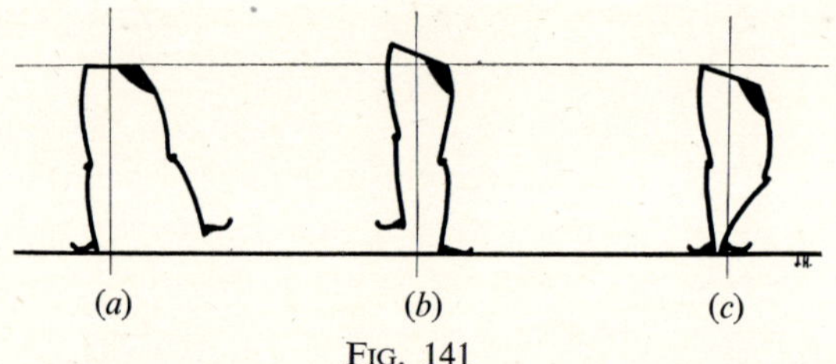

FIG. 141

To illustrate the early stages of tuberculosis of the hip.

position of maximum capacity of the joint). The muscles around the joint maintain the hip in this position with the result that in order to stand upon the affected limb the child must necessarily tilt the pelvis upwards on the opposite side in order to preserve the angle of abduction (Fig. 141 *b*). This posture

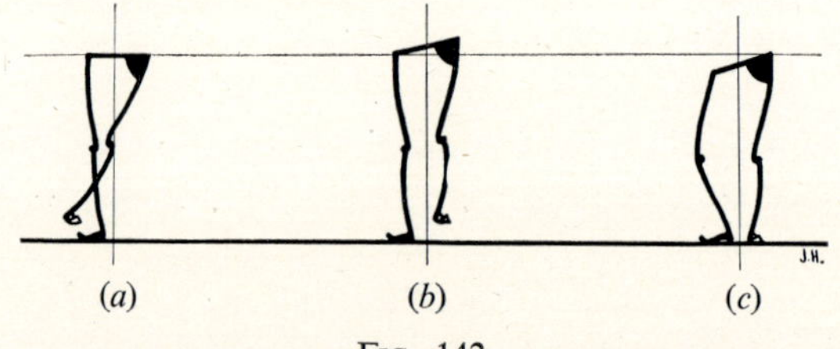

FIG. 142

To illustrate the flexion-adduction deformity.

therefore gives the impression of apparent lengthening of the affected limb, and in order to stand with both feet to the ground the knee on the same side must necessarily be bent (Fig. 141 *c*), and it is this state of affairs that causes the child to exhibit the characteristic limp. If the disease is allowed to progress beyond this stage then erosion of the articular surfaces occurs and initiates the most pronounced muscle spasm in all the muscles around the joint. Now as the *adductor* muscles of the thigh are considerably stronger than the *abductor* group, the continual muscle spasm of the stronger muscles pulling

against the weaker ones will slowly and inexorably pull the limb into the position of a fixed adduction. In this way the obtuse angle of abduction which characterized the previous stage will become replaced by the acute angle of fixed *adduction* (Fig. 142 *a*). Thus in order to keep both legs parallel whilst walking, the child will have to tilt the pelvis upwards on the *diseased* side (Fig. 142 *b*), and in order to place both feet on the floor whilst standing, the knee on the *sound* side will have to be bent (Fig. 142 *c*) thus giving the impression of apparent shortening of the diseased limb. If the disease is still allowed to progress in spite of this obvious deformity, then destruction of the head and neck of the femur with subsequent dislocation of the joint, accompanied by pronounced muscle wasting and abscess formation will inevitably ensue.

Treatment

During the stage of activity of the infection, rest of the hip is achieved by immobilization on a Robert Jones abduction frame in order to assist the process of resolution and allow fibrous ankylosis to take place without deformity. In addition, light skin extension should be applied to the affected limb in order to prevent distortion of the softened head of the femur by pressure against the acetabulum. Anti-tuberculous drugs are administered in the first place for a period of between three and six months and in some cases a second course of similar duration may become necessary. Immobilization is continued until such time as regression of the infection is evidenced by the criteria that we have previously mentioned and when the stage of repair is well advanced the child may be removed from the frame, and most authorities continue immobilization in a double plaster of Paris hip spica for a further month or so. Once ambulation is allowed it is customary to fit a weight relieving caliper to the affected limb in order to afford continual protection to the diseased joint against the strains of weight bearing.

The decision as to the advisability of subsequent extra-articular arthrodesis is a difficult one to make and is conditioned by a number of factors which are not within the scope of this work. It would appear, however, that with the ever increasing knowledge and experience in the use of anti-tuberculous drugs, arthrodesis will become less frequently indicated in the future

than it has been in the past, and it may well be that the standard form of treatment that we have just described may become considerably shortened in duration by surgical excision of the diseased tissues during the stage of activity; a procedure which, in the past, has always been fraught with many dangers but which, under the protection of the anti-tuberculous drugs, may in the future become a safe and commonplace form of treatment.

Tuberculosis of the Knee-joint

In tuberculous diseases of the knee-joint the infection not uncommonly commences in the synovial membrane, and in a certain proportion of cases it may remain localized to this structure and fail to involve the other articular tissues. In this event fibrous ankylosis may not follow regression of the infection and a reasonable degree of function in the joint may ultimately be obtained.

Clinical Features

Swelling of the joint, which is produced both by thickening of the synovial membrane and by distension of the joint cavity with tuberculous material, is often the earliest clinical manifestation of the disease and is usually thrown into ever greater relief by the pronounced wasting of the surrounding thigh and calf muscles. A limp is also a common presenting sign and is caused by fixation of the joint in a few degrees of flexion by spasm in the hamstring group of muscles, and as the disease progresses this flexion deformity is liable to increase in extent. Pain is seldom severe and is usually only present when movement at the joint is attempted. Occasionally there may be little more than a mild synovial swelling or an effusion into the joint, and in this event great difficulty may be experienced in deciding whether in fact the condition is tuberculous in origin or is merely due to some other form of chronic synovitis. In such an instance, biopsy of the synovial membrane or of an inguinal lymph node may succeed in proving the diagnosis but the child should be treated as a case of tuberculous disease from the first, until such time as either the opposite is proved or persistently negative results to investigations and the absence of progressive clinical signs render the diagnosis of tuberculosis increasingly unlikely.

Treatment

Immobilization of the joint is most satisfactorily obtained in a Thomas' splint which is easily applied and which also permits easy inspection of the joint. Light skin traction should be applied in order to overcome any flexion deformity that may be present, and immobilization should be continued until the stage of activity has passed and healing is well advanced. When ambulation is allowed a weight relieving caliper should be worn for a few months in order to protect the diseased joint against the stresses and strains of walking, and as a rule when this is discarded a moulded leather knee splint is worn in its place. As tuberculosis of the knee-joint is notorious for its liability to reactivation even years after the original infection, arthrodesis of the joint often becomes a necessary insurance. Authorities differ both as to the advisability of this procedure and as to the time it should be carried out; whereas some prefer early operation others consider it best delayed until the child has finished growing.

TUBERCULOUS DACTYLITIS

Unlike the conditions we have considered so far, tuberculous dactylitis is primarily a disease of bone in which secondary involvement of the joint structures is an unusual feature. The infection commences within the medulla of a phalanx or metacarpal bone and the subsequent formation of tuberculous granulation tissue and caseous material causes destruction of the cortex and considerable increase in the girth of the bone. Treatment consists of prolonged immobilization of the wrist and affected finger in a plaster of Paris cast but if, in spite of these measures, the disease process continues to progress, incision of the affected bone with thorough evacuation of its contents should be carried out. In some instances the whole of the diseased bone may be removed intact.

AF412770

supplement the intake by the administration of water or saline by the rectal route, given either by continuous infusion or by the injection of 1 to 2 ounces at six-hourly intervals.

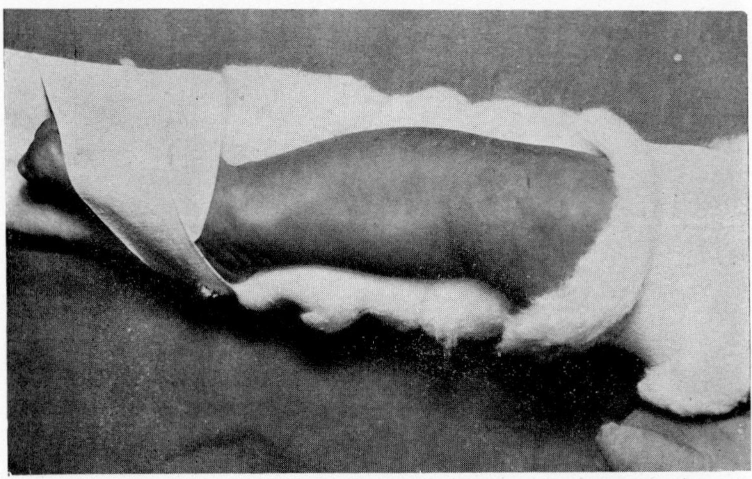

FIG. 2
To demonstrate a satisfactory method of immobilizing the leg.

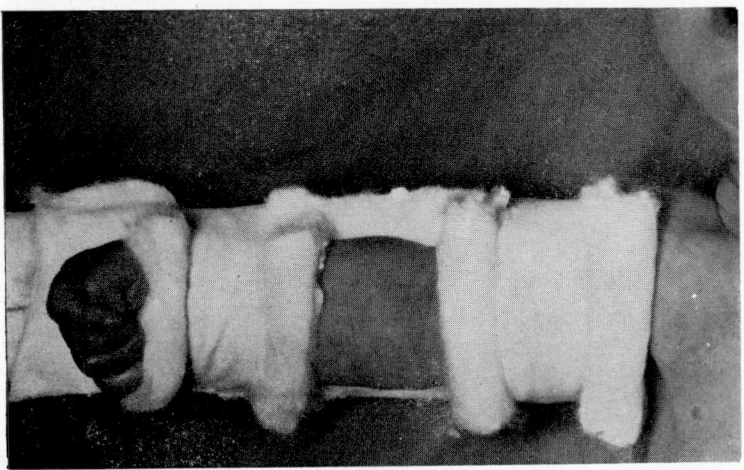

FIG. 3
Immobilization of the arm.

If the degree of dehydration is more severe, then the urgency of the situation demands that fluid be replaced via the intravenous route. Owing to the small size of the superficial veins in children it is usually impossible to introduce a needle directly into them through the skin, and for this reason it is necessary to expose a vein under local anaesthetic. You will come across a wide variety of cannulae and special needles which are used

WESTMINSTER CHILDREN'S HOSPITAL INTRAVENOUS FLUID CHART

Name... Birth Weight .... Present Weight ....
Date...

TIME	PULSE	AMOUNT IN HOUR	RATE OF DRIP	READING ON SCALE	REMARKS	FEEDS BY MOUTH	VOMITS	STOOLS	URINE	
a.m. 1										
2										
3										
4										
5										
6										
7										
8										
9										
10										
11										
12										
p.m. 1										
2										
3										
4										
5										
6										
7										
8										
9										
10										
11										
12										
TOTALS										

TOTAL INTAKE FOR 24 HOURS

FIG. 4

The intravenous fluid administration chart.

for intravenous infusions but quite the most satisfactory expedient is a short length of polythene tubing which after being connected to a standard drip apparatus (Fig. 1) may be introduced an inch or so into the vein and secured to the limb with adhesive strapping. In infants and very young children the

THE
SURGERY OF CHILDHOOD
FOR NURSES

BY

RAYMOND FARROW

M.A., B.M., B.Ch. (Oxon), F.R.C.S. (Eng.)

Late Surgical Registrar, the Westminster Children's Hospital, London

E. & S. LIVINGSTONE LTD.

EDINBURGH AND LONDON

1956

TO
MY WIFE

PRINTED IN GREAT BRITAIN AT
THE UNIVERSITY PRESS
ABERDEEN

PREFACE

In the writing of this book I have attempted at all times to direct the nurse's attention to the *fundamental* features of those surgical conditions of childhood with which she will most commonly have to deal. Thus, in the consideration of congenital abnormalities I have, for the sake of clarity, deliberately simplified some of the more confusing points of embryology in order to present a straightforward and uncomplicated picture of the *basic* problem which is in need of correction. When dealing with the clinical appearances of the various conditions, I have laid greater stress on the pre-operative and the post-operative state and care, rather than on diagnosis, for it is in these respects that the nurse's responsibility is most directly applied.

With regards to treatment, it is essential that the nurse, whose care is imperative for the ultimate success of any surgical operation, should have a clear understanding of *why* a particular procedure is undertaken. For this reason I have not, I hope, entered into controversy but have merely tried to explain to her the accepted forms of treatment in which she will most commonly be expected to participate.

I am most grateful to Mr. David Levi, M.S., F.R.C.S., for the loan of Figs. 8, 16, 18, 19, 35, 36, 44, 55, 56, 132, 136 and 138; to Mr. George MacNab, F.R.C.S., for the loan of Figs. 7, 9, 17, 75, 87, 92, 93 and 95; to Mr. J. S. Batchelor, F.R.C.S., for Figs. 102 and 104; to Mr. Miles Foxen, F.R.C.S., for Figs. 60 and 61 ; to Mr. J. Crawford Adams, M.D., F.R.C.S., for Fig. 106 ; to Mr. George Bonney, M.S., F.R.C.S., for Fig. 115; to Mr. Stanley Aylett, M.B.E., F.R.C.S., for Fig. 117; to Mr. J. P. Reidy, F.R.C.S., for Figs. 24, 25 and 26; to the Hon. Mrs. Noel Richards, M.D., F.R.C.P., for Figs. 46 and 84; to Dr. Ian Anderson, M.D., M.R.C.P., for Fig. 137; to Her Majesty's Stationery Office for permission to reproduce Figs. 2 and 3; to the Management Committee of the Westminster Children's Hospital for permission to reproduce Figs. 4 and 49 ; to Miss Campbell, S.R.N., R.S.C.N., for her help in reading the original drafts; to Dr. Peter Hansell and the staff of the Westminster Hospital Photographic Department for their splendid photographs ; to Miss Jill Hassell, the medical artist, the excellence of whose work stands out for itself; to Miss Sylvia Sherry and Miss June Hood for their assistance in preparing the typescript; to Mr. Charles Macmillan for his constant encouragement and help, and finally to Mr. and Mrs. George Mayne without whose generous sacrifice of time and convenience, a start upon the writing of this book might not have been made.

R. F.

London, *April*, 1956.

THE
SURGERY OF CHILDHOOD
FOR NURSES